Preclinical Rheumatic Disease

Editors

VIVIAN P. BYKERK
KAREN H. COSTENBADER
KEVIN DEANE

RHEUMATIC DISEASE CLINICS OF NORTH AMERICA

www.rheumatic.theclinics.com

Consulting Editor
MICHAEL H. WEISMAN

November 2014 • Volume 40 • Number 4

ELSEVIER

1600 John F. Kennedy Boulevard • Suite 1800 • Philadelphia, Pennsylvania, 19103-2899
http://www.theclinics.com

RHEUMATIC DISEASE CLINICS OF NORTH AMERICA Volume 40, Number 4
November 2014 ISSN 0889-857X, ISBN 13: 978-0-323-32024-5

Editor: Jennifer Flynn-Briggs
Developmental Editor: Casey Jackson

Rheumatic Disease Clinics of North America (ISSN 0889-857X) is published quarterly by Elsevier Inc., 360 Park Avenue South, New York, NY 10010-1710. Months of issue are February, May, August, and November. Business and editorial offices: 1600 John F. Kennedy Boulevard, Suite 1800, Philadelphia, PA 19103-2899. Periodicals postage paid at New York, NY and additional mailing offices. Subscription prices are USD 335.00 per year for US individuals, USD 579.00 per year for US institutions, USD 165.00 per year for US students and residents, USD 395.00 per year for Canadian individuals, USD 722.00 per year for Canadian institutions, USD 465.00 per year for international individuals, USD 722.00 per year for international institutions, and USD 230.00 per year for Canadian and foreign students/residents. To receive student/resident rate, orders must be accompanied by name of affiliated institution, date of term, and the *signature* of program/residency coordinator on institution letterhead. Orders will be billed at individual rate until proof of status received. Foreign air speed delivery is included in all *Clinics* subscription prices. All prices are subject to change without notice. **POSTMASTER:** Send address changes to *Rheumatic Disease Clinics of North America,* Elsevier Health Sciences Division, Subscription Customer Service, 3251 Riverport Lane, Maryland Heights, MO 63043. **Customer Service: 1-800-654-2452 (US and Canada). From outside of the US and Canada: 314-447-8871. Fax: 314-447-8029. For print support, e-mail: JournalsCustomerService-usa@elsevier.com. For online support, e-mail: JournalsOnline Support-usa@elsevier.com.**

Reprints. For copies of 100 or more of articles in this publication, please contact the Commercial Reprints Department, Elsevier Inc., 360 Park Avenue South, New York, New York, 10010-1710; Tel.: +1-212-633-3874, Fax: +1-212-633-3820, and E-mail: reprints@elsevier.com.

Rheumatic Disease Clinics of North America is covered in *MEDLINE/PubMed (Index Medicus), Current Contents/Clinical Medicine, Science Citation Index, ISI/BIOMED,* and *EMBASE/Excerpta Medica.*

Contributors

CONSULTING EDITOR

MICHAEL H. WEISMAN, MD
Director, Division of Rheumatology; Professor of Medicine, Cedars-Sinai Medical Center, Los Angeles, California

EDITORS

VIVIAN P. BYKERK, MD
Associate Professor of Medicine, Weill Cornell Medical College, Director of the Inflammatory Arthritis Center, Hospital for Special Surgery, New York, New York

KAREN H. COSTENBADER, MD, MPH
Associate Professor of Medicine, Harvard Medical School, Co-Director, Lupus Center, Division of Rheumatology, Immunology and Allergy, Brigham and Women's Hospital, Boston, Massachusetts

KEVIN DEANE, MD, PhD
Associate Professor of Medicine, Division of Rheumatology, University of Colorado School of Medicine, Aurora, Colorado

AUTHORS

HELEN BENHAM, B.App.Sci, MBBS (Hons), FRACP, PhD
Translational Research Institute, The University of Queensland Diamantina Institute, Woolloongabba, Queensland, Australia; The University of Queensland School of Medicine, Brisbane, Queensland, Australia

VIVIAN P. BYKERK, MD, FRCPC
Associate Professor of Medicine, Division of Rheumatology, Hospital for Special Surgery, Weill Cornell Medical College, New York, New York

NED CALONGE, MD, MPH
President and CEO, The Colorado Trust; Associate Professor, Department of Family Medicine, University of Colorado School of Medicine; Associate Professor, Department of Epidemiology, Colorado School of Public Health, Denver, Colorado

ROWLAND W. CHANG, MD, MPH
Professor in Medicine, Division of Rheumatology; Department of Preventive Medicine, Northwestern University Feinberg School of Medicine, Chicago, Illinois

KAREN H. COSTENBADER, MD, MPH
Division of Rheumatology, Immunology and Allergy, Department of Medicine, Brigham and Women's Hospital, Harvard Medical School, Boston, Massachusetts

KEVIN D. DEANE, MD, PhD
Division of Rheumatology, University of Colorado School of Medicine, Aurora, Colorado

M. KRISTEN DEMORUELLE, MD
Assistant Professor of Medicine, Division of Rheumatology, University of Colorado School of Medicine, Aurora, Colorado

DAVID T. FELSON, MD, MPH
Professor of Medicine and Epidemiology, Medicine, Boston University School of Medicine, Boston, Massachusetts; Professor of Medicine and Public Health, University of Manchester, Manchester, Lancashire, United Kingdom; Clinical Epidemiology Unit, Boston University, Boston, Massachusetts; NIHR Biomedical Research Unit, University of Manchester, Manchester, United Kingdom

AXEL FINCKH, MD
Division of Rheumatology, University Hospital of Geneva, Genève, Switzerland

DANIELLE M. GERLAG, MD, PhD
Division of Clinical Immunology and Rheumatology, Academic Medical Center, University of Amsterdam, Amsterdam, The Netherlands; GlaxoSmithKline, Cambridge, United Kingdom

RICHARD HODGSON, BM, PhD
NIHR Biomedical Research Unit, University of Manchester, Manchester, United Kingdom

V. MICHAEL HOLERS, MD
Professor of Medicine and Immunology, Division of Rheumatology, University of Colorado School of Medicine, Aurora, Colorado

ROBERT D. INMAN, MD
Professor of Medicine/Immunology, Division of Rheumatology, Toronto Western Hospital, University of Toronto, Toronto, Ontario, Canada

JUDITH A. JAMES, MD, PhD
Lou Kerr Chair in Biomedical Research; Program Head, Arthritis and Clinical Immunology Research Program, Oklahoma Medical Research Foundation; Associate Vice Provost of Clinical and Translational Science and Professor, Departments of Medicine, Pathology, Microbiology and Immunology, Oklahoma Clinical and Translational Science Institute, University of Oklahoma Health Sciences Center, Oklahoma City, Oklahoma

SEOYOUNG C. KIM, MD, ScD, MSCE
Divisions of Pharmacoepidemiology and Pharmacoeconomics and of Rheumatology, Allergy and Immunology, Brigham and Women's Hospital, Boston, Massachusetts

KRISTINE A. KUHN, MD, PhD
Assistant Professor of Medicine, Division of Rheumatology, University of Colorado School of Medicine, Aurora, Colorado

TABITHA N. KUNG, MD, MPH, FRCPC
Clinical Associate, Department of Medicine, Mount Sinai Hospital, University of Toronto, Toronto, Ontario, Canada

SOI-CHENG LAW, BSc (Hons)
Translational Research Institute, The University of Queensland Diamantina Institute, Woolloongabba, Queensland, Australia

LINDSEY A. MACFARLANE, MD
Department of Medicine, Brigham and Women's Hospital, Boston, Massachusetts

DARCY S. MAJKA, MD, MS
Assistant Professor in Medicine, Division of Rheumatology; Department of Preventive Medicine, Northwestern University Feinberg School of Medicine, Chicago, Illinois

LISA A. MANDL, MD, MPH
Assistant Research Professor of Medicine and Public Health, Weill Cornell Medical School; Hospital for Special Surgery, New York City, New York

DANIEL P. MARCUSA, BA
Hospital for Special Surgery, New York City, New York

AARON W. MICHELS, MD
Assistant Professor of Pediatrics and Medicine, Barbara Davis Center for Childhood Diabetes, University of Colorado School of Medicine, Aurora, Colorado

ISABEL PEDRAZA, MD
Assistant Professor of Medicine, Division of Pulmonary/Critical Care Medicine, Cedars-Sinai Medical Center, Los Angeles, California

KARIM RAZA, FRCP, PhD
Professor, School of Immunity and Infection, College of Medical and Dental Sciences, University of Birmingham; Department of Rheumatology, Sandwell and West Birmingham Hospitals NHS Trust, Birmingham, United Kingdom

HUGH H. REID, BSc (Hons), PhD
Department of Biochemistry and Molecular Biology, School of Biomedical Sciences, Monash University, Clayton, Victoria, Australia

JULIE M. ROBERTSON, PhD
Arthritis and Clinical Immunology Research Program, Oklahoma Medical Research Foundation, Oklahoma City, Oklahoma

JAMIE ROSSJOHN, BSc (Hons), PhD
Professor, Department of Biochemistry and Molecular Biology, School of Biomedical Sciences, Monash University, Clayton, Victoria, Australia; Institute of Infection and Immunity, School of Medicine, Cardiff University, Cardiff, United Kingdom

KIMBER SIMMONS, MD
Barbara Davis Center for Childhood Diabetes, University of Colorado School of Medicine, Aurora, Colorado

JEFFREY A. SPARKS, MD, MMSc
Division of Rheumatology, Immunology and Allergy, Department of Medicine, Brigham and Women's Hospital, Harvard Medical School, Boston, Massachusetts

RANJENY THOMAS, MBBS, MD
Professor, Translational Research Institute, The University of Queensland Diamantina Institute, Woolloongabba, Queensland, Australia

SAMINA A. TURK, MD
Jan van Breemen Research Institute/Reade, Amsterdam, The Netherlands

MARIAN H. VAN BEERS-TAS, MD
Jan van Breemen Research Institute/Reade, Amsterdam, The Netherlands

DIRKJAN VAN SCHAARDENBURG, MD, PhD
Jan van Breemen Research Institute/Reade, Amsterdam, The Netherlands

DINNY WALLIS, MBChB
Specialty Registrar, Department of Rheumatology, Royal Hampshire County Hospital, Winchester, United Kingdom

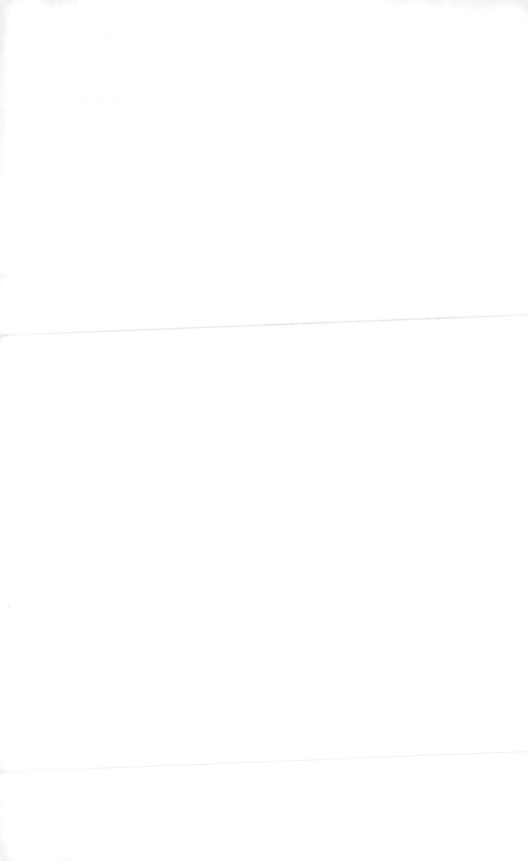

Contents

Chronic inflammatory and autoimmune conditions result from an interplay between genetic and environmental factors culminating in the phenotypes of established disease. The transition from health to established disease is relatively well understood in rheumatoid arthritis (RA), which provides an exemplar for other diseases. This article addresses terminologies to describe the phases of disease leading to RA, disease initiation and the point from which disease duration should be timed, the future research agenda suggested by this approach to the definition of phases of disease, and the importance of capturing the patient perspective in research into the earliest phases of disease.

Gout is a common inflammatory arthritis triggered by the crystallization of uric acid within the joints. Gout affects millions worldwide and has an increasing prevalence. Recent research has been carried out to better qualify and quantify the risk factors predisposing individuals to gout. These can largely be broken into nonmodifiable risk factors, such as gender, age, race, and genetics, and modifiable risk factors, such as diet and lifestyle. Increasing knowledge of factors predisposing certain individuals to gout could potentially lead to improved preventive practices. This review summarizes the nonmodifiable and modifiable risk factors associated with development of gout.

Rheumatoid arthritis (RA) develops through a series of stages. In the seropositive subset of classified RA patients, a preclinical stage is present for years before the onset of clinically apparent disease. Relevant preclinical biomarkers include autoantibodies, alterations of lymphoid populations, elevated cytokines/chemokines, genetic/genomic factors, imaging studies, clinical findings, dietary and environmental biomarkers, cardiovascular disease risk assessment, microbiome analyses, and metabolomic changes.

Identifying the population of asymptomatic subjects at sufficiently high risk for disease to be informative and representative of "preclinical patients" is a challenge. This article reviews the results of analyses that have been undertaken in these "at-risk" subjects.

Preclinical lupus encompasses a spectrum from enhanced SLE risk without clinical symptoms to individuals with autoantibodies and some SLE clinical features without meeting ACR classification. Studies have identified antibody and serological biomarkers years before disease onset. Incomplete lupus and undifferentiated connective tissue disease may occur during preclinical disease periods, but only 10–20% of these individuals transition to SLE and many have a mild disease course. Further studies are warranted to characterize biomarkers of early disease, identify individuals in need of close monitoring or preventive interventions, and elucidate mechanisms of disease pathogenesis without confounding factors of immunosuppressive medications or organ damage.

Rheumatic diseases offer distinct challenges to researchers because of heterogeneity in disease phenotypes, low disease incidence, and geographic variation in genetic and environmental factors. Emerging research areas, including epigenetics, metabolomics, and the microbiome, may provide additional links between genetic and environmental risk factors in the pathogenesis of rheumatic disease. This article reviews the methods used to establish genetic and environmental risk factors and studies gene-environment interactions in rheumatic diseases, and provides specific examples of successes and challenges in identifying gene-environment interactions in rheumatoid arthritis, systemic lupus erythematosus, and ankylosing spondylitis. Emerging research strategies and future challenges are discussed.

Although there are many examples of autoantibodies in disease-free individuals, they can be a preclinical phenomenon heralding future autoimmune rheumatic disease. They may be a marker for autoreactive B-cell activation and other inflammatory autoimmune processes. The increased prevalence of cardiovascular disease (CVD) in autoimmune rheumatic diseases such as rheumatoid arthritis and systemic lupus erythematosus, and the increased risk of CVD in patients with rheumatic disease with autoantibodies, suggest that CVD may have autoimmune features. Autoantibodies might be risk markers for subclinical and clinical CVD development not only in patients with rheumatic diseases but in the general population as well.

Signs and symptoms often occur well in advance of a formal diagnosis of rheumatoid arthritis (RA). However, these do not necessarily represent symptoms that are included in classification criteria. Their intensity, frequency, and persistence over time seem to be important in the spectrum from preclinical autoimmunity to classifiable RA. Prospective study of signs and symptoms in individuals at risk for RA will help to determine their onset and relationship with epitope spreading, cytokine evolution, sensitive imaging, and their usefulness in discriminating between individuals patients who will develop incident inflammatory arthritis versus normal controls.

In recent years the early identification of axial spondyloarthritis has become a high priority area of research. Evidence that therapy may slow radiographic progression of disease has heightened the importance of recognition of early disease. However, the concept of early axial spondyloarthritis and natural history of early disease are not fully understood. Future strategies to detect early and preclinical disease may incorporate clinical information, radiographic, serologic, and genetic testing. The risks and benefits of screening and early identification of disease need careful consideration.

Studies suggest that many persons with painful osteoarthritis already have extensive structural disease including malalignment, which may preclude successful stabilization or reversal of disease; this provides a strong rationale for developing strategies to prevent disease or to identify and treat it early. This article reviews a variety of approaches likely to capture those at high risk of or with early disease. However, given the absence of effective treatments, it is unclear whether structural disease could be successfully slowed or prevented in those with early symptoms or at high risk of disease.

The etiology of most systemic autoimmune diseases remains unknown. There is often a preclinical period of systemic autoimmunity prior to the onset of clinically classifiable disease; established and emerging data suggest that dysregulated immune interactions with commensal microbiota may play a role in the initial generation of autoimmunity in this preclinical period. This article reviews potential mechanisms by which alterations of healthy microbiota may induce autoimmunity as well as mucosal microbial associations with autoimmune diseases. If mucosal microbiota lead to the development of autoimmunity, these mucosal sites, microorganisms, and immunologic mechanisms can be targeted to prevent the onset of systemic autoimmune disease.

There exists a preclinical phase to the disease progression of rheumatoid arthritis, in which there is evidence of autoimmunity but no overt clinical arthritis. Identifying patients in this phase would allow for early treatment, to potentially halt manifestation of the disease. Imaging, because it is noninvasive, provides an appealing alternative to gold-standard synovial biopsies for identification of these preclinical patients. Ultrasonography, magnetic resonance imaging, and positron emission tomography all have their advantages and disadvantages as imaging modalities in this regard. Further research into alternative imaging modalities with larger cohorts is required to determine the most effective technique.

Despite treatment advances, rheumatoid arthritis (RA) is still associated with significant disability, decreased work capacity, and reduced life expectancy. Effective immunotherapies to restore immune tolerance promise greater specificity, lower toxicity, and a longer-term solution to controlling and preventing RA. Design of effective therapies requires a fundamental understanding of the critical immunopathogenetic pathways in RA. This article reviews advances in the understanding of self-antigen-specific T cells in autoimmune diseases including RA and type 1 diabetes, which bring exciting insights to the mechanisms underpinning loss of tolerance and how tolerance could be restored for disease prevention in the preclinical or recent-onset period.

Rheumatoid arthritis (RA) results from an interaction between genetic susceptibility and environmental factors. Several of these factors are known, such as family history of RA, high birth weight, smoking, silica exposure, alcohol nonuse, obesity, diabetes mellitus, rheumatoid factor, anti-citrullinated protein antibody, and genetic variants such as the shared epitope and protein tyrosine phosphatase nonreceptor type 22. The impact of these factors can be modeled in the 2 main groups at risk of RA: family members of patients with RA and seropositive persons with or without arthralgia. Current models have the potential to select individuals for preventive strategies.

Rheumatic diseases affect a significant portion of the population and lead to increased health care costs, disability, and premature mortality; effective preventive measures for these diseases could lead to substantial improvements in public health. Natural history studies show that for most rheumatic diseases there is a period of preclinical disease development during which abnormal biomarkers or other processes can be detected. These changes are useful to understand mechanisms of disease pathogenesis; in addition, they may be applied to estimate a personal risk of future disease while individuals are still relatively asymptomatic and ultimately be used to identify individuals who may be targeted for preventive interventions.

Screening for presymptomatic disease provides the potential for early intervention and improved outcomes. However, although this practice has potential benefits, it also has potential harms that must be considered. The U.S. Preventive Services Task Force (USPSTF) is a nonfederal panel of experts convened by the Agency for Health Research and Policy to systematically review the evidence for preventive services, including disease screening, and to create evidence-based recommendations for primary care practice in the United States. As rheumatologists contemplate the potential of screening for preclinical disease, understanding the process used by the USPSTF can help guide research efforts supporting such screening.

Type 1 diabetes (T1D) is a chronic autoimmune disorder resulting from immune-mediated destruction of insulin-producing beta cells within the pancreatic islets. Prediction of T1D is now possible, as having 2 or more islet autoantibodies confers a 100% risk of diabetes development. With the ability to predict disease development, clinical trials to prevent diabetes onset have been completed and are currently under way. This review focuses on the natural history, prediction, and prevention trials in T1D. We review the lessons learned from these attempts at preventing a chronic autoimmune disease and apply the paradigm from T1D prevention to other autoimmune disorders.

RHEUMATIC DISEASE CLINICS OF NORTH AMERICA

DOWNLOAD
Free App!

Review Articles
THE CLINICS

NOW AVAILABLE FOR YOUR iPhone and iPad

Foreword

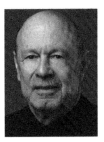

Michael H. Weisman, MD
Consulting Editor

Never make predictions, especially about the future
—*Casey Stengel*

This volume is dedicated to finding out why Casey Stengel gave us his remarkable insight—the absolute need to make predictions about the future simply because the future is now. We have been enormously successful in treating rheumatic disease patients with safer and now easily tolerated interventions once the diseases are recognized clinically. This success has moved the needle closer and closer to finding the earliest predictive signs and symptoms for later clinical disease, leading to much debate on when these diseases actually start. Therefore it is feasible to even think about disease prevention, and it is not much of a leap to consider finding those most at risk and considering an early intervention.

By looking at several diseases addressed in this volume, we can begin to focus on the interaction of the environment and genetic risk specific to each disease, whether it is osteoarthritis, ankylosing spondylitis, lupus, or rheumatoid arthritis. With the identification of biomarkers and pathways from studies of the earliest features of disease, we may be able to target interventions toward disease mechanisms with the ultimate goal of halting and even preventing the perpetuation of a chronic illness. The expansion of our knowledge about the microenvironment (as well as the macroenvironment) we encounter on a daily basis has made this possible.

What this editor is most cognizant of in this volume is the confluence of experts from population science, genetics, immunology, biochemistry, and clinical medicine addressing this vital issue. Drs Bykerk, Costenbader, and Deane have done a remarkable job.

Michael H. Weisman, MD
Division of Rheumatology
Cedars-Sinai Medical Center
8700 Beverly Boulevard
Los Angeles, CA 90024, USA

E-mail address:
michael.weisman@cshs.org

Rheum Dis Clin N Am 40 (2014) xiii
http://dx.doi.org/10.1016/j.rdc.2014.09.002
0889-857X/14/$ – see front matter © 2014 Published by Elsevier Inc.

rheumatic.theclinics.com

Preface

Preclinical Rheumatic Disease

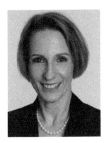 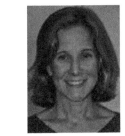 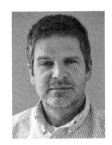

Vivian P. Bykerk, MD   Karen H. Costenbader, MD, MPH   Kevin Deane, MD, PhD

Editors

The ability to intervene at the earliest phases in the pathogenesis of a chronic rheumatic disease caused by auto-inflammatory, autoimmune, or tissue injury mechanisms has the potential to prevent disease manifestations and consequences, limiting loss of quality of life, comorbidity, and costs to society. This issue is dedicated to exploring the stages of rheumatic disease, biologic mechanisms contributing to the pathogenesis, along with possible ways to study and screen for persons at risk with the ultimate goal of finding ways to prevent these devastating diseases.

Despite modification of classification and diagnostic criteria to identify diseases earlier, and the emergence of very effective targeted therapies used in conjunction with early diagnosis and treatment, this has not yet resulted in cures for or prevention of these diseases, or even successful drug-free remission in most cases. In rheumatoid arthritis (RA), for example, very few persons affected can succeed in maintaining drug-free remission over an extended period of time. As such, the ability to identify and screen for these diseases very early on in the preclinical phases may yield the best chance of successful intervention to prevent full manifestations of disease. Efforts aimed at finding the earliest point in pathogenesis, when there is evidence of autoimmunity but no expression of overt disease, are underway for many rheumatic diseases. These include studies by many researchers, applying a variety of methods, including analyses of populations who are at high risk for future rheumatic disease such as first-degree relatives and people who may be in the very early phases of rheumatic disease based on the presence of specific symptoms and/or laboratory tests indicating the presence of autoimmunity.

In this issue, several scientists and clinical researchers renowned for their work to progress in understanding of the very early phases of so-called preclinical rheumatic disease have generously given their time and expertise to provide their perspective of what is known about the evolutions of rheumatic diseases and clinical arthritis. The issues are complex and have started with a common way of thinking about the stages

Rheum Dis Clin N Am 40 (2014) xv–xviii
http://dx.doi.org/10.1016/j.rdc.2014.09.001
rheumatic.theclinics.com

of preclinical disease as so eloquently described by Drs Raza and Gerlag. Their overview describes consensus among researchers in this field about the perspectives of these stages. Briefly, in almost all rheumatic diseases, one can think of the preclinical phase as occurring in several stages. These include a period of genetic risk, exposure to environmental factors, followed by development of asymptomatic autoimmunity, development of nonspecific symptoms, elaboration of an immune or inflammatory response, and ultimately, definitive clinical manifestations.

Clinicians frequently see patients with evidence of autoimmunity with nonspecific manifestations and have no evidence based on clinical studies to guide them regarding management. Drs Kung and Turk have thoroughly researched and described the approaches to and challenges of interpreting symptoms and signs in the preclinical phases using preclinical RA as an example. They highlight the numerous studies ongoing to date and argue for the case that a combination of symptoms and tests that demonstrate signs of active autoimmunity is needed to implement any form of secondary prevention. They also note that symptoms at this phase may not necessarily reflect those in classification criteria. Dr Turk and coauthors, in summarizing results from an extensive systematic review of this topic, contend that given the currently available evidence for identifying those at highest risk for evolving into classifiable **RA, screening is best performed in relatives of patients with established disease or in those with symptoms and positive blood tests. Even with this approach, the odds of developing disease within a year are still low. Both Dr Willis and Dr Mandl delve into the need to consider advanced imaging to detect the earliest sign of disease because abnormal findings in high-resolution imaging often occur before an inflammatory disease is classifiable. They caution, however, that this approach is not yet ready for clinical use as the specificity of these tests can be poor.

Drs Finckh and Deane further note that to prevent overt expression and persistence of autoimmune disease it is possible to intervene at varying stages. In some situations, the best approach could ultimately be through primary prevention of initial autoimmunity or tissue injury, although at present most are approaching this through secondary prevention in which attempts to halt progression of a disease would be implemented in those already into the earliest phases of pathogenesis. Ideally, screening and prevention should occur while subjects are still in an asymptomatic or minimally symptomatic stage. However, as Dr Colange highlights, primary or secondary screening tests to identify those at risk must balance the risks and harms of intervention when considering any modification of risk factors, such as induction of tolerance, or pharmacologic interventions.

In rheumatic diseases, such as osteoarthritis (OA) or gout, not all the same stages apply. For both, there may be genetic susceptibility and environmental risk factors. However, the mechanisms of disease pathogenesis differ. In OA, this involves tissue injury as described by Dr Felson in his review of the earliest phases of OA. In gout, the earliest phases involve metabolic mechanisms. Drs MacFarlane and Kim note there are now clear associations of specific genetic polymorphisms associated with gout that are linked to altered uric acid metabolism. Thus, primary prevention by genetic manipulation could be a viable option in the future. Importantly, gout pathogenesis is often accompanied by dietary and personal factors, including obesity, before leading to the overt expression of chronic gout, making the case that risk modification is possible. This is not the case, however, for most other rheumatic diseases. For example, although much is also known about many genetic polymorphisms associated with the development of RA, the interrelation of these environmental triggers at the earliest phases of autoimmunity is only just being explored. Drs Sparks and

Costenbader review data from the study of gene–environment interactions that may to lead to insights for the primary prevention of many of these diseases. They have described several of these advances in the context of a path forward to understanding the role of gene–environment interactions in inflammatory arthritis and how these might explain the biologic mechanisms underpinning the onset of autoimmunity. They provide examples that have already been worked out in the development of RA and spondyloarthropathy.

Basic scientists are looking to identify novel mechanisms of disease pathogenesis. Dr Holers describes how these may be working in the pathogenesis of RA, suggesting that the disease may originate and evolve in tissues other than joints, specifically, the oral mucosa or lungs, given recent evidence of small airways disease in individuals at risk for developing RA. In one example of pathogenesis, he describes the role of microorganisms found in the oral mucosa because they give rise to citrullinated peptide antigens. In susceptible individuals, it results in the generation of anticitrullinated peptide antibodies that expand in their repertoire with epitope spreading of new antibodies to other citrullinated protein antigens, followed by elevated cytokines and chemokines, and subsequent systemic synovial inflammation. Drs Kuhn and Demourelle expand this perspective by considering the role of altered microbiota in varying mucosal tissues because they may contribute to autoimmunity or auto-inflammatory diseases. Newer hypotheses of biologic mechanisms invoke an altered microbiome as being key to disease pathogenesis. Microbial dysbiosis is also being explored in spondyloarthropathies, which are highly associated with gut inflammation, as noted in the review by Drs Willis and Inman. Auto-antibody formation is has been considered to play a critical role in the pathogenesis of systemic lupus erythematosus (SLE). Clinicians and researchers alike are aware they are present in the earliest expression of this disease. However, as Drs Robertson and James point out, the complexity of this illness, even with newer classification criteria, hampers a simple understanding of the mechanisms leading from preclinical genetic risk to autoimmunity and overt disease in SLE.

As you will appreciate by reading each of these articles, the authors tackle the issues of preclinical rheumatic disease from a different perspective. Clinical researchers are still finding ways to better understand and to identify those at risk for autoimmunity, inflammation, and tissue injury. The understanding of genetic risk and epigenetic modifications triggered by environmental factors is far from complete.

Advances toward achieving this understanding have progressed further for some diseases than others, and in particular, clinical prevention trials in type 1 diabetes have been underway for some years. Drs Simon and Michaels have aptly described how advances in this field have combined the understanding of genetic risk, use of natural history studies, and discoveries that antibodies against islet cell antigens are predictive of young children developing type 1 diabetes. When these antibodies are detected in children under the age of 2, they are highly associated with T-cell-mediated destruction islet cells and ultimate failure to produce insulin. This understanding has led to trials of secondary prevention using immunotherapy. Results of the success of this approach have not yet been realized; however, if any are effective, this will generate the first evidence that supports the rationale of secondary prevention of autoimmune disease. For most rheumatic diseases, scientists are still exploring ways to identify early expression of autoimmunity and how this may relate to genetic polymorphisms and environmental exposures.

We sincerely thank our colleagues for providing their insights and contributions to this issue. As you see, each has contributed a different perspective as to how we as clinicians, researchers, and scientists can work toward preventing the very rheumatic diseases that cause so much suffering for our patients.

Vivian P. Bykerk, MD
Weill Cornell Medical College
Inflammatory Arthritis Center
Hospital for Special Surgery
535 East 70th Street
New York, NY 10021, USA

Karen H. Costenbader, MD, MPH
Harvard Medical School
Lupus Center
Division of Rheumatology, Immunology, and Allergy
Brigham and Women's Hospital
75 Francis Street
Boston, MA 02115, USA

Kevin Deane, MD, PhD
Division of Rheumatology
University of Colorado School of Medicine
1775 Aurora Court, Mail Stop B-115
Aurora, CO 80045, USA

E-mail addresses:
bykerkv@hss.edu (V.P. Bykerk)
KCOSTENBADER@PARTNERS.ORG (K.H. Costenbader)
Kevin.Deane@ucdenver.edu (K. Deane)

Preclinical Inflammatory Rheumatic Diseases
An Overview and Relevant Nomenclature

Karim Raza, FRCP, PhD[a,b,*], Danielle M. Gerlag, MD, PhD[c,d]

KEYWORDS

- Rheumatoid arthritis • Preclinical • Early • Risk • Prediction • Prevention

KEY POINTS

- Terminologies have been developed to describe the preclinical and clinically apparent phases of disease leading to rheumatoid arthritis (RA).
- Disease duration in research studies should be timed from the points of onset of the clinically apparent phases: the onset of phase D (symptoms without clinical arthritis), the onset of phase E (clinical arthritis), and the onset of phase F (RA).
- The future research agenda should include identifying and understanding (1) additional environmental risk factors for RA, (2) gene-environment interactions, (3) the full extent of immune abnormalities that characterize the preclinical phase of disease and the site of initiation of these immune responses, (4) processes that lead to the localization of the disease to the joints, and (5) the range of symptoms that characterize the early clinical phases of disease.

BACKGROUND

Inflammatory rheumatic diseases are common and are associated with significant morbidity, as a consequence of articular and extra-articular manifestations, as well as reduced life expectancy.

Disclosures: D.M. Gerlag is currently employed by GlaxoSmithKline. K. Raza has received honoraria from Pfizer, UCB, AbbVie, and BMS and meeting expenses from Pfizer and Roche. Work by K Raza and and DM Gerlag in the field of RA risk is supported through the European Union's FP7 Health Programme, under the grant agreement FP7-HEALTH-F2-2012-305549 (Euro-TEAM).
[a] School of Immunity and Infection, College of Medical and Dental Sciences, University of Birmingham, Birmingham B15 2TT, UK; [b] Department of Rheumatology, Sandwell and West Birmingham Hospitals NHS Trust, Birmingham B18 7QH, UK; [c] Academic Medical Center, Division of Clinical Immunology & Rheumatology F4-105, Meibergdreef 9, 1105 AZ Amsterdam, The Netherlands; [d] Clinical Unit Cambridge, GlaxoSmithKline, Addenbrooke's Centre for Clinical Investigation, Box 128, Hills Road, Cambridge CB2 0GG, UK
* Corresponding author. Rheumatology Research Group, Centre for Transitional Inflammation Research, University of Birmingham Research Laboratories, New Queen Elizabeth Hospital, Birmingham B15 2WD, UK.
E-mail address: k.raza@bham.ac.uk

Rheum Dis Clin N Am 40 (2014) 569–580
http://dx.doi.org/10.1016/j.rdc.2014.07.001
0889-857X/14/$ – see front matter © 2014 Elsevier Inc. All rights reserved.

rheumatic.theclinics.com

In patients with rheumatoid arthritis (RA), a considerable body of research has shown that early treatment leads to significantly improved outcomes. For example, the initiation of disease-modifying antirheumatic drug therapy within the first 12 weeks of the onset of symptoms significantly reduces the rate of radiological progression compared with treatments started later,[1] with patients with more aggressive disease benefiting most from early therapy.[2] Although data are most robust for RA, there are data for other inflammatory rheumatic diseases suggesting that early treatment may also improve long-term outcomes.[3] However, treatments in the established phases of disease, even if given early, are rarely curative.

A desire to cure and even prevent disease has led to increased interest in the earliest phases of the inflammatory rheumatic diseases, including both the earliest phases of clinically apparent disease (before patients have developed the full set of characteristics that allow them to be classified as having the disease in question), and the phases of disease before the onset of symptoms.

This article focuses on RA, although many of the concepts discussed are equally relevant to other inflammatory rheumatic (eg, systemic sclerosis and systemic lupus erythematosus) and nonrheumatic (eg, type 1 diabetes) diseases.

THE INITIAL IDENTIFICATION OF A PRECLINICAL PHASE OF RHEUMATOID ARTHRITIS

Although understanding of the preclinical phase of RA has increased considerably in the last few years, the existence of such a phase was first appreciated in the 1980s. Pioneering work from Finland made use of serum samples from individuals participating in a series of community-based cardiovascular studies, because it was possible to identify those who had developed RA after sample collection.[4] Of 30 subjects who developed seropositive RA (between a few months and 9 years after the collection of serum samples), 16 were positive for rheumatoid factor with the frequency of positivity being greater in those nearer the onset of clinically manifest arthritis.[4] The presence of antiperinuclear and antikeratin antibodies in individuals before the onset of RA was subsequently reported.[5,6] Research in this area grew rapidly through the 1990s and 2000s and was the subject of a recent review by van Steenbergen and colleagues.[7]

As research interest increased, so did the number of terms used by researchers to describe the earliest phases of RA, including pre-RA, preclinical RA, autoantibody-positive arthralgia, early RA, very early RA, and extremely early RA. A lack of consistency regarding terminology made it difficult to compare results between studies and a paucity of information regarding the terminologies used in original articles made it difficult to understand what phase of disease individual researchers were reporting on. In order to develop an agreed set of terminologies regarding the phases of disease leading up to the development of RA, the EULAR (European League Against Rheumatism) Standing Committee for Investigative Rheumatology established the Study Group for Risk Factors for RA. Many of the principles underlying the nomenclature developed by this Study Group are applicable to the earliest phases of other chronic autoimmune/chronic inflammatory diseases.

TERMINOLOGIES TO DESCRIBE INDIVIDUALS IN PHASES LEADING UP TO THE DEVELOPMENT OF RHEUMATOID ARTHRITIS

In order to develop a set of terminologies to describe individuals in phases leading up to the development of RA, a multidisciplinary group including rheumatologists, laboratory scientists, and a patient representative reviewed and provided descriptive terms for the phases that individuals may pass through before the development of RA and commented on terms and phrases widely used in the literature to describe these phases. Proposals for new terminologies were discussed during a 2-day workshop, at the end of which consensus was reached.[8] It was recommended that, in prospective studies, individuals at risk of developing RA would be described as having:

1. Genetic risk factors for RA
2. Environmental risk factors for RA
3. Systemic autoimmunity associated with RA
4. Symptoms without clinical arthritis (the term arthritis being used to denote clinically apparent soft tissue swelling or fluid and not bony overgrowth alone)
5. Unclassified arthritis
6. RA

This nomenclature is illustrated in **Fig. 1**. Recognizing that individuals typically progress through these phases, an important aspect of these terminologies was that A to E could be used in a combinatorial manner if appropriate. Thus, for example, a study of asymptomatic individuals who were anti-citrullinated protein/peptide antibody (ACPA) positive would be capturing individuals at phase C, whereas a study of patients who were ACPA positive but who also had inflammatory-sounding musculoskeletal symptoms (but without a clinically swollen joint) would be capturing individuals in phase C and D. The combinatorial nature of this system of terminology is also an acknowledgment that:

1. An individual does not necessarily move through all phases in turn before developing RA (see dashed lines in **Fig. 1**). For example, an individual in phase D may never have had detectable systemic autoimmunity associated with RA, particularly for example in the case of autoantibody-negative individuals.
2. The phases do not necessarily occur in the same order in all patients. For example, some patients may develop autoantibodies before the development of inflammatory joint symptoms and other patients may develop these after the onset of such symptoms.

The terms used to describe the different phases before the development of RA are intentionally broad. Thus "Genetic risk factors for RA" and "Environmental risk factors for RA" deliberately did not define any particular genetic or environmental risk factors. "Systemic autoimmunity associated with RA" did not define any specific immune

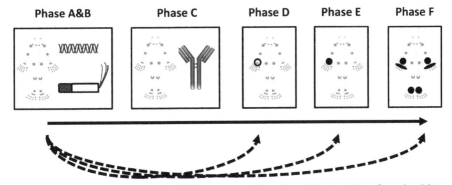

Fig. 1. The 5 phases (A–E) an individual may pass through in the transition from health to the development of RA (phase F). The open circle in phase D represents a painful but non-swollen joint. The filled shapes in phases E and F represent joints with clinically apparent soft tissue swelling.

abnormalities, such as any specific autoantibody, and "Symptoms without clinical evidence of arthritis" did not define any specific symptoms. This was a very conscious decision, because restricting these categories by specifying risk factors and features known at the time of the development of the terminologies would have rendered the nomenclature rapidly redundant in this advancing field. It was recognized that future research would define additional risk factors and features relevant to each of these phases, beyond current knowledge, and would assess the predictive utility of each of these. In addition, there are currently recognized biomarkers that are known to be present before the development of RA and that are not specifically reflected in the nomenclature. The presence of synovitis on imaging, but not clinically, is an example of this.[9] This is not to suggest that the study group viewed this as an unimportant biomarker. Rather, the nomenclature should provide a framework for future research to assess at which phases, and for transit to which phases, this, like other biomarkers, is useful.

Defining these phases should facilitate the study of mechanisms underlying the transitions between each of these phases and the biomarkers that predict these transitions; critical issues if interventions are to be implemented to prevent progression to RA in at-risk individuals.

PRE-RHEUMATOID ARTHRITIS

At the time these terminologies were developed, the phrase pre-RA was widely used, with many investigators describing individuals in phase C, for example, as having pre-RA. The recommendations suggested that the prefix "pre-RA with" could be used before any one or any combination combinations of A to E but only to retrospectively describe a phase an individual was in once it is known that they had developed RA. For example, given that healthy individuals who are ACPA positive do not necessarily develop RA, it was thought inappropriate to label them as being, or refer to them having, pre-RA. The personal implications (including emotional and financial) of a diagnosis of RA were recognized to be such that the inevitability of developing RA suggested by the phrase pre-RA was thought to be inappropriate. In contrast, in a prospective study of individuals RA-at risk phase C in which some patients did develop RA it was thought appropriate to use the phrase "pre-RA with" to describe phases in which the patient (now known to have RA) had previously been.

Avoiding the phrase pre-RA unless it is known that the individual is going to develop RA is also an acknowledgment that individuals may follow a backward disease course. For example, some individuals present with an unclassified arthritis (phase E) that entirely resolves without specific therapy. The study of patients with resolving outcomes will potentially provide new data on proresolution mechanisms[10] and may provide novel proresolution biomarkers and treatment approaches that can be used to prevent progression in patients at risk.

PRECLINICAL DISEASE

The phrase "preclinical" RA is also widely used, often to describe all phases before the development of a disease classifiable as RA. The terminologies recommended by the EULAR study group effectively divide at-risk phases into those that are asymptomatic (A, B, and C) and those that are symptomatic (D and E). The term preclinical disease is recommended to be used for patients in phases A to C, with patients in phases D and E being in clinically apparent at-risk phases.

THE MEASUREMENT OF DISEASE DURATION

Disease duration is a frequently reported variable in studies of disease mechanisms, observation studies addressing predictors of outcome, and in intervention studies in patients with early disease. However, the definition of disease duration is usually ignored and depends on the point of onset from which disease duration is being reported.

The identification of a point of onset is difficult because it is currently not know where, let alone when, disease begins. Furthermore, in patients who progress through phase C toward the development of RA, it is impossible to define the time of onset of phase C outside the context of a prospective study of at-risk individuals in phases A and B who are subjected to frequent follow-up. However, as individuals move through the preclinical phases of disease to the clinical disease phases, points can be identified more easily from which duration could be timed. Historically, in those studies that have reported the point from which disease duration is being timed, there has been a diversity of approaches to the dating of onset, including from (1) onset of any joint symptoms related to the current episode, including arthralgia/morning stiffness; (2) onset of self-reported joint swelling; (3) onset of clinically observed swelling; (4) time of fulfillment of classification criteria for RA.[11] However, because an evolution of pathologic processes during the clinically apparent at-risk phases would suggest that treatments need to be tailored depending on symptom duration, it is important to understand whether pathologic processes change following the onset of symptomatic disease (phase C onward). It is therefore important that the duration of symptoms, and a description of the symptoms from which duration is timed, be made more explicit in studies of at-risk individuals.

The EULAR study group has recommended that, as best practice, the following dates are recorded in prospective cohort studies and that disease duration is timed for each of them:

1. First musculoskeletal symptoms relevant (in the opinion of the assessing rheumatologist) to the current complaint
2. First persistent (ie, chronic until presentation) patient-reported joint swelling
3. Initial fulfillment of criteria for RA (1987 American College of Rheumatology [ACR][12] and 2010 ACR EULAR[13]) based on data obtained retrospectively from the patient's history
4. Initial fulfillment of criteria for RA (1987 ACR and 2010 ACR EULAR) based on the rheumatologist's assessment

Of these 4, the first is perhaps the most contentious because it can sometimes be difficult to identify which of a patient's symptoms were related to, and marked the onset of, inflammatory joint disease. Recent data suggest that the spectrum of symptoms that mark the onset of phase C is varied.[14,15] Ongoing research is designed to identify those symptoms with the highest predictive value of the future development of RA; these data will help define the subset of symptoms that should most appropriately mark the onset of time point 1 (as listed earlier).

AN OVERVIEW OF THE TRANSITIONS FROM HEALTH TO DISEASE IN INDIVIDUALS AT RISK OF RHEUMATOID ARTHRITIS

More than 100 genetic loci have now been associated with RA. Twin studies have shown that the hereditability of RA is approximately 60%, suggesting that a large proportion of the disease risk results from environmental factors that likely interact with genetic risk factors. The largest genetic risk factor for RA lies within the human leukocyte antigen (HLA) class II region, which encodes the HLA-DRB1 molecule; specific alleles associated with RA share a conserved amino acid sequence referred to as the shared epitope.[16] The largest genetic association with RA outside the HLA region lies within the protein tyrosine phosphatase nonreceptor 22 (PTPN22) gene.[17] The risk genes within the HLA class II locus, the risk variant of the PTPN22 gene, and the best characterized environmental risk factor for RA (smoking) all interact to increase the risk of seropositive RA.[18–20]

Division of the phases of RA into those detailed earlier helps to focus attention on the transitions for which the known genetic and environmental factors are risk factors. This is a critically important question from the perspective of approaches to disease prevention because modulation of an environmental risk factor relevant for the transition from one phase to another may not have the same effect for other transitions. For example, recent evidence suggests that the HLA class II locus is associated less with the risk of developing ACPA and more with the risk of progression from a state of ACPA positivity (phase C) to having RA[21]; by contrast, environmental factors including smoking may be more important in transition from phase A to phase C.[21,22] From the perspective of preventing RA, smoking cessation campaigns may therefore more effectively be targeted at first-degree relatives of those with RA (phase A and B) than patients with positive ACPA and musculoskeletal symptoms (phase B, C, and D).

Although many genetic factors are known to be risk factors for RA, some are known to be protective. For example, HLA-DRB1*13 is associated with protection against ACPA-positive RA.[23] Understanding the full extent of genetic protective factors, and the transitions at which their protective effects operate, will be important in understanding the transitions to RA. Additional areas that need to be explored include the full extent of genetic, epigenetic, and environmental risk factors for both autoantibody-positive and autoantibody-negative RA as well as gene-environment interactions.

Although the synovium is the principal site of disorder in the established phase of disease, it may not be the site at which the disease is initiated. Systemic immune abnormalities in individuals without joint symptoms, and a lack of immune infiltrates in the synovium during the earliest phase before clinical signs and symptoms of arthritis,[24] point to other tissues (in particular the mucosal sites of the lung, gastrointestinal tract, and periodontium) as being important in the initiation of adaptive immune reactions.[25–29] Important for the research agenda is an understanding of the site of disease initiation, and the influence of environmental exposure including the microbiome at these sites as triggers for the development of systemic autoimmunity. Furthermore, the full extent of RA-related autoimmunity needs to be addressed. With the recent identification of immunity against carbamylated residues it has become clear that autoreactivity is seen against a range of posttranslational modifications[30]; an understanding of the drivers toward specific breakages in tolerance should provide data on disease mechanisms operating in at-risk individuals.

It has been widely suggested that there is a second hit that triggers the switch from systemic autoimmunity to a joint-centric disease.[24,31] Understanding the causal factors relevant to this transition will be critical to further understandings of transitions from phase C to the clinical phases of disease and to develop secondary prevention approaches.

PREDICTING AND PREVENTING RHEUMATOID ARTHRITIS

Several algorithms have been developed to predict RA development in individuals in different at-risk phases, such as phase A,[32,33] phase C and D,[34] and phase E.[35,36] An understanding of risk factors for progression to RA has been central to the development of all these algorithms. However, in all cases, validation and optimization of the algorithms is required, necessitating the identification of additional risk factors for and biomarkers of the development of RA. The research agenda in this area will need to focus on (1) the role of tissue-based biomarkers in the prediction of outcome, recognizing that it is becoming easier to access synovial tissue[37] and other potentially relevant tissues[38] using minimally invasive approaches. (2) The role of imaging-based biomarkers, including imaging of the synovium.[39–42] (3) The assessment of the relative values of a broad range of biomarkers, including those derived from an understanding of genetic and environmental risk factors, measures of systemic autoimmunity, measures of pathologic processes operating at a tissue level, and measures of clinical features with the aim of developing an optimal prediction model that may incorporate variables from all these domains.

A critical aim of being able to identify groups at high risk for the development of RA is the ability to intervene to reduce the risk of RA development. In the context of the development of seropositive RA, prevention can be considered as primary or secondary, with primary prevention involving prevention of development of RA-related systemic autoimmunity (ie, prevention of development of phase C) and secondary prevention involving prevention of development of clinically apparent arthritis in individuals with preexisting systemic autoimmunity (ie, prevention of transition from phase C onward). Several approaches have been proposed to reduce the risk of RA. These approaches include those targeting known environmental risk factors by lifestyle modification (eg, smoking cessation[43] and weight loss in patients with obesity[44]). As discussed earlier, smoking cessation is most likely to be effective as a primary prevention strategy; the most appropriate phase in which to intervene with weight loss measures is currently unclear. Pharmacologic approaches for primary prevention, for example with vitamin D and omega 3, are also currently being investigated.[45] Although no data are yet available regarding approaches to secondary prevention, a study assessing the effects of rituximab on the development of RA in individuals in phase C and D has recently finished recruitment, with outcome data expected in 2018 (Prevention of RA by B cell directed therapy (Prairi) trial' NTR1969; www.trialregister.nl). An understanding of mechanisms involved in transitions to and from phase C will inform the choice of therapeutic approach for future prevention studies, and predictive algorithms will help define appropriate at-risk populations in which to test these approaches.

THE IMPORTANCE OF ENGAGING THE PATIENT PERSPECTIVE IN THE CONTEXT OF RESEARCH INTO AT-RISK PHASES OF DISEASE

The value of capturing the patient perspective in the context of research in RA is well recognized.[46,47] As understanding of disease mechanisms and predictive and therapeutic strategies evolves into earlier phases of RA, the ethics of research in these area and ways of effectively communicating with individuals to allow them to make informed choices, understand the implications of test results, and effect appropriate behavioral change need to be researched and developed. Conducting this research with the support of research partners who have the lived experience of RA, or who may be at risk of RA, will help ensure that the research recognizes and takes account of the perspectives of the end users and will facilitate the translation of research findings into tests and preventive strategies that can be implemented in an effective and ethical manner.

The challenge faced in the context of this is illustrated by the fact that international guidelines for the management of RA highlight the importance of early treatment, ideally within the first 3 months of symptom onset.[48] Multiple studies have shown that this is not achieved, often as a consequence of patients not seeking help rapidly when their symptoms occur.[49,50] Central to this is a widespread lack of public understanding that RA is a serious disease with significant morbidity and mortality, that effective therapies are available, and that rapid presentation and referral are critical to improve outcomes.[51–53] This poor RA-related health literacy in the general public is an important challenge in the context of the development of implementable predictive and preventive strategies. The effective implementation of screening tools and strategies for people at risk of RA requires a willingness of individuals to undergo assessments and to understand the implications of test results as a guide for modifying behavior. It is important that the information given to people encouraging them to participate in assessments and treatments is designed and tailored to communicate effectively. Such information should communicate risks, the importance of assessment, and ways in which lifestyle choice may influence risk, while avoiding psychological distress or misunderstandings (eg, believing that having risk factors for RA equates to a diagnosis of RA).

LESSONS FOR OTHER CHRONIC AUTOIMMUNE DISEASES

The approach described earlier for RA can readily be applied to other chronic autoimmune disease, both nonrheumatic (eg, type 1 diabetes[54–56]) and rheumatic. For example, in the case of systemic sclerosis, the presence of presclerodermatous disease is well recognized and is typically characterized by the presence of autoantibodies (eg, antinuclear antibody), Raynaud phenomenon, and nail fold capillary dilatation,[57] which are analogous to phase C and D in the context of RA. As we have proposed for RA, current efforts in systemic sclerosis include an attempt to define the features that identify individuals who are at the highest risk of progressing.[58] We believe that the use of standard terminologies by those working in RA will facilitate research in a range of areas, including etiology and predictive and preventive strategies. We also suggest that the use of equivalent terminologies to describe the at-risk phases of other chronic autoimmune diseases will provide information on similarities and difference between diseases. This information in turn may enhance our understanding of approaches to prediction and prevention, informing decision making regarding the strategies that, having been shown to be effective in one disease, should be explored in another disease, and the strategies that should not.

ACKNOWLEDGMENT

This research was supported by the Innovative Medicines Initiative project BTCure (grant agreement number 115142-1), European Union Seventh Framework Programme project EuroTEAM, Grant Number FP7-HEALTH-F2-2012-305549.

REFERENCES

1. van der Linden MP, le Cessie S, Raza K, et al. Long-term impact of delay in assessment of patients with early arthritis. Arthritis Rheum 2010;62(12): 3537–46.
2. Finckh A, Liang MH, van Herckenrode CM, et al. Long-term impact of early treatment on radiographic progression in rheumatoid arthritis: a meta-analysis. Arthritis Rheum 2006;55(6):864–72.

3. Tillett W, Jadon D, Shaddick G, et al. Smoking and delay to diagnosis are associated with poorer functional outcome in psoriatic arthritis. Ann Rheum Dis 2013; 72(8):1358–61.
4. Aho K, Palosuo T, Raunio V, et al. When does rheumatoid disease start? Arthritis Rheum 1985;28(5):485–9.
5. Kurki P, Aho K, Palosuo T, et al. Immunopathology of rheumatoid arthritis. Antikeratin antibodies precede the clinical disease. Arthritis Rheum 1992;35(8):914–7.
6. Aho K, von Essen R, Kurki P, et al. Antikeratin antibody and antiperinuclear factor as markers for subclinical rheumatoid disease process. J Rheumatol 1993; 20(8):1278–81.
7. van Steenbergen HW, Huizinga TW, van der Helm-van Mil AH. The preclinical phase of rheumatoid arthritis: what is acknowledged and what needs to be assessed? Arthritis Rheum 2013;65(9):2219–32.
8. Gerlag DM, Raza K, van Baarsen LG, et al. EULAR recommendations for terminology and research in individuals at risk of rheumatoid arthritis: report from the Study Group for Risk Factors for Rheumatoid Arthritis. Ann Rheum Dis 2012; 71(5):638–41.
9. Rakieh C, Nam JL, Hunt L, et al. Predicting the development of clinical arthritis in anti-CCP positive individuals with non-specific musculoskeletal symptoms: a prospective observational cohort study. Ann Rheum Dis 2014. [Epub ahead of print].
10. Buckley CD, Gilroy DW, Serhan CN, et al. The resolution of inflammation. Nat Rev Immunol 2013;13(1):59–66.
11. Raza K, Saber TP, Kvien TK, et al. Timing the therapeutic window of opportunity in early rheumatoid arthritis: proposal for definitions of disease duration in clinical trials. Ann Rheum Dis 2012;71(12):1921–3.
12. Arnett FC, Edworthy SM, Bloch DA, et al. The American Rheumatism Association 1987 revised criteria for the classification of rheumatoid arthritis. Arthritis Rheum 1988;31(3):315–24.
13. Aletaha D, Neogi T, Silman AJ, et al. 2010 Rheumatoid arthritis classification criteria: an American College of Rheumatology/European League Against Rheumatism collaborative initiative. Ann Rheum Dis 2010;69(9):1580–8.
14. Stack RJ, Sahni M, Mallen CD, et al. Symptom complexes at the earliest phases of rheumatoid arthritis: a synthesis of the qualitative literature. Arthritis Care Res (Hoboken) 2013;65(12):1916–26.
15. Stack RJ, van Tuyl LH, Sloots M, et al. Symptom complexes in patients with seropositive arthralgia and in patients newly diagnosed with rheumatoid arthritis: a qualitative exploration of symptom development. Rheumatology (Oxford) 2014;53(9):1646–53.
16. Gregersen PK, Silver J, Winchester RJ. The shared epitope hypothesis. An approach to understanding the molecular genetics of susceptibility to rheumatoid arthritis. Arthritis Rheum 1987;30(11):1205–13.
17. Begovich AB, Carlton VE, Honigberg LA, et al. A missense single-nucleotide polymorphism in a gene encoding a protein tyrosine phosphatase (PTPN22) is associated with rheumatoid arthritis. Am J Hum Genet 2004;75(2):330–7.
18. Padyukov L, Silva C, Stolt P, et al. A gene-environment interaction between smoking and shared epitope genes in HLA-DR provides a high risk of seropositive rheumatoid arthritis. Arthritis Rheum 2004;50(10):3085–92.
19. Klareskog L, Stolt P, Lundberg K, et al. A new model for an etiology of rheumatoid arthritis: smoking may trigger HLA-DR (shared epitope)-restricted immune reactions to autoantigens modified by citrullination. Arthritis Rheum 2006;54(1): 38–46.

20. Kallberg H, Padyukov L, Plenge RM, et al. Gene-gene and gene-environment interactions involving HLA-DRB1, PTPN22, and smoking in two subsets of rheumatoid arthritis. Am J Hum Genet 2007;80(5):867–75.

21. Bos WH, Ursum J, de Vries N, et al. The role of the shared epitope in arthralgia with anti-cyclic citrullinated peptide antibodies (anti-CCP), and its effect on anti-CCP levels. Ann Rheum Dis 2008;67(9):1347–50.

22. Haj Hensvold A, Magnusson PK, Joshua V, et al. Environmental and genetic factors in the development of anticitrullinated protein antibodies (ACPAs) and ACPA-positive rheumatoid arthritis: an epidemiological investigation in twins. Ann Rheum Dis 2013. [Epub ahead of print].

23. van der Woude D, Lie BA, Lundstrom E, et al. Protection against anti-citrullinated protein antibody-positive rheumatoid arthritis is predominantly associated with HLA-DRB1*1301: a meta-analysis of HLA-DRB1 associations with anti-citrullinated protein antibody-positive and anti-citrullinated protein antibody-negative rheumatoid arthritis in four European populations. Arthritis Rheum 2010;62(5):1236–45.

24. van de Sande MG, de Hair MJ, van der Leij C, et al. Different stages of rheumatoid arthritis: features of the synovium in the preclinical phase. Ann Rheum Dis 2011;70(5):772–7.

25. de Pablo P, Chapple IL, Buckley CD, et al. Periodontitis in systemic rheumatic diseases. Nat Rev Rheum 2009;5(4):218–24.

26. Scher JU, Bretz WA, Abramson SB. Periodontal disease and subgingival microbiota as contributors for rheumatoid arthritis pathogenesis: modifiable risk factors? Curr Opin Rheum 2014;26(4):424–9.

27. Mikuls TR, Thiele GM, Deane KD, et al. Porphyromonas gingivalis and disease-related autoantibodies in individuals at increased risk of rheumatoid arthritis. Arthritis Rheum 2012;64(11):3522–30.

28. Willis VC, Demoruelle MK, Derber LA, et al. Sputum autoantibodies in patients with established rheumatoid arthritis and subjects at risk of future clinically apparent disease. Arthritis Rheum 2013;65(10):2545–54.

29. Brusca SB, Abramson SB, Scher JU. Microbiome and mucosal inflammation as extra-articular triggers for rheumatoid arthritis and autoimmunity. Curr Opin Rheum 2014;26(1):101–7.

30. Shi J, Knevel R, Suwannalai P, et al. Autoantibodies recognizing carbamylated proteins are present in sera of patients with rheumatoid arthritis and predict joint damage. Proc Natl Acad Sci U S A 2011;108(42):17372–7.

31. McInnes IB, Schett G. Cytokines in the pathogenesis of rheumatoid arthritis. Nat Rev Immunol 2007;7(6):429–42.

32. Yarwood A, Han B, Raychaudhuri S, et al. A weighted genetic risk score using all known susceptibility variants to estimate rheumatoid arthritis risk. Ann Rheum Dis 2013. [Epub ahead of print].

33. Sparks JA, Chen CY, Jiang X, et al. Improved performance of epidemiologic and genetic risk models for rheumatoid arthritis serologic phenotypes using family history. Ann Rheum Dis 2014. [Epub ahead of print].

34. van de Stadt LA, Witte BI, Bos WH, et al. A prediction rule for the development of arthritis in seropositive arthralgia patients. Ann Rheum Dis 2013;72(12):1920–6.

35. van der Helm-van Mil AH, le Cessie S, van Dongen H, et al. A prediction rule for disease outcome in patients with recent-onset undifferentiated arthritis: how to guide individual treatment decisions. Arthritis Rheum 2007;56(2):433–40.

36. van der Helm-van Mil AH, Detert J, Cessie S, et al. Validation of a prediction rule for disease outcome in patients with recent-onset undifferentiated arthritis: moving toward individualized treatment decision-making. Arthritis Rheum 2008; 58(8):2241–7.
37. Kelly S, Humby F, Filer A. Ultrasound-guided synovial biopsy: a safe, well-tolerated and reliable technique for obtaining high-quality synovial tissue from both large and small joints in early arthritis patients. Ann Rheum Dis 2013. [Epub ahead of print].
38. de Hair MJ, Zijlstra IA, Boumans MJ, et al. Hunting for the pathogenesis of rheumatoid arthritis: core-needle biopsy of inguinal lymph nodes as a new research tool. Ann Rheum Dis 2012;71(11):1911–2.
39. Filer A, de Pablo P, Allen G, et al. Utility of ultrasound joint counts in the prediction of rheumatoid arthritis in patients with very early synovitis. Ann Rheum Dis 2011;70(3):500–7.
40. van Steenbergen HW, van Nies JA, Huizinga TW, et al. Characterising arthralgia in the preclinical phase of rheumatoid arthritis using MRI. Ann Rheum Dis 2014. [Epub ahead of print].
41. van Steenbergen HW, van Nies JA, Huizinga TW, et al. Subclinical inflammation on MRI of hand and foot of anti-citrullinated peptide antibody-negative arthralgia patients at risk for rheumatoid arthritis. Arthritis Res Ther 2014;16(2):R92.
42. van de Stadt LA, Bos WH, Meursinge Reynders M, et al. The value of ultrasonography in predicting arthritis in auto-antibody positive arthralgia patients: a prospective cohort study. Arthritis Res Ther 2010;12(3):R98.
43. Kallberg H, Ding B, Padyukov L, et al. Smoking is a major preventable risk factor for rheumatoid arthritis: estimations of risks after various exposures to cigarette smoke. Ann Rheum Dis 2011;70(3):508–11.
44. de Hair MJ, Landewe RB, van de Sande MG, et al. Smoking and overweight determine the likelihood of developing rheumatoid arthritis. Ann Rheum Dis 2013;72(10):1654–8.
45. Manson JE, Bassuk SS, Lee IM, et al. The VITamin D and OmegA-3 TriaL (VITAL): rationale and design of a large randomized controlled trial of vitamin D and marine omega-3 fatty acid supplements for the primary prevention of cancer and cardiovascular disease. Contemp Clin Trials 2012;33(1):159–71.
46. de Wit M, Abma T, Koelewijn-van Loon M, et al. Involving patient research partners has a significant impact on outcomes research: a responsive evaluation of the international OMERACT conferences. BMJ Open 2013;3(5). pii:e002241.
47. Hewlett S, Wit M, Richards P, et al. Patients and professionals as research partners: challenges, practicalities, and benefits. Arthritis Rheum 2006;55(4): 676–80.
48. Combe B, Landewe R, Lukas C, et al. EULAR recommendations for the management of early arthritis: report of a task force of the European Standing Committee for International Clinical Studies Including Therapeutics (ESCISIT). Ann Rheum Dis 2007;66(1):34–45.
49. Kumar K, Daley E, Carruthers DM, et al. Delay in presentation to primary care physicians is the main reason why patients with rheumatoid arthritis are seen late by rheumatologists. Rheumatology (Oxford) 2007;46(9):1438–40.
50. Raza K, Stack R, Kumar K, et al. Delays in assessment of patients with rheumatoid arthritis: variations across Europe. Ann Rheum Dis 2011;70(10):1822–5.
51. Sheppard J, Kumar K, Buckley CD, et al. 'I just thought it was normal aches and pains': a qualitative study of decision-making processes in patients with early rheumatoid arthritis. Rheumatology (Oxford) 2008;47(10):1577–82.

52. Kumar K, Daley E, Khattak F, et al. The influence of ethnicity on the extent of, and reasons underlying, delay in general practitioner consultation in patients with RA. Rheumatology (Oxford) 2010;49(5):1005–12.
53. Stack RJ, Shaw K, Mallen C, et al. Delays in help seeking at the onset of the symptoms of rheumatoid arthritis: a systematic synthesis of qualitative literature. Ann Rheum Dis 2012;71(4):493–7.
54. Atkinson MA, Eisenbarth GS, Michels AW. Type 1 diabetes. Lancet 2014; 383(9911):69–82.
55. Ziegler AG, Rewers M, Simell O, et al. Seroconversion to multiple islet autoantibodies and risk of progression to diabetes in children. JAMA 2013;309(23): 2473–9.
56. Skyler JS, Greenbaum CJ, Lachin JM, et al. Type 1 Diabetes TrialNet–an international collaborative clinical trials network. Ann N Y Acad Sci 2008;1150:14–24.
57. Matucci-Cerinic M, Allanore Y, Czirjak L, et al. The challenge of early systemic sclerosis for the EULAR Scleroderma Trial and Research group (EUSTAR) community. It is time to cut the Gordian knot and develop a prevention or rescue strategy. Ann Rheum Dis 2009;68(9):1377–80.
58. Minier T, Guiducci S, Bellando-Randone S, et al. Preliminary analysis of the Very Early Diagnosis of Systemic Sclerosis (VEDOSS) EUSTAR multicentre study: evidence for puffy fingers as a pivotal sign for suspicion of systemic sclerosis. Ann Rheum Dis 2013. [Epub ahead of print].

Gout

A Review of Nonmodifiable and Modifiable Risk Factors

Lindsey A. MacFarlane, MD[a], Seoyoung C. Kim, MD, ScD, MSCE[b,c],*

KEYWORDS

- Gout • Risk factors • Race • Sex • Genetics • Diet

KEY POINTS

- The prevalence of gout and hyperuricemia increases with age; women tend to be affected by gout at an older age than their male counterparts.
- Genome-wide association studies (GWAS) have identified several genetic polymorphisms, mainly affecting renal urate excretion, which alter serum uric acid levels and subsequently the risk of developing gout.
- Alcohol, purines from meat and seafood, and fructose- or sugar-sweetened beverages have been associated with increased risk of incident gout, whereas dairy products, coffee, vitamin C, and cherries may protect patients from developing hyperuricemia and gout.
- Obesity and weight gain of 13.6 kg or greater is associated with risk of incident gout.

INTRODUCTION

Gout is one of the most common inflammatory arthritides, caused by hyperuricemia, with an increasing prevalence. Hyperuricemia is often a consequence of renal underexcretion of uric acid; more than 70% of urate is excreted via the kidney primarily through the proximal tubule.[1] Hyperuricemia is proved positively associated with incident gout in a dose-dependent manner as seen in both the Normative Aging Study and Framingham Heart Study.[2–4] According to data from 2007 to 2008, approximately 8.3 million US adults were affected by gout, reflecting a 1.2% increase in prevalence from data approximately 20 years prior.[2,5] Gout is associated with high economic burden, resulting in 5 more absence days from work and more than $3000 in additional annual

Disclosures: S.C. Kim is supported by the National Institutes of Health grant K23 AR059677. She received a research grant from Pfizer.

a Department of Medicine, Brigham and Women's Hospital, 75 Francis Street, Boston, MA 02115, USA; b Division of Pharmacoepidemiology and Pharmacoeconomics, Brigham and Women's Hospital, 1620 Tremont Street, Suite 3030, Boston, MA 02120, USA; c Division of Rheumatology, Allergy and Immunology, Brigham and Women's Hospital, 75 Francis Street, Boston, MA 02115, USA
* Corresponding author. 1620 Tremont Street, Suite 3030, Boston, MA 02120.
E-mail address: skim62@partners.org

cost compared with patients without gout.[6] Given the burden of gout on society, factors that predispose to hyperuricemia and gout have been of keen interest, but there is a paucity of clinical trials for the primary prevention of gout.[7]

Nonmodifiable risk factors, including gender, age, and race or ethnicity, have been under investigation for potential roles in gout development.[4,8,9] More recently, GWAS have revealed genetic variants primarily involving renal urate transport that may explain certain individuals' propensity for developing hyperuricemia and gout.[10,11] In addition to these nonmodifiable risk factors, modifiable or lifestyle factors play a significant role in reducing or increasing the risk of gout.[2,12]

This review focuses on the nonmodifiable and modifiable risk factors of gout. With the increasing prevalence of gout, a strong knowledge of these risk factors for preclinical gout and hyperuricemia is important so that at-risk individuals can be identified and appropriately counseled. The linkage between gout and comorbidities, including cardiovascular disease and metabolic syndrome, as well as the role of medications, is beyond the scope of this review.

DEMOGRAPHIC FACTORS
Gender

In the population under 65 years of age, men have a 4-fold higher prevalence of gout than do women; however, this male-to-female ratio reduces to 3:1 over 65 years.[8] For women as for men, higher levels of uric acid confer an increase in risk of gout. Prospective cohort data suggest the incidence of gout in women increases with serum uric acid levels but at a lower rate of this increase, such that women with a uric acid level greater than 5 mg/dL have a significantly lower risk of gout than male counterparts.[4]

The mean age of gout onset is approximately 10 years older in women than in men.[13–15] This delayed onset has been attributed to estrogen's enhancement of renal tubular urate excretion leading to the reduced risk of hyperuricemia and gout in premenopausal women.[16] Prior work reports increased risk of hyperuricemia and incident gout in both natural and surgical (removal of ovaries prior to cessation of menses) menopause after adjusting for age, body mass index (BMI), smoking, hypertension, and diet but decreased uric acid levels and risk of incident gout in postmenopausal women taking hormone therapy.[16,17] The risk of incident gout was higher among women with surgical menopause and premature menopause (age <45 years) in comparison to those with natural and average age of menopause.[17]

Mechanistic data for this association were provided via research on ovariectomized mice with and without hormone replacement. Estrogen and progesterone decreased posttranslational expression of the urate reabsorption system, including urate transporter 1 (URAT1), glucose transporter type 9 (GLUT9), sodium-coupled monocarboxylate transporter 1 (Smct1), and urate efflux transporter ATP-binding cassette subfamily G member 2 (ABCG2), thus reducing renal urate reabsorption.[18] A second potential mechanism for the increased risk in postmenopausal women compared with premenopausal women arises from the increased prevalence of insulin resistance in the postmenopausal population.[14] Elevated insulin levels are known to reduce renal urate excretion; this effect is more pronounced in women than men and is likely mediated through sex hormones.[14,19]

Age

Increasing age is strongly associated with an increased risk of hyperuricemia and gout. Cross-sectional data from the National Health and Nutrition Examination Survey

(NHANES) and a claims database demonstrated increasing prevalence of gout or serum uric acid with increasing age groups.[8,20] Prevalence of other factors associated with gout, such as hypertension, diabetes, and diuretic use, also increases with age.[21] Evidence from the Framingham Heart Study demonstrates increased risk of incident gout with age, obesity, alcohol, diuretic use, and hypertension, with age the only variable to have a different strength of association between women and men.[4] In both the Normative Aging Study and a Japanese population, age was a predictor for incident gout or hyperuricemia along with BMI, hypertension, cholesterol, and alcohol.[3,22] **Table 1** outlines characteristics of the selected studies on the effect of gender and age on gout.

Race/Ethnicity

The risk of developing hyperuricemia and gout varies across populations according to race and ethnicity. A comparison of African American and white male physicians revealed that African Americans had a 2-fold increased risk of gout, with a respective incidence rate of 3.11 and 1.82 per 1000 person-years, which was partially attributed to increased incidence of hypertension in African Americans.[23] Further longitudinal evidence from the Atherosclerosis Risk in Communities demonstrated an increased risk of incident gout in African Americans with hazard ratio (HR) of 1.62 (95% CI, 1.24–2.12) for women and HR 1.49 (95% CI, 1.11–2.00) for men, which persisted after adjustment for uric acid level, BMI, diet, diabetes, hypertension, and diuretic use.[9] In contrast, evidence from the Coronary Artery Risk Development in Young Adults (CARDIA) cohort showed that young African American women and men (mean age 24) had lower uric acid levels than white women and men after adjusting for BMI, glomerular filtration rate, medications, and diet.[24] Over the 20 years of follow-up, African American and white men had similar risk of incident hyperuricemia (HR 1.12; 95% CI, 0.88–1.40), but African American women had 2.3 times the risk of hyperuricemia (95% CI, 1.34–3.99) in comparison with white women.[24] This study supports previous data from NHANES, which found that white adolescents of both genders had higher uric acid levels than both African Americans and Hispanics.[25] Factors, including sugar intake, BMI, onset of puberty, and glomerular filtration rate, did not seem to account for the noted variance, leading both investigators to consider genetics a potential contributor to the different uric acid levels by race.[24,25]

The Maori population in New Zealand has been the focus of several population-based gout studies.[26] Work from Klemp and colleagues[26] noted hyperuricemia was more common in the Maori than Europeans—27.1% versus 9.4% in men and 26.6% versus 10.5% in women, respectively. Being Maori also conferred a higher prevalence (6.4%) of gout compared with Europeans (2.9%). The high prevalence of elevated uric acid and gout has been confirmed in subsequent studies and is attributed to the high prevalence of comorbidities, such as obesity, diabetes, and hypertension, in the Maori potentially stemming from underlying genetic predisposition exacerbated by European introduction of alcohol and protein-rich diet.[27–30]

The Hmong, a group originating in southern China, have also displayed a propensity for gout, with a prevalence of 6.1% in Minnesota Hmong men versus 2.5% in non-Hmong men.[31] The unique, abrupt introduction of this population to a purine-heavy Western diet and alcohol after the Vietnam conflict was thought to have some responsibility for the results.[31] In a retrospective study of Hmong versus white patients in Minnesota, the Hmong were found significantly younger at gout onset (37.4 vs 55 years) and to have higher uric acid levels at disease onset yet had fewer comorbid diseases, including hypertension, chronic kidney disease, obesity, and diuretic or heavy alcohol use, also leading to speculation on genetic predisposition.[32]

Table 1
Study design and populations from selected citations pertaining to age and gender in gout

Study	Analysis	Population	Outcome
Campion et al,[3] 1987	Prospective cohort	Normative Aging Study, United States 2046 Men	Incident gout predicted by BMI ($P<.01$), age ($P<.01$), hypertension ($P<.05$), and cholesterol level ($P<.05$)
Puig et al,[15] 1991	Cross-sectional	Chart review of Spanish patients 45 Women and 220 men	Mean age at time of gout diagnosis 60.9 y for women and 51.2 y for men ($P<.001$)
Fang & Alderman,[20] 2000	Cross-sectional	First NHANES 5926 Women and men	Increase in uric acid from 5.3 mg/dL in patients <45 y to 5.7 mg/dL in those >65 y ($P<.001$)
Kuzuya et al,[22] 2002	Prospective cohort	Japanese health center data 30,349 Women and 50,157 men	Serum uric acid increases with age. Association with age persists after controlling for BMI and alcohol
Wallace et al,[8] 2004	Cross-sectional	Claims database for 8,000,000 patients in United States from 1990 to 1999	Increase in gout or hyperuricemia with increasing age groups 45–64 (14 per 1000 persons), 65–74 (31 per 1000 persons), and 75+ (41 per 1000 persons)
Harrold et al,[120] 2006	Cross-sectional	7 Managed care plans, United States 1158 Women and 4975 men	Women with gout have a mean age of 70 y vs 58 y for men ($P<.001$). Women more likely to have hypertension, dyslipidemia, coronary heart disease, diabetes mellitus, peripheral arterial disease, renal insufficiency, renal failure than men. Women received diuretics more often than men 77% vs 40% ($P<.001$).
Hak & Choi,[16] 2008	Cross-sectional	Third NHANES, United States 7662 Women	Serum uric acid levels in women with natural and surgical menopause were higher than in premenopausal women by 0.34 mg/dL (95% CI, 0.19–0.49) and 0.36 mg/dL (95% CI, 0.14–0.57). In comparison to untreated postmenopausal women, postmenopausal hormone use associated with a lower serum uric acid level 0.24 mg/dL (95% CI, 0.11–0.36).
Bhole et al,[4] 2010	Prospective cohort	Framingham Heart Study, United States 2476 Women and 1951 men	Increasing age, obesity, alcohol, diuretic use, and hypertension increase incident gout in women (all $P<.05$). Magnitude of associations differed from men for age only (P for interaction = .02)

(continued on next page)

Table 1 *(continued)*			
Study	**Analysis**	**Population**	**Outcome**
Hak et al,[17] 2010	Prospective cohort	Nurses' Health Study, United States 92,535 Women	Postmenopausal women have increased risk of incident gout, RR = 1.26 (95% CI, 1.03–1.55), compared with premenopausal women. In comparison with untreated postmenopausal women, postmenopausal hormone users have a reduced risk of gout, RR = 0.82 (95% CI, 0.70–0.96).
Chen et al,[14] 2012	Prospective cohort	Outcome database from Taiwan's National Health Insurance 265 Women and 1,341 men	Mean age for diagnosis of gout 62.2 y in women and 54 y for men ($P<.001$).
Öztürk et al,[13] 2013	Cross-sectional	Multicenter population in Turkey 55 Women and 257 men	Mean age for symptoms of gout 60.4 y in women and 50.6 y in men ($P<.001$)

A recent review of gout in the Filipino population reported that Filipinos are also at a higher risk of elevated uric acid levels and gout, with mean serum urate levels among US Filipinos approximately 1 mg/dL higher than other US races and Filipinos in the Philippines.[33] The possibility that the purine-heavy Western diet was at play was considered, but discrepancy persisted even after controlling for diet; furthermore, Filipinos in the United States continued to have lower purine diets that their non-Filipino counterparts.[33] Ultimately, the variation was thought secondary to a potential combination of comorbidities, including obesity, hypertension, diabetes, renal impairment, and heart disease as well as genetic cofactors.[33]

GENETIC FACTORS
Heritability

In the early 1990s, Emmerson and colleagues[34] sought to explain a genetic predisposition for gout through renal urate clearance. In studying 37 pairs of normouricemic twins, they found that monozygotic twins had more similar values of urate clearance and fractional excretion of urate than dizygotes. They calculated the heritability of renal urate clearance to be 60%, whereas the heritability of the fractional excretion of urate was 87%.[34] Further investigation through segregation analysis on serum uric acid found a significant correlation in between siblings (r = 0.19) and parent-offspring (r = 0.22).[35] The segregation analysis was not consistent, however, with a major mendelian gene, leading the investigators to conclude that uric acid levels were likely multifactorial with contribution from several genetic as well as environmental factors, such as diet and menopausal status.[35] The first GWAS for potential genes associated with uric acid used a cohort from the Framingham Heart Study. Evidence of linkage to uric acid was found on chromosome 15 and suggested on chromosomes 2 and 8.[36] Further interest in defining a role for genetics in gout has since culminated in many GWAS, which have identified genetic polymorphisms associated with uric acid and gout.[10] Many of the uncovered genes code for proteins essential to renal urate reabsorption and secretion (discussed later) (**Fig. 1**).[1]

Specific Genetic Factors

SLC22A12

SLC22A12 encodes URAT1, which is located on the brush border of the proximal tubules and is integral in urate absorption. URAT1 was first identified in 2002 by Enomoto and colleagues[37] and was pivotal from a clinical standpoint because analysis of a Japanese patient with idiopathic renal hypouricemia showed mutations in SLC22A12. Furthermore, oocytes with mutated URAT1 complementary RNA had abolished urate transport ability.[37] SLC22A12 variants have since been observed in additional patients with low serum urate levels and low susceptibility to gout.[38,39] SLC22A12 alleles have also been associated with hyperuricemia and decreased fractional excretion of uric acid (FEUA) in Chinese and German populations, respectively.[40,41] Further work in a cohort of 69 patients with gout showed that 23% had mutations in the SLC22A12 gene.[42] Differing polymorphisms in SLC22A12 have been shown to have various effects on renal urate excretion through URAT1 and, therefore, influence serum urate levels and corresponding gout risk. A summary of studies and outcomes is in **Table 2**.

SLC2A9

SLC2A9 encodes GLUT9, a urate uniporter, initially thought to be a glucose or fructose transporter located on the basolateral membrane of the proximal tubule. Data from GWAS have elucidated its role, however, as a urate transporter and demonstrated its inhibition with known uricosuric agents, such as probenecid, losartan, and benzbromarone.[10,43-45] GLUT9 is responsible for a large portion of urate reabsorption, such that complete loss of GLUT9 leads to dramatic urate excretion more so than seen with URAT1.[1] As with SLC22A12, mutations in SLC2A9 were initially described in patients with idiopathic renal hypouricemia without mutation in SLC22A12.[44,46] Many studies have correlated polymorphisms in SLC2A9 with uric acid levels and gout, as listed in **Table 3**. Of the genetic loci, SLC2A9 has perhaps the strongest

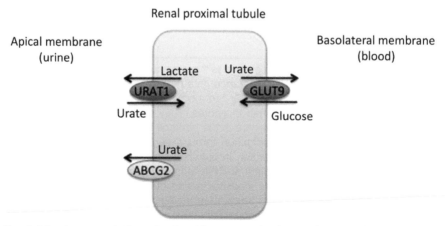

Fig. 1. Visual representation of uric acid transport in the renal proximal tubule. URAT1 (SLC22A12) and GLUT9 (SLC2A9) function to reabsorb uric acid whereas ABCG2 acts to secrete uric acid.

Table 2
Studies pertaining to *SLC22A12* polymorphisms and effect on serum uric acid and gout

Study	Population	Polymorphism	Outcome
Iwai et al,[39] 2004	Japanese	Multiple missense, nonsense, and deletion mutations	Mutations associated with decreased SUA
Taniguchi et al,[38] 2005	Japanese	Mutation in exon 4	Alleles associated with decreased SUA and protection from gout
Graessler et al,[40] 2006	German	rs3825016 rs7932775 rs11231825 rs11602903	Alleles associated with SUA levels and varying risk for reduced FEUA
Shima et al,[121] 2006	Japanese	rs893006	Alleles associated with varying range of SUA levels
Vazquez-Mellado et al,[42] 2007	Mexican	Mutations in exons 4 and 5	Mutations found in patients with gout
Jang et al,[122] 2008	Korean	rs1529909	Alleles associated with decreased SUA and increased FEUA[a]
Guan et al,[123] 2009	Chinese	rs893006	Alleles associated with varying range of SUA levels
Kolz et al,[49] 2009	European	rs505802	Alleles associated with decreased SUA
Li et al,[41] 2010	Chinese	rs382507 rs57606 rs7932775 rs11231825 rs11602903	Alleles associated with increased SUA
Tu et al,[124] 2010	Chinese, Solomon Islanders	rs475688 rs7932775	Alleles associated with increased SUA, gout risk, and tophi
Tin et al,[59] 2011	African American	rs12800450	Alleles associated with decreased SUA and gout risk
Karns et al,[50] 2012	Croatian	rs17300741	Alleles associated with increased SUA

Abbreviation: SUA, serum uric acid.
[a] Significant association in men only.

association with uric acid levels and also seems to exert a greater effect in women as discerned by several studies.[45,47–51] *SLC2A9* is estimated to explain the 3.4% to 8.8% of serum uric acid variance in women and 0.5% to 2.0% in men.[10] Certain *SLC2A9* alleles have been linked to tophaceous gout,[52] which is notable because GLUT9 is found on chondrocytes.[53] Because evidence is lacking for why certain patients develop tophi, GLUT9, with its presence on chondrocytes, becomes an enticing target.[52]

Table 3
Studies pertaining to *SLC2A9* polymorphisms and effect on serum uric acid and gout

Study	Population	Polymorphism	Outcome
Li et al,[125] 2007	Sardinian, Chianti	rs6855911 rs7442295	Alleles associated with varying range of SUA levels[a]
Brandstätter et al,[51] 2008	American, Italian	rs6449213 rs6855911 rs7442295 rs12510549	Alleles associated with decreased SUA[a]
Dehghan et al,[55] 2008	American, Dutch	rs6449213 rs16890979	Alleles associated with SUA and gout risk[a]
Doring et al,[47] 2008	German, Austrian, Polish	rs6449213 rs7442295 rs6855911 rs12510549	Alleles associated with varying SUA levels and gout[a]
McArdle et al,[126] 2008	Amish American	rs10489070 rs16890979	Alleles associated with decreased SUA[a]
Stark et al,[127] 2008	German	rs6449213 rs6855911 rs7442295 rs12510549	Alleles associated with predisposition to and protection from gout[b]
Wallace et al,[48] 2008	European	rs6449213 rs7442295	Alleles associated with increased SUA
Hollis-Moffatt et al,[128] 2009	New Zealand: Maori, Pacific Island, white	rs5028843 rs11942223 rs12510549 rs16890979	Alleles associated with predisposition to and protection from gout
Kolz et al,[49] 2009	European	rs734553 rs12498742	Alleles associated with decreased SUA[a]
Vitart et al,[45] 2008	Croatian, Scottish, German	rs6449213 rs737267 rs1014290	Alleles associated with SUA, FEUA, and gout[a]
Tu et al,[129] 2010	Chinese, Solomon Islanders	rs3733589 rs3733591 rs1014290 rs10939650	Alleles associated with increased SUA, gout risk, and tophi
Urano et al,[130] 2010	Japanese	rs1014290 rs3733591	Alleles associated with predisposition to and protection from gout
Yang et al,[131] 2010	American, Dutch, Icelandic	rs13129697	Alleles associated with decreased SUA and gout risk
Charles et al,[132] 2011	African American	rs3775948 rs6449213 rs6856396 rs7663032	Alleles associated with SUA[a]
Hamajima et al,[133] 2011	Japanese	rs11722228	Alleles associated with varying range of SUA levels[a]
Hollis-Moffatt et al,[52] 2011	New Zealand: Maori, Pacific Island, white	rs3733591	Allele associated with tophi in Maori but not gout in populations studied
Sulem et al,[134] 2011	Icelandic	rs734553	Alleles associated with SUA and gout risk

(continued on next page)

Table 3
(continued)

Study	Population	Polymorphism	Outcome
Tin et al,[59] 2011	African American	rs13129697 rs7663032	Alleles associated with increased SUA and gout risk
Li et al,[135] 2012	Chinese	rs6850166 rs13124007	Alleles associated with predisposition to and protection from gout and risk of tophi
Karns et al,[50] 2012	Croatian	rs737267 rs3775948 rs6855911 rs717615 rs7442295 rs13129697 rs16890979	Alleles associated with decreased SUA[a]
Voruganti et al,[136] 2013	Mexican American	rs737267 rs6449213 rs6832439 rs13131257	Alleles associated with decreased SUA
Voruganti et al,[137] 2014	American Indian	rs737267 rs6449213 rs6832439 rs10805346 rs12498956 rs13131257 rs16890979	Alleles associated with varying SUA levels

Abbreviation: SUA, serum uric acid.
[a] Association stronger in women then men.
[b] Association stronger in men then women.

ABCG2

ABCG2 encodes the ABCG2, a multidrug resistance transporter that mediates urate secretion across the apical membrane of the proximal tubule. *ABCG2* was identified through GWAS and its functionality proved by demonstrating a 53% reduction in urate transport rate with mutation.[54] Population studies confirmed a linkage with both serum uric acid and gout, although the association was stronger in men than women.[54,55] Variants in *ABCG2* are thought responsible for 10% of gout in whites, in concordance another finding that 10% of Japanese gout patients had genotypes causing a 75% reduction in ABCG2 function.[54,56] Patients with severe ABCG2 dysfunction were found to have symptom onset 6.5 years earlier than those with normal function, providing further clinical relevance to these polymorphisms.[57] *ABCG2* may have a role in gout severity; a recent study found a variant of *ABCG2* associated with a 50% increase in tophaceous gout compared with nontophaceous gout.[58] Moreover, these investigators discovered a gene-environment interaction, reporting an additive effect of alcohol and the Q141K (rs2231142) variant—patients with Q141K and current alcohol use had an odds ratio (OR) for tophaceous gout of 12.69 (95% CI, 2.88–55.86) in comparison to an OR of 6.21 (95% CI, 2.47–15.64) for Q141K alone.[58] Studies pertaining to *ABCG2* are listed in **Table 4**.

Genetic studies demonstrate both homogeneity and heterogeneity among populations. Certain polymorphisms have a level of concordance: for instance, of the 11 loci

Table 4
Studies pertaining to *ABCG2* polymorphisms and effect on serum uric acid and gout

Study	Population	Polymorphism	Outcome
Dehghan et al,[55] 2008	American, Dutch	rs2231142	Alleles associated with increased SUA and gout risk[a]
Kolz et al,[49] 2009	European	rs2231142 rs2199936	Alleles associated with increased SUA[a]
Matsuo et al,[56] 2009	Japanese	rs2231142 rs72552713	Alleles associated with increased SUA and gout risk
Woodward et al,[54] 2009	American	rs2231142	Alleles Associated with increased SUA levels and gout risk[a]
Phipps-Green et al,[138] 2010	New Zealand: Maori, Pacific Island, white	rs2231142	Associated with increased risk of gout. Association not seen in Maori
Wang et al,[139] 2010	Chinese	rs2231142	Associated with increased risk of gout[b]
Yamagishi et al,[140] 2010	Japanese	rs2231142	Alleles associated with increased SUA and gout risk
Yang et al,[131] 2010	American, Dutch, Icelandic	rs2199936	Alleles associated with increased SUA and gout risk
Matsuo et al,[141] 2011	Japanese	rs2231142 rs72552713	Alleles associated with increased SUA and gout risk
Matsuo et al,[142] 2011	Japanese	rs2231142 rs72552713	Alleles associated with increased SUA and gout risk
Sulem et al,[134] 2011	Icelandic	rs2231142	Alleles associated with SUA and gout
Karns et al,[50] 2012	Croatian	rs2231142 rs2199936	Alleles associated with increased SUA[a]
Matsuo et al,[57] 2013	Japanese	rs22311423 rs72552713	Associated with early onset gout
Tu et al,[58] 2014	Taiwanese	rs2231137 rs2231142 rs72552713	Alleles associated with tophaceous gout Alcohol consumption exerts an additive risk in patients with rs2231142

Abbreviation: SUA, serum uric acid.
[a] Association stronger in men than women.
[b] Nonsignificant association with elevated SUA.

associated with uric acid in Europeans, 10 of these were replicated in African Americans.[11,59] Other alleles, however, seem population specific, notably the *SLC2A9* variant associated with gout in Chinese and Japanese populations could not be replicated in New Zealanders.[52] As Dehghan and colleagues[55] concluded, although the risk of individual genetic variants may be unimpressive, allelic combinations and the prevalence of some alleles in a population may compound into a larger effect on uric acid and gout. The overall genetic risk score from this study indicated a 40-fold risk of incident gout, which is purportedly higher than the risk conferred by environmental factors. Studies have continued to define new reproducible variants and confirm those previously discovered.[49,60] A recent study by Kottgen and colleagues[60] found 28 loci associated with uric acid concentrations; 18 of these loci were novel. The novel loci seemed associated with carbohydrate metabolism but not urate transport. Deeper understanding of genetic polymorphisms and their role in gout may shed light on individuals' susceptibility to gout and lead to more targeted therapy.

DIETARY FACTORS
Alcohol

Since antiquity, alcohol consumption has been linked to gout. More formal research from the 1960s demonstrated that alcohol administration caused decreased uric acid excretion and hyperuricemia.[61] Ethanol ingestion increases serum lactate levels, which inhibit uric acid excretion at the renal tubule; however, this has not been confirmed in subsequent studies.[62] In terms of the production theory, ethanol prompts ATP consumption, leading to purine degradation, yielding an increase in plasma oxypurines and uric acid.[62,63] Longitudinal studies in beer consumption confirmed increased plasma uric acid levels and attributed this to production via ethanol but failed to find increased plasma levels of oxypurines, suggesting this was a short-term consequence.[64,65] Some investigators have instead posited that the guanosine purine load in beer specifically may cause increase in uric acid synthesis.[66]

The above studies spurred further consideration as to whether the purine components of beer augmented the hyperuricemic effects of ethanol. A comparison of alcoholic beer to nonalcoholic beer found that plasma uric acid levels increased 6.5% and 4.4% ($P<.05$), respectively, suggesting that purine load alone had a significant effect on uric acid.[67] With regard to hyperuricemia, beer poses the greatest threat with the combine effects of ethanol and purine. A cross-sectional NHANES study showed serum uric acid levels significantly increased with greater beer and liquor intake after adjustment for age.[68] Uric acid increased per serving per day 0.46 mg/dL (95% CI, 0.32–0.60) with beer and 0.29 mg/dL (95% CI, 0.14–0.45) with liquor. The effect was lessened but remained significant after adjustment for diet, diuretics, hypertension, BMI, and creatinine. No association was seen with wine.[68] A subsequent cross-sectional analysis using the CARDIA cohort found high uric acid levels with increased beer intake. The effect was strongest in women, with uric acid increase of 0.03 mg/dL per each additional weekly serving of beer.[69] In terms of incident gout, a prospective cohort study of men found that 2 or more beers per day increased the risk of gout by 2.5, with a multivariate relative risk (RR) per 355 ml serving per day of 1.49 (95% CI, 1.32–1.70). A similar amount of spirits increased risk by 1.6 in comparison to none with an RR per drink or shot per day of 1.15 (95% CI, 1.04–1.28).[70] Less common is moonshine; in addition to its ethanol load, its distillation often leads to lead contamination. Chronic moonshine imbibers are at risk for lead toxicity and concomitant saturnine gout due to lead-induced renal dysfunction, decreased urate excretion, and potentially an increase in urate production.[71,72] The associations of other alcoholic beverage, such as liquor and wine, have also been investigated (outlined in **Table 5**). Although the definitive verdict on the contribution of wine to gout risk is still unclear, this evidence confirms a longstanding suspicion for alcohol, especially beer, as a gout risk factor. A meta-analysis of 17 observational studies did show an increased risk of gout associated with alcohol consumption and recommended reducing alcohol intake for the primary prevention of gout.[73]

Purine-Rich Food

Food rich in purines, including meats, seafood, some vegetables, and animal protein, have been theorized to lead to gout, because uric acid is the end product of purine degradation. Skepticism existed because protein can have a uricosuric effect, which would actually lower urate levels.[74] Recent NHANES data demonstrated increased

Table 5
Summary of the effects of beer, liquor, and wine on SUA or gout by study

Study	Design	Population	Beer SUA	Beer Gout	Liquor SUA	Liquor Gout	Wine SUA	Wine Gout
Eastmond et al,[143] 1995	Pre–post comparison	4 Gout patients	↑	—	↔	—	—	—
van der Gaag et al,[144] 2000	Randomized crossover trial	11 Men	↑	—	↑	—	↑	—
Choi et al,[70] 2004	Prospective cohort	47,150 Men without history of gout	—	↑	—	↑	—	↔
Choi et al,[68] 2004	Cross-sectional	14,809 Men and women	↑	—	↑[a]	—	↔	—
Zhang et al,[145] 2006	Case-crossover	197 Gout patients	—	↑	—	↑	—	↑
Yu et al,[78] 2008	Cross-sectional	2176 Men and women	↑[b]	—	—	—	—	—
Gaffo et al,[69] 2010	Cross-sectional	3123 Men and women	↑[a]	—	↑[b]	—	↔	—
Neogi et al,[146] 2014	Case-crossover	724 Gout patients	—	↑	—	↑	—	↑

Abbreviation: SUA, serum uric acid.
[a] Effect stronger in women.
[b] Effect noted only in men.

uric acid levels in association with greater meat and seafood consumption but not with total protein intake.[75] The elevation in uric acid levels between the 1st and 5th quintiles of meat intake was 0.11 mg/dL (95% CI, 0.01–0.22), and 0.10 mg/dL for seafood (95% CI, 0.02–0.18) after adjustment for age, gender, BMI, creatinine, medication, hypertension, and diet.[75] Another prospective study by Choi and colleagues[76] found that each additional daily serving of meat increased the incident risk of gout by 21% with a multivariate RR of 1.41 (95% CI, 1.07–1.86) between the lowest and highest quintiles of meat intake. Each additional weekly serving of seafood increased risk by 7%, with an RR of 1.51 (95% CI, 1.17–1.95) between the highest and lowest consumers. No effect was seen with purine-rich vegetables; however, those in the highest quintile of vegetable protein intake had an RR of 0.73 (95% CI, 0.56–0.96) in comparison to the lowest quintile. These differences were thought secondary to the differing types, quantity, and bioavailability of purines found in various foods.[76] Despite moderate purine content in soy, soy has not been shown associated with gout and may be inversely associated with hyperuricemia.[77–79] An absolute low purine diet may not be necessary in the primary prevention of gout, because many purine-containing foods do not contribute to hyperuricemia or gout and may be protective.[80]

Fructose/Sugar-Sweetened Beverages

Because diets have come to include increasing quantities of fructose- and sugar-sweetened beverages (the main sweetener being fructose), these additives have come under investigation for their contribution to gout. Initial studies on these sweeteners found increased plasma uric acid and lactate levels probably driven either by purine nucleotide degradation or de novo purine synthesis.[81–83] Fructose is the only known carbohydrate to increase uric acid levels, which is thought secondary to degradation of ATP. Because fructose phosphorylation depletes phosphate, a path toward uric acid formation is favored instead of regeneration of ATP. Additionally, de novo purine synthesis from these beverages is still considered to have a role in increased uric acid. Lastly, fructose may increase the risk of insulin resistance and subsequent hyperinsulinemia, decreasing uric acid excretion and further promoting hyperuricemia.[19,84–86] Several groups have linked the handling of fructose- and sugar-sweetened beverages to genetic polymorphisms in SLC2A9 and ABCG2. Data suggest that different alleles influence serum urate responses to a fructose or sucrose load.[87–90]

Cross-sectional NHANES data showed an increase in uric acid of 0.33 mg/dL (95% CI, 0.11–0.73) in participants drinking 1 to 3.9 sugar-sweetened servings per day in comparison with those drinking none after adjustment for diet, including total energy intake, age, gender, medications, hypertension, and glomerular filtration rate.[84] In these moderate users, the OR for hyperuricemia (defined as serum uric acid level >7.0 mg/dL in men and >5.7 mg/dL in women) was 1.51 (P = .003 for trend) in comparison with no intake,[84] which was in accordance with prior NHANES data showing that men had increased uric acid levels with increased added sugar or sugar-sweetened beverages in their diet.[91] Prospective cohort studies have also shown that those consuming 2 or more sugar-sweetened beverages per day had an increased risk of incident gout (RR 1.85; 95% CI, 1.08–3.16) in comparison with those drinking less than 1 sugar-sweetened beverage a month.[85] Men in the highest 5th of fructose ingestion incurred double the risk of gout than those in the lowest (RR 2.02; 95% CI, 1.49–2.75) after adjustment for total carbohydrate intake.[85] These associations were confirmed in a prospective cohort study of women, showing that 1 serving of sugar-sweetened beverage per day increased the risk of incident gout (RR 1.74; 95% CI, 1.19–2.25) compared with less than 1 serving per day. An increased gout risk was also found with fructose intake with an RR for the highest quintile of 1.62 (95% CI, 1.20–2.19) in comparison with the lowest after adjustment for total carbohydrate intake.[86]

The role of fructose in gout has been contested in the literature. A meta-analysis of controlled fructose feeding trials and uric acid levels among diabetics and nondiabetics reported that isocaloric fructose intake did not alter uric acid levels; only the hypercaloric (fructose levels double the 95th percentile for fructose intake) increased uric acid. It is not clear that all previous observational studies had appropriately adjusted for total energy and carbohydrate intake.[92] Several studies did not find an association with fructose and hyperuricemia, including 1 cross-sectional analysis finding and association with sugar-sweetened beverages but not with fructose.[93,94] Whether or not fructose itself is the responsible component for hyperuricemic effects of sugar-sweetened beverages is debatable. Current data suggest, however, that heavy utilization of these food items is not advisable for those at risk of hyperuricemia and gout.

Dairy Products

Initial studies demonstrated decrease in serum uric acid levels after milk protein (casein and lactalbumin) ingestion secondary to a presumed uricosuric effect of the protein load.[95] In a cross-sectional NHANES study, Choi and colleagues[75] found an inverse association for uric acid and dairy, with a decrease in uric acid of 0.21 mg/dL (95% CI, −0.37 to −0.04) between the highest and lowest total dairy intake quintiles. This effect remained significant after adjustment for covariates. Prospective data on incident gout showed that men in the highest quintile of dairy intake had an RR of 0.56 (95% CI, 0.42–0.74) compared with the lowest quintile.[76] This inverse correlation of dairy and uric acid has been observed in the Scottish and Korean populations as well.[94,96] A randomized controlled trial (RCT) found that milk consumption lead to an acute 10% decrease in serum uric acid (P<.0001) and an increase in FEUA.[97] Additional work in both cellular and murine acute gout models showed that the dairy fractions glycomacropeptide (GMP) and G600 milk fat extract had antiinflammatory effects causing a decrease in interleukin (IL)-1β expression, thus providing a second protective mechanism for dairy.[98] This knowledge was applied to a second RCT investigating skim milk enriched with GMP and G600 in patients with gout. Although all patients received milk products and had a decrease in gout flares, those in the group supplemented with GMP and G600 had a greater decrement in number of flares and increase in FEUA.[99] Dairy products have been shown protective in terms of gout from a urate-lowering and potentially antiinflammatory standpoint.

Coffee

Due to caffeine-induced diuresis and the hypothesis that uric acid excretion would increase with increased renal blood flow, coffee versus green tea consumption was studied in Japanese men. Uric acid decreased as coffee intake rose, a correlation not seen with green tea.[100] A second study in Japanese men and women confirmed this association and found it stronger in men than women.[101] Cross-sectional studies in a US population also document an inverse association with uric acid and coffee consumption but not with tea or total caffeine.[102] Subjects drinking 4 to 5 cups of coffee a day had a significant uric acid decrement of 0.26 mg/dL (95% CI, −0.41 to −0.11) in comparison with those not drinking coffee after adjustment for age and gender. A moderate inverse correlation was seen with decaffeinated coffee, leading to the conclusion that the effect was due to factors outside of caffeine.[102] A prospective cohort study found that the risk of incident gout was inversely associated with daily intake of 4 to 5 cups of coffee (RR 0.60; 95% CI, 0.41–0.87) and 4 or more cups of decaffeinated coffee (RR 0.73; 95% CI, 0.46–1.17) but not with total caffeine (RR 0.83; 95% CI, 0.64–1.08).[103] Similar results regarding coffee consumption and incident gout were noted in the Nurses' Health Study.[104] It was postulated that the antioxidant properties, including those of phenol chlorogenic acid, might increase insulin sensitivity and decrease serum insulin; as discussed previously, insulin levels have a positive correlation with uric acid due to decreased renal excretion. Furthermore, xanthines, either in caffeine or in coffee itself, could inhibit xanthine oxidase, acting in a manner similar to allopurinol.[101–104] Coffee represents another potentially protective beverage for those at risk for gout.

Vitamin C

Vitamin C has been touted as protective against gout; ingestion of ascorbic acid was found to increase the fractional clearance of uric acid resulting in a reduction of serum uric acid.[105] Supplementation with 500 mg/d of vitamin C significantly reduced serum uric acid levels in an RCT, with a mean uric acid reduction of 0.5 mg/dL (95% CI, −0.6 to −0.3).[106] Observational data in men demonstrated an inverse relationship for vitamin C doses and serum uric acid, with levels that remained significant after adjustment for covariates, including BMI, blood pressure, medications, and diet.[107] A prospective cohort study of male health professionals reported a decreased risk of incident gout in patients taking 1500 mg/d of vitamin C (RR 0.55; 95% CI, 0.38–0.80) compared with those with intake less than 250 mg/d.[108] A meta-analysis of 13 RCTs on vitamin C and uric acid in patients without gout confirmed the inverse association and suggested that the combined effect demonstrated a serum uric acid reduction of 0.35 mg/dL (95% CI, −0.66 to −0.03).[109] The uricosuric effects of vitamin C have been explained by its ability to compete with uric acid for reabsorption at the proximal tubule. Evidence suggests this competitive inhibition may be occurring at

URAT1 and a sodium-dependent anion cotransporter. It has also been postulated that vitamin C improves renal function, further augmenting the uricosuric effect, and functions as an antioxidant-reducing inflammation.[107,108]

Cherries

A few studies have addressed the role of cherries in gout. The first by Jacob and colleagues[110] sought to follow-up on prior reports from the 1950s in light of antioxidant and antiinflammatory effects of polyphenols, including anthocyanins, and vitamin C found in the fruit. Cherry consumption was found to acutely lower serum uric acid in healthy women ages 22 to 40 years old.[110] To date, there are no studies on the risk of incident gout related to cherry consumption, but cherry consumption was found to lower recurrent gout attacks by 35% in a case-crossover study.[111] The effect of cherries on glomerular filtration rate and xanthine oxidase as well as their antioxidant effects were all taken into consideration as reasoning for the beneficial outcome on gout.[111] A prospective RCT of cherry juice, available regardless of season, found a significant reduction in gout flares after 4 months with 55% free of attack.[112] Although the effects on preclinical gout have yet to be elucidated, cherries may lower uric acid levels and decrease the risk of incident gout. There is an ongoing RCT that determines the effect of blueberries on uric acid in hyperuricemic patients who are not on pharmacotherapy (ClinicalTrials.gov Identifier: NCT01532622). **Fig. 2** Summarizes the effects of diet on gout.

OTHER LIFESTYLE FACTORS

Few studies examined the role of physical activity and body weight on the risk of gout. A study of male runners found that men who ran over 4 km/d or faster than 4.0 m/s had a lower incidence of gout, although this was partially attributable to their leaner frames and BMI.[113] In a prospective cohort of men, Choi and colleagues[114] found that greater BMI correlated with increased age-adjusted RR of incident gout, BMI of 25 to 29.9

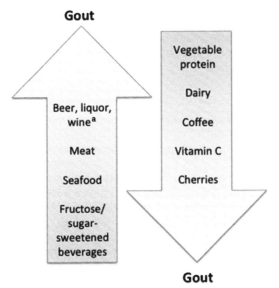

Fig. 2. Summary of the effects of diet on risk of gout. [a] Discrepancy surrounding effect.

(RR 1.95; 95% CI, 1.44–2.65), BMI of 30 to 34.9 (RR 2.33; 95% CI, 1.62–3.36), and BMI of 35 or greater (RR 2.97; 95% CI, 1.73–5.10) compared with men with a BMI of 21 to 22.9. Additionally, men who gained 13.6 kg or more since 21 years of age had an RR of 1.99 (95% CI, 1.49–2.66) versus men who had stable weight within 1.8 kg. The RR was attenuated but remained significant for after adjustment for diet, hypertension, and chronic renal failure.[114] Because many turn to surgical means of weight loss, it is encouraging that a recent prospective study of 60 patients with type 2 diabetes and BMI greater than or equal to 35 kg/m^2 found clinically significant reductions in serum uric acid levels 1 year after bariatric surgery.[115] Uric acid levels and gout attacks initially increase perioperatively secondary in part to the catabolic effect of surgery, rapid weight loss, and renal impairment.[115,116] Patients with weight loss post–bariatric surgery, however, ultimately benefit from reduced inflammation and show decreased production of ILs, including IL-1β, IL-6, and IL-8, in response to monosodium urate crystals.[117] Weight reduction is encouraged for many disease processes and may help stave off the risk of incident gout as well.

Little investigation has been done on smoking and risk for gout. A study by Hanna and colleagues[118] actually reported lower serum uric acid levels in chronic smokers, although data were not adjusted for potential confounders, such as BMI.[116] This confirmed findings from a prior crossover study reporting decreased uric acid levels after smoking a cigarette.[119] Because uric acid is a potent antioxidant, the reduction was thought a testament to the oxidative stress caused by cigarette use.[118] From a health standpoint, smoking is clearly not a viable mechanism for uric acid reduction. It raises a question, however, as to whether susceptible individuals who cease smoking are at risk for increasing uric acid levels and subsequently incident gout.

SUMMARY

There is robust evidence for nonmodifiable and modifiable risk factors and their contribution to incident gout. Although a patient's individual risk likely represents a complex interplay between factors outside of their control, such as age, gender, race, and genetics, and modifiable factors, such as diet and lifestyle, patients at risk for hyperuricemia or gout should be educated on modifiable factors to reduce the risk. With the current knowledge in the literature, it is conceivable that a risk score could be developed to better predict an individual's risk for developing gout. Despite a large body of data for gout summarized in this review, further work in risk stratification and primary prevention of gout is needed.

REFERENCES

1. Lipkowitz MS. Regulation of uric acid excretion by the kidney. Curr Rheumatol Rep 2012;14(2):179–88.
2. Roddy E, Choi HK. Epidemiology of Gout. Rheum Dis Clin North Am 2014;40(2): 155–75.
3. Campion EW, Glynn RJ, DeLabry LO. Asymptomatic hyperuricemia. Risks and consequences in the Normative Aging Study. Am J Med 1987;82(3):421–6.
4. Bhole V, de Vera M, Rahman MM, et al. Epidemiology of gout in women: fifty-two-year followup of a prospective cohort. Arthritis Rheum 2010;62(4):1069–76.
5. Zhu Y, Pandya BJ, Choi HK. Prevalence of gout and hyperuricemia in the US general population: the National Health and Nutrition Examination Survey 2007-2008. Arthritis Rheum 2011;63(10):3136–41.
6. Wertheimer A, Morlock R, Becker MA. A revised estimate of the burden of illness of gout. Curr Ther Res Clin Exp 2013;75:1–4.

7. Singh JA, Reddy SG, Kundukulam J. Risk factors for gout and prevention: a systematic review of the literature. Curr Opin Rheumatol 2011;23(2):192–202.
8. Wallace KL, Riedel AA, Joseph-Ridge N, et al. Increasing prevalence of gout and hyperuricemia over 10 years among older adults in a managed care population. J Rheumatol 2004;31(8):1582–7.
9. Maynard JW, McAdams-Demarco MA, Law A, et al. Racial differences in gout incidence in a population-based cohort: Atherosclerosis Risk in Communities Study. Am J Epidemiol 2014;179(5):576–83.
10. Reginato AM, Mount DB, Yang I, et al. The genetics of hyperuricaemia and gout. Nat Rev Rheumatol 2012;8(10):610–21.
11. Merriman TR, Choi HK, Dalbeth N. The genetic basis of gout. Rheum Dis Clin North Am 2014;40(2):279–90.
12. Choi HK, Mount DB, Reginato AM. Pathogenesis of gout. Ann Intern Med 2005; 143(7):499–516.
13. Öztürk MA, Kaya A, Senel S, et al. Demographic and clinical features of gout patients in Turkey: a multicenter study. Rheumatol Int 2013;33(4):847–52.
14. Chen JH, Yeh WT, Chuang SY, et al. Gender-specific risk factors for incident gout: a prospective cohort study. Clin Rheumatol 2012;31(2):239–45.
15. Puig JG, Michan AD, Jimenez ML, et al. Female gout. Clinical spectrum and uric acid metabolism. Arch Intern Med 1991;151(4):726–32.
16. Hak AE, Choi HK. Menopause, postmenopausal hormone use and serum uric acid levels in US women–the Third National Health and Nutrition Examination Survey. Arthritis Res Ther 2008;10(5):R116.
17. Hak AE, Curhan GC, Grodstein F, et al. Menopause, postmenopausal hormone use and risk of incident gout. Ann Rheum Dis 2010;69(7):1305–9.
18. Takiue Y, Hosoyamada M, Kimura M, et al. The effect of female hormones upon urate transport systems in the mouse kidney. Nucleosides Nucleotides Nucleic Acids 2011;30(2):113–9.
19. Choi HK, Ford ES. Haemoglobin A1c, fasting glucose, serum C-peptide and insulin resistance in relation to serum uric acid levels–the Third National Health and Nutrition Examination Survey. Rheumatology (Oxford) 2008;47(5):713–7.
20. Fang J, Alderman MH. Serum uric acid and cardiovascular mortality the NHANES I epidemiologic follow-up study, 1971-1992. National Health and Nutrition Examination Survey. JAMA 2000;283(18):2404–10.
21. Saag KG, Choi H. Epidemiology, risk factors, and lifestyle modifications for gout. Arthritis Res Ther 2006;8(Suppl 1):S2.
22. Kuzuya M, Ando F, Iguchi A, et al. Effect of aging on serum uric acid levels: longitudinal changes in a large Japanese population group. J Gerontol A Biol Sci Med Sci 2002;57(10):M660–4.
23. Hochberg MC, Thomas J, Thomas DJ, et al. Racial differences in the incidence of gout. The role of hypertension. Arthritis Rheum 1995;38(5):628–32.
24. Gaffo AL, Jacobs DR Jr, Lewis CE, et al. Association between being African-American, serum urate levels and the risk of developing hyperuricemia: findings from the Coronary Artery Risk Development in Young Adults cohort. Arthritis Res Ther 2012;14(1):R4.
25. DeBoer MD, Dong L, Gurka MJ. Racial/ethnic and sex differences in the relationship between uric acid and metabolic syndrome in adolescents: an analysis of National Health and Nutrition Survey 1999-2006. Metabolism 2012;61(4):554–61.
26. Klemp P, Stansfield SA, Castle B, et al. Gout is on the increase in New Zealand. Ann Rheum Dis 1997;56(1):22–6.

27. Rose BS. Gout in Maoris. Semin Arthritis Rheum 1975;5(2):121–45.
28. Singh JA. Racial and gender disparities among patients with gout. Curr Rheumatol Rep 2013;15(2):307.
29. Winnard D, Wright C, Taylor WJ, et al. National prevalence of gout derived from administrative health data in Aotearoa New Zealand. Rheumatology (Oxford) 2012;51(5):901–9.
30. Stamp LK, Wells JE, Pitama S, et al. Hyperuricaemia and gout in New Zealand rural and urban Maori and non-Maori communities. Intern Med J 2013;43(6):678–84.
31. Portis AJ, Laliberte M, Tatman P, et al. High prevalence of gouty arthritis among the Hmong population in Minnesota. Arthritis Care Res (Hoboken) 2010;62(10): 1386–91.
32. Waheddduddin S, Singh JA, Culhane-Pera KA, et al. Gout in the Hmong in the United States. J Clin Rheumatol 2010;16(6):262–6.
33. Prasad P, Krishnan E. Filipino gout: a review. Arthritis Care Res (Hoboken) 2014; 66(3):337–43.
34. Emmerson BT, Nagel SL, Duffy DL, et al. Genetic control of the renal clearance of urate: a study of twins. Ann Rheum Dis 1992;51(3):375–7.
35. Wilk JB, Djousse L, Borecki I, et al. Segregation analysis of serum uric acid in the NHLBI Family Heart Study. Hum Genet 2000;106(3):355–9.
36. Yang Q, Guo CY, Cupples LA, et al. Genome-wide search for genes affecting serum uric acid levels: the Framingham Heart Study. Metabolism 2005;54(11): 1435–41.
37. Enomoto A, Kimura H, Chairoungdua A, et al. Molecular identification of a renal urate anion exchanger that regulates blood urate levels. Nature 2002;417(6887): 447–52.
38. Taniguchi A, Urano W, Yamanaka M, et al. A common mutation in an organic anion transporter gene, SLC22A12, is a suppressing factor for the development of gout. Arthritis Rheum 2005;52(8):2576–7.
39. Iwai N, Mino Y, Hosoyamada M, et al. A high prevalence of renal hypouricemia caused by inactive SLC22A12 in Japanese. Kidney Int 2004;66(3):935–44.
40. Graessler J, Graessler A, Unger S, et al. Association of the human urate transporter 1 with reduced renal uric acid excretion and hyperuricemia in a German Caucasian population. Arthritis Rheum 2006;54(1):292–300.
41. Li C, Han L, Levin AM, et al. Multiple single nucleotide polymorphisms in the human urate transporter 1 (hURAT1) gene are associated with hyperuricaemia in Han Chinese. J Med Genet 2010;47(3):204–10.
42. Vazquez-Mellado J, Jimenez-Vaca AL, Cuevas-Covarrubias S, et al. Molecular analysis of the SLC22A12 (URAT1) gene in patients with primary gout. Rheumatology (Oxford) 2007;46(2):215–9.
43. Caulfield MJ, Munroe PB, O'Neill D, et al. SLC2A9 is a high-capacity urate transporter in humans. PLoS Med 2008;l(10):e197.
44. Anzai N, Ichida K, Jutabha P, et al. Plasma urate level is directly regulated by a voltage-driven urate efflux transporter URATv1 (SLC2A9) in humans. J Biol Chem 2008;283(40):26834–8.
45. Vitart V, Rudan I, Hayward C, et al. SLC2A9 is a newly identified urate transporter influencing serum urate concentration, urate excretion and gout. Nat Genet 2008;40(4):437–42.
46. Matsuo H, Chiba T, Nagamori S, et al. Mutations in glucose transporter 9 gene SLC2A9 cause renal hypouricemia. Am J Hum Genet 2008;83(6):744–51.
47. Doring A, Gieger C, Mehta D, et al. SLC2A9 influences uric acid concentrations with pronounced sex-specific effects. Nat Genet 2008;40(4):430–6.

48. Wallace C, Newhouse SJ, Braund P, et al. Genome-wide association study identifies genes for biomarkers of cardiovascular disease: serum urate and dyslipidemia. Am J Hum Genet 2008;82(1):139–49.
49. Kolz M, Johnson T, Sanna S, et al. Meta-analysis of 28,141 individuals identifies common variants within five new loci that influence uric acid concentrations. PLoS Genet 2009;5(6):e1000504.
50. Karns R, Zhang G, Sun G, et al. Genome-wide association of serum uric acid concentration: replication of sequence variants in an island population of the Adriatic coast of Croatia. Ann Hum Genet 2012;76(2):121–7.
51. Brandstatter A, Kiechl S, Kollerits B, et al. Sex-specific association of the putative fructose transporter SLC2A9 variants with uric acid levels is modified by BMI. Diabetes Care 2008;31(8):1662–7.
52. Hollis-Moffatt JE, Gow PJ, Harrison AA, et al. The SLC2A9 nonsynonymous Arg265His variant and gout: evidence for a population-specific effect on severity. Arthritis Res Ther 2011;13(3):R85.
53. Mobasheri A, Neama G, Bell S, et al. Human articular chondrocytes express three facilitative glucose transporter isoforms: GLUT1, GLUT3 and GLUT9. Cell Biol Int 2002;26(3):297–300.
54. Woodward OM, Kottgen A, Coresh J, et al. Identification of a urate transporter, ABCG2, with a common functional polymorphism causing gout. Proc Natl Acad Sci U S A 2009;106(25):10338–42.
55. Dehghan A, Kottgen A, Yang Q, et al. Association of three genetic loci with uric acid concentration and risk of gout: a genome-wide association study. Lancet 2008;372(9654):1953–61.
56. Matsuo H, Takada T, Ichida K, et al. Common defects of ABCG2, a high-capacity urate exporter, cause gout: a function-based genetic analysis in a Japanese population. Sci Transl Med 2009;1(5):5ra11.
57. Matsuo H, Ichida K, Takada T, et al. Common dysfunctional variants in ABCG2 are a major cause of early-onset gout. Sci Rep 2013;3:2014.
58. Tu HP, Ko AM, Chiang SL, et al. Joint effects of alcohol consumption and ABCG2 Q141K on chronic tophaceous gout risk. J Rheumatol 2014;41(4):749–58.
59. Tin A, Woodward OM, Kao WH, et al. Genome-wide association study for serum urate concentrations and gout among African Americans identifies genomic risk loci and a novel URAT1 loss-of-function allele. Hum Mol Genet 2011;20(20): 4056–68.
60. Kottgen A, Albrecht E, Teumer A, et al. Genome-wide association analyses identify 18 new loci associated with serum urate concentrations. Nat Genet 2013; 45(2):145–54.
61. Maclachlan MJ, Rodnan GP. Effect of food, fast and alcohol on serum uric acid and acute attacks of gout. Am J Med 1967;42(1):38–57.
62. Faller J, Fox IH. Ethanol-induced hyperuricemia: evidence for increased urate production by activation of adenine nucleotide turnover. N Engl J Med 1982; 307(26):1598–602.
63. Faller J, Fox IH. Ethanol induced alterations of uric acid metabolism. Adv Exp Med Biol 1984;165(Pt A):457–62.
64. Moriwaki Y, Ka T, Takahashi S, et al. Effect of beer ingestion on the plasma concentrations and urinary excretion of purine bases: one-month study. Nucleosides Nucleotides Nucleic Acids 2006;25(9–11):1083–5.
65. Ka T, Moriwaki Y, Takahashi S, et al. Effects of long-term beer ingestion on plasma concentrations and urinary excretion of purine bases. Horm Metab Res 2005;37(10):641–5.

66. Gibson T, Rodgers AV, Simmonds HA, et al. Beer drinking and its effect on uric acid. Br J Rheumatol 1984;23(3):203–9.
67. Yamamoto T, Moriwaki Y, Takahashi S, et al. Effect of beer on the plasma concentrations of uridine and purine bases. Metabolism 2002;51(10):1317–23.
68. Choi HK, Curhan G. Beer, liquor, and wine consumption and serum uric acid level: the Third National Health and Nutrition Examination Survey. Arthritis Rheum 2004;51(6):1023–9.
69. Gaffo AL, Roseman JM, Jacobs DR Jr, et al. Serum urate and its relationship with alcoholic beverage intake in men and women: findings from the Coronary Artery Risk Development in Young Adults (CARDIA) cohort. Ann Rheum Dis 2010;69(11):1965–70.
70. Choi HK, Atkinson K, Karlson EW, et al. Alcohol intake and risk of incident gout in men: a prospective study. Lancet 2004;363(9417):1277–81.
71. Dalvi SR, Pillinger MH. Saturnine gout, redux: a review. Am J Med 2013;126(5):450.e1–8.
72. Krishnan E, Lingala B, Bhalla V. Low-level lead exposure and the prevalence of gout: an observational study. Ann Intern Med 2012;157(4):233–41.
73. Wang M, Jiang X, Wu W, et al. A meta-analysis of alcohol consumption and the risk of gout. Clin Rheumatol 2013;32(11):1641–8.
74. Matzkies F, Berg G, Madl H. The uricosuric action of protein in man. Adv Exp Med Biol 1980;122A:227–31.
75. Choi HK, Liu S, Curhan G. Intake of purine-rich foods, protein, and dairy products and relationship to serum levels of uric acid: the Third National Health and Nutrition Examination Survey. Arthritis Rheum 2005;52(1):283–9.
76. Choi HK, Atkinson K, Karlson EW, et al. Purine-rich foods, dairy and protein intake, and the risk of gout in men. N Engl J Med 2004;350(11):1093–103.
77. Villegas R, Xiang YB, Elasy T, et al. Purine-rich foods, protein intake, and the prevalence of hyperuricemia: the Shanghai Men's Health Study. Nutr Metab Cardiovasc Dis 2012;22(5):409–16.
78. Yu KH, See LC, Huang YC, et al. Dietary factors associated with hyperuricemia in adults. Semin Arthritis Rheum 2008;37(4):243–50.
79. Messina M, Messina VL, Chan P. Soyfoods, hyperuricemia and gout: a review of the epidemiologic and clinical data. Asia Pac J Clin Nutr 2011;20(3):347–58.
80. Choi HK. A prescription for lifestyle change in patients with hyperuricemia and gout. Curr Opin Rheumatol 2010;22(2):165–72.
81. Fox IH, Kelley WN. Studies on the mechanism of fructose-induced hyperuricemia in man. Metabolism 1972;21(8):713–21.
82. Raivio KO, Becker A, Meyer LJ, et al. Stimulation of human purine synthesis de novo by fructose infusion. Metabolism 1975;24(7):861–9.
83. Emmerson BT. Effect of oral fructose on urate production. Ann Rheum Dis 1974;33(3):276–80.
84. Choi JW, Ford ES, Gao X, et al. Sugar-sweetened soft drinks, diet soft drinks, and serum uric acid level: the Third National Health and Nutrition Examination Survey. Arthritis Rheum 2008;59(1):109–16.
85. Choi HK, Curhan G. Soft drinks, fructose consumption, and the risk of gout in men: prospective cohort study. BMJ 2008;336(7639):309–12.
86. Choi HK, Willett W, Curhan G. Fructose-rich beverages and risk of gout in women. JAMA 2010;304(20):2270–8.
87. Dalbeth N, House ME, Gamble GD, et al. Population-specific influence of SLC2A9 genotype on the acute hyperuricaemic response to a fructose load. Ann Rheum Dis 2013;72(11):1868–73.

88. Dalbeth N, House ME, Gamble GD, et al. Influence of the ABCG2 gout risk 141 K allele on urate metabolism during a fructose challenge. Arthritis Res Ther 2014;16(1):R34.

89. Batt C, Phipps-Green AJ, Black MA, et al. Sugar-sweetened beverage consumption: a risk factor for prevalent gout with SLC2A9 genotype-specific effects on serum urate and risk of gout. Ann Rheum Dis 2013. [Epub ahead of print].

90. Jeroncic I, Mulic R, Klismanic Z, et al. Interactions between genetic variants in glucose transporter type 9 (SLC2A9) and dietary habits in serum uric acid regulation. Croat Med J 2010;51(1):40–7.

91. Gao X, Qi L, Qiao N, et al. Intake of added sugar and sugar-sweetened drink and serum uric acid concentration in US men and women. Hypertension 2007;50(2):306–12.

92. Wang DD, Sievenpiper JL, de Souza RJ, et al. The effects of fructose intake on serum uric acid vary among controlled dietary trials. J Nutr 2012;142(5): 916–23.

93. Sun SZ, Flickinger BD, Williamson-Hughes PS, et al. Lack of association between dietary fructose and hyperuricemia risk in adults. Nutr Metab (Lond) 2010;7:16.

94. Zgaga L, Theodoratou E, Kyle J, et al. The association of dietary intake of purine-rich vegetables, sugar-sweetened beverages and dairy with plasma urate, in a cross-sectional study. PLoS One 2012;7(6):e38123.

95. Garrel DR, Verdy M, PetitClerc C, et al. Milk- and soy-protein ingestion: acute effect on serum uric acid concentration. Am J Clin Nutr 1991;53(3):665–9.

96. Ryu KA, Kang HH, Kim SY, et al. Comparison of nutrient intake and diet quality between hyperuricemia subjects and controls in Korea. Clin Nutr Res 2014;3(1): 56–63.

97. Dalbeth N, Wong S, Gamble GD, et al. Acute effect of milk on serum urate concentrations: a randomised controlled crossover trial. Ann Rheum Dis 2010;69(9): 1677–82.

98. Dalbeth N, Gracey E, Pool B, et al. Identification of dairy fractions with antiinflammatory properties in models of acute gout. Ann Rheum Dis 2010;69(4): 766–9.

99. Dalbeth N, Ames R, Gamble GD, et al. Effects of skim milk powder enriched with glycomacropeptide and G600 milk fat extract on frequency of gout flares: a proof-of-concept randomised controlled trial. Ann Rheum Dis 2012;71(6): 929–34.

100. Kiyohara C, Kono S, Honjo S, et al. Inverse association between coffee drinking and serum uric acid concentrations in middle-aged Japanese males. Br J Nutr 1999;82(2):125–30.

101. Pham NM, Yoshida D, Morita M, et al. The relation of coffee consumption to serum uric Acid in Japanese men and women aged 49-76 years. J Nutr Metab 2010;2010.

102. Choi HK, Curhan G. Coffee, tea, and caffeine consumption and serum uric acid level: the third national health and nutrition examination survey. Arthritis Rheum 2007;57(5):816–21.

103. Choi HK, Willett W, Curhan G. Coffee consumption and risk of incident gout in men: a prospective study. Arthritis Rheum 2007;56(6):2049–55.

104. Choi HK, Curhan G. Coffee consumption and risk of incident gout in women: the Nurses' Health Study. Am J Clin Nutr 2010;92(4):922–7.

105. Stein HB, Hasan A, Fox IH. Ascorbic acid-induced uricosuria. A consequence of megavitamin therapy. Ann Intern Med 1976;84(4):385–8.

106. Huang HY, Appel LJ, Choi MJ, et al. The effects of vitamin C supplementation on serum concentrations of uric acid: results of a randomized controlled trial. Arthritis Rheum 2005;52(6):1843–7.

107. Gao X, Curhan G, Forman JP, et al. Vitamin C intake and serum uric acid concentration in men. J Rheumatol 2008;35(9):1853–8.

108. Choi HK, Gao X, Curhan G. Vitamin C intake and the risk of gout in men: a prospective study. Arch Intern Med 2009;169(5):502–7.

109. Juraschek SP, Miller ER 3rd, Gelber AC. Effect of oral vitamin C supplementation on serum uric acid: a meta-analysis of randomized controlled trials. Arthritis Care Res (Hoboken) 2011;63(9):1295–306.

110. Jacob RA, Spinozzi GM, Simon VA, et al. Consumption of cherries lowers plasma urate in healthy women. J Nutr 2003;133(6):1826–9.

111. Zhang Y, Neogi T, Chen C, et al. Cherry consumption and decreased risk of recurrent gout attacks. Arthritis Rheum 2012;64(12):4004–11.

112. Schlesinger N, Schlesinger M. Previously reported prior studies of cherry juice concentrate for gout flare prophylaxis: comment on the article by Zhang et al. Arthritis Rheum 2013;65(4):1135–6.

113. Williams PT. Effects of diet, physical activity and performance, and body weight on incident gout in ostensibly healthy, vigorously active men. Am J Clin Nutr 2008;87(5):1480–7.

114. Choi HK, Atkinson K, Karlson EW, et al. Obesity, weight change, hypertension, diuretic use, and risk of gout in men: the health professionals follow-up study. Arch Intern Med 2005;165(7):742–8.

115. Dalbeth N, Chen P, White M, et al. Impact of bariatric surgery on serum urate targets in people with morbid obesity and diabetes: a prospective longitudinal study. Ann Rheum Dis 2014;73(5):797–802.

116. Antozzi P, Soto F, Arias F, et al. Development of acute gouty attack in the morbidly obese population after bariatric surgery. Obes Surg 2005;15(3):405–7.

117. Dalbeth N, Pool B, Yip S, et al. Effect of bariatric surgery on the inflammatory response to monosodium urate crystals: a prospective study. Ann Rheum Dis 2013;72(9):1583–4.

118. Hanna BE, Hamed JM, Touhala LM. Serum uric Acid in smokers. Oman Med J 2008;23(4):269–74.

119. Tsuchiya M, Asada A, Kasahara E, et al. Smoking a single cigarette rapidly reduces combined concentrations of nitrate and nitrite and concentrations of antioxidants in plasma. Circulation 2002;105(10):1155–7.

120. Harrold LR, Yood RA, Mikuls TR, et al. Sex differences in gout epidemiology: evaluation and treatment. Ann Rheum Dis 2006;65(10):1368–72.

121. Shima Y, Teruya K, Ohta H. Association between intronic SNP in urate-anion exchanger gene, SLC22A12, and serum uric acid levels in Japanese. Life Sci 2006;79(23):2234–7.

122. Jang WC, Nam YH, Park SM, et al. T6092C polymorphism of SLC22A12 gene is associated with serum uric acid concentrations in Korean male subjects. Clin Chim Acta 2008;398(1–2):140–4.

123. Guan M, Zhang J, Chen Y, et al. High-resolution melting analysis for the rapid detection of an intronic single nucleotide polymorphism in SLC22A12 in male patients with primary gout in China. Scand J Rheumatol 2009;38(4):276–81.

124. Tu HP, Chen CJ, Lee CH, et al. The SLC22A12 gene is associated with gout in Han Chinese and Solomon Islanders. Ann Rheum Dis 2010;69(6):1252–4.

125. Li S, Sanna S, Maschio A, et al. The GLUT9 gene is associated with serum uric acid levels in Sardinia and Chianti cohorts. PLoS Genet 2007;3(11):e194.

126. McArdle PF, Parsa A, Chang YP, et al. Association of a common nonsynonymous variant in GLUT9 with serum uric acid levels in old order amish. Arthritis Rheum 2008;58(9):2874–81.
127. Stark K, Reinhard W, Neureuther K, et al. Association of common polymorphisms in GLUT9 gene with gout but not with coronary artery disease in a large case-control study. PLoS One 2008;3(4):e1948.
128. Hollis-Moffatt JE, Xu X, Dalbeth N, et al. Role of the urate transporter SLC2A9 gene in susceptibility to gout in New Zealand Maori, Pacific Island, and Caucasian case-control sample sets. Arthritis Rheum 2009;60(11):3485–92.
129. Tu HP, Chen CJ, Tovosia S, et al. Associations of a non-synonymous variant in SLC2A9 with gouty arthritis and uric acid levels in Han Chinese subjects and Solomon Islanders. Ann Rheum Dis 2010;69(5):887–90.
130. Urano W, Taniguchi A, Anzai N, et al. Association between GLUT9 and gout in Japanese men. Ann Rheum Dis 2010;69(5):932–3.
131. Yang Q, Kottgen A, Dehghan A, et al. Multiple genetic loci influence serum urate levels and their relationship with gout and cardiovascular disease risk factors. Circ Cardiovasc Genet 2010;3(6):523–30.
132. Charles BA, Shriner D, Doumatey A, et al. A genome-wide association study of serum uric acid in African Americans. BMC Med Genomics 2011;4:17.
133. Hamajima N, Okada R, Kawai S, et al. Significant association of serum uric acid levels with SLC2A9 rs11722228 among a Japanese population. Mol Genet Metab 2011;103(4):378–82.
134. Sulem P, Gudbjartsson DF, Walters GB, et al. Identification of low-frequency variants associated with gout and serum uric acid levels. Nat Genet 2011;43(11):1127–30.
135. Li C, Chu N, Wang B, et al. Polymorphisms in the presumptive promoter region of the SLC2A9 gene are associated with gout in a Chinese male population. PLoS One 2012;7(2):e24561.
136. Voruganti VS, Kent JW Jr, Debnath S, et al. Genome-wide association analysis confirms and extends the association of SLC2A9 with serum uric acid levels to Mexican Americans. Front Genet 2013;4:279.
137. Voruganti VS, Franceschini N, Haack K, et al. Replication of the effect of SLC2A9 genetic variation on serum uric acid levels in American Indians. Eur J Hum Genet 2014;22(7):938–43.
138. Phipps-Green AJ, Hollis-Moffatt JE, Dalbeth N, et al. A strong role for the ABCG2 gene in susceptibility to gout in New Zealand Pacific Island and Caucasian, but not Maori, case and control sample sets. Hum Mol Genet 2010;19(24):4813–9.
139. Wang B, Miao Z, Liu S, et al. Genetic analysis of ABCG2 gene C421A polymorphism with gout disease in Chinese Han male population. Hum Genet 2010;127(2):245–6.
140. Yamagishi K, Tanigawa T, Kitamura A, et al. The rs2231142 variant of the ABCG2 gene is associated with uric acid levels and gout among Japanese people. Rheumatology (Oxford) 2010;49(8):1461–5.
141. Matsuo H, Takada T, Ichida K, et al. Identification of ABCG2 dysfunction as a major factor contributing to gout. Nucleosides Nucleotides Nucleic Acids 2011;30(12):1098–104.
142. Matsuo H, Takada T, Ichida K, et al. ABCG2/BCRP dysfunction as a major cause of gout. Nucleosides Nucleotides Nucleic Acids 2011;30(12):1117–28.
143. Eastmond CJ, Garton M, Robins S, et al. The effects of alcoholic beverages on urate metabolism in gout sufferers. Br J Rheumatol 1995;34(8):756–9.

144. van der Gaag MS, van den Berg R, van den Berg H, et al. Moderate consumption of beer, red wine and spirits has counteracting effects on plasma antioxidants in middle-aged men. Eur J Clin Nutr 2000;54(7):586–91.
145. Zhang Y, Woods R, Chaisson CE, et al. Alcohol consumption as a trigger of recurrent gout attacks. Am J Med 2006;119(9):800.e13–8.
146. Neogi T, Chen C, Niu J, et al. Alcohol quantity and type on risk of recurrent gout attacks: an internet-based case-crossover study. Am J Med 2014;127(4):311–8.

Insights from Populations at Risk for the Future Development of Classified Rheumatoid Arthritis

V. Michael Holers, MD

KEYWORDS

- Preclinical rheumatoid arthritis • Epidemiology • Biomarkers • Autoantibodies
- Dietary factors • Prediction • Prevention • Imaging

KEY POINTS

- Seropositive rheumatoid arthritis (RA) typically begins with a prolonged preclinical period characterized by circulating autoantibodies in the absence of clinically apparent inflammatory arthritis.
- As the point of clinically apparent disease approaches, preclinical RA is characterized by increasing epitope spreading of new antibodies to citrullinated protein antigens peptide specificities, elevated cytokines and chemokines, alterations in autoantibody avidity, and G0 carbohydrate content.
- Subjects at increased risk for developing classified RA based on the presence of RA-related autoantibodies demonstrate autoimmune and inflammatory characteristics similar to individuals with existing RA and those known by retrospective analyses to have been in the preclinical RA period.
- At-risk individuals are characterized by the increased prevalence of asymptomatic small airways disease that may play a key role in initiation of the disease.
- Further studies of at-risk individuals have the potential to deepen the understanding of the initiation and propagation of RA.

INTRODUCTION
Stages in the Evolution of Rheumatoid Arthritis

Rheumatoid arthritis (RA) encompasses 2 major subsets of disease, seropositive and seronegative.[1,2] Seropositive individuals exhibit RA-related autoantibodies, which

Disclosure: Dr V.M. Holers receives royalty payments for a licensed patent for the use of biomarker patterns in the diagnosis of rheumatoid arthritis.
Division of Rheumatology, University of Colorado School of Medicine, Room 3102E, 1775 Aurora Court, Aurora, CO 80045, USA
E-mail address: Michael.Holers@ucdenver.edu

Rheum Dis Clin N Am 40 (2014) 605–620
http://dx.doi.org/10.1016/j.rdc.2014.07.003
0889-857X/14/$ – see front matter

rheumatic.theclinics.com

include antibodies to citrullinated protein antigens (ACPAs), with this posttranslational modification most commonly found in an antigenic form on fibrinogen, vimentin, type II collagen, and enolase.[3,4] In addition, antibodies to the Fc domains of self-immunoglobulin (Ig) molecules that are designated rheumatoid factors (RF) are also found.[5] Based on clinical comparisons as well as studies of environmental and genetic associations, it is considered that seropositive and seronegative forms of RA likely exhibit overlapping but distinct pathogenic mechanisms.[6,7]

The current understanding of the natural history of seropositive RA is summarized in **Fig. 1**. In this regard, one might consider that the onset of RA occurs around the time that clinically apparent arthritis appears. However, there is a prolonged period characterized by the presence of highly specific RA-related autoimmunity, including both ACPA and RF, in patients that typically begins 3 to 5 years[8–16] before the onset of clinically apparent disease (reviewed by Deane and colleagues[17]). Although this period is defined retrospectively as the "preclinical" period of RA in subjects who eventually develop the disease, it is perhaps best designated an "ACPA and/or RF+ at-risk" status in the populations being studied in cross-sectional or prospective studies, because the eventual outcome in individual subjects is yet unknown.[18] Subjects may progressively develop further immune alterations and then clinically apparent arthritis. It is considered possible to "reverse" the disease course at these early points,[18,19] although it is uncertain as to the proportion of subjects who do so and the primary determinants of such a change.

Herein, evidence is presented addressing the question of whether intensive studies and deep phenotyping of individuals in the ACPA+ and/or RA-related autoantibody positive at-risk status can inform the field with regard to the mechanisms by which the earliest immunologic abnormalities develop and what biologic processes may be the early "drivers" of disease. As outlined herein, the results in aggregate of these studies of at-risk individuals do provide such insights and strongly suggest that the initiation RA likely involves an extraarticular, and most likely a mucosal, inflammatory process and/or dysbiosis.

Early Stage Studies of Rheumatoid Arthritis Natural History Utilize Several Approaches to Define the "At-Risk" Population

At-risk populations have been defined based on several characteristics, with the most commonly utilized being a close familial relationship, usually at the first-degree relative

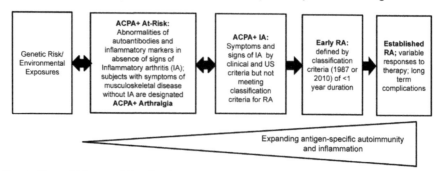

Fig. 1. Natural history of RA development. RA progresses through a series of stages first identified and characterized by detectable circulating RA-specific autoimmunity (ACPA+ At-Risk), with or without "arthralgia," followed by progression through symptoms, signs and clinically apparent and classifiable disease. The presence of bidirectional arrows at early stages indicates that subjects with early disease may resolve the findings and return to an earlier state.

(FDR) level. FDRs are studied because these individuals exhibit a 3- to 5-fold increase in lifetime risk for the development of classified RA.[20,21] Additionally, however, at-risk individuals can be identified by the carriage of the shared epitope (SE)-containing HLA alleles, which are overrepresented within RA populations.[22,23] A third approach is the identification of subjects who present to health care settings with RA-related autoantibodies and nonspecific musculoskeletal symptoms without arthritis, designated as an "arthralgia" population.[24–26] Finally, at-risk subjects can be identified through large health fair screenings primarily designed to identify clinically active but undiagnosed RA, and wherein RA-related autoantibody-positive subjects without arthritis or signs or symptoms of classified RA are also found.[27]

For practical reasons relating to the lack of ability to accurately classify individuals who do not elaborate RA-related autoantibodies, many studies of at-risk individuals have largely focused on the RA-related autoantibody-positive population. However, because there are also immune abnormalities associated with the autoantibody negative FDR population,[22,28] as well as modest increases in cytokines and chemokines as the onset of clinically apparent seronegative disease approaches,[8] utilizing a more inclusive definition of the at-risk population is also useful for studies.

PRESENCE OF BIOMARKERS IN THE PRECLINICAL PERIOD AND IMPLICATIONS FOR DISEASE PATHOGENESIS
Autoantibodies

Findings in classified rheumatoid arthritis
ACPA and RF are commonly found in RA and indeed are components of the definition of seropositive disease.[29,30] As a practical matter, ACPA are typically measured using commercial enzyme-linked immunosorbent assay-based tests that are certified and approved for clinical use, and when assessed using these methods are designated anti-cyclic citrullinated peptide (anti-CCP) antibodies.[31,32] Anti-CCP antibodies have been described in subjects with classified RA as demonstrating a sensitivity of 60% to 70% with a specificity of approximately 98%,[3,33] improving substantially over the approximate 80% to 85% specificity of RFs.[5] However, the specificity of ACPAs differs by the specific anti-CCP commercial test utilized, the control population against which the test is compared, and the stage of disease being evaluated.[34] In addition to enzyme-linked immunosorbent assays, there are an increasing number of peptide- and protein-based array methods that can be used to refine the epitope specificity of ACPAs, which demonstrate a very wide variety of non–cross-reactive citrullinated peptide specificities in patients with classified RA.[35,36]

In addition to ACPA and RFs, several other autoantigens are recognized by smaller subgroups of patients with classified RA. These autoantibodies have been reported to recognize carbamylated proteins antigens (anti-CarP) wherein arginine is converted to homocitrulline,[37] mutated citrullinated vimentin,[38] RA-33,[39] and peptidyl arginine deiminase type 4,[40] among others.

Findings in at-risk populations
Using stored serum banks to study the evolution of autoantibodies in the preclinical period, both increase in titers and epitope spreading have been found to occur that encompasses a wider variety of targets as the clinical onset nears.[8,35,41] With regard to assessment of subjects in real time, a subset of FDR elaborate RA-related autoantibodies, analyzed as anti-CCP2, anti-CCP3.1, RF by nephelometry, and RF by isotype positivity. When analyzed, a largely non-Hispanic white FDR population was found to exhibit an approximately 16% positivity inclusive of this range of autoantibodies [(23), and updated], and the North American Native population was reported to exhibit

anti-CCP antibodies in 17% of FDR, 11% of more distant relatives, and 3% in controls.[42] In FDR within multicase families in Sweden, concentrations and frequencies of anti-CCP and RF isotypes were also significantly increased. Of note, in that population the distribution of IgA and IgM isotypes was higher than IgG in the relatives, whereas the IgG isotype dominated in probands with RA.[43]

FDRs have also been studied to determine whether there are similar increases in epitope spreading associated with an anti-CCP–positive test. One study showed that anti-CCP–positive FDRs elaborate a substantially increased number of ACPA than control FDRs without RA-related autoantibodies, with a subset being positive for 9 or more ACPA in a pattern typical for classified RA.[44] An increasing number of positive ACPAs was also associated with the presence of a tender joint on examination. In another independent study of an FDR population using a 6-member ACPA panel, a high prevalence of ACPAs (48%) and was found as compared with controls (10%), with citrullinated vimentin most commonly targeted.[45] Of note, a high proportion of ACPAs in that study were of the IgA isotype.

Thus, RA-free FDRs show reactivity to multiple ACPA, demonstrating that both an anti-CCP positivity in this population is not likely to be a "false positive," but rather is similar in nature to subjects with classified RA, and that there is evidence of genetic and/or familial effects within the FDR population. What is as yet unknown is whether other anti-CCP characteristics found in patients with classified RA, such as increased avidity,[46] substantial complement activating potential,[47] and altered G0 carbohydrates that promote IgG effector functions,[48,49] are also present in samples from these real-time at-risk populations, although these questions are under study. Additionally, because only 3% to 5% of FDRs will ultimately develop RA, the high proportion of immune abnormalities in FDRs must either not be a stable phenotype, reflect early immune dysregulation that progresses to other autoimmune diseases in this population, or that the individuals elaborating the immune dysregulation do not all progress through additional stages of disease. Although limited in scope, evidence for both conclusions is present. Finally, reflecting clinical variability in early arthritis, in subjects enrolled in the Canadian Early Arthritis Cohort who underwent baseline and at least the 12-month follow-up studies, both RF and ACPA were found to fluctuate, with approximately 10% of subjects converting from ACPA negative to ACPA positive, and vice versa.[50]

Alterations of Antigen-specific and Innate Lymphocyte Populations

Findings in classified rheumatoid arthritis

CD4 T cells specific for citrullinated synovial antigens have been identified and quantitated through the use of major histocompatibility class II tetramers, whereas samples from patients with classified RA display an increased frequency of citrullinated peptide (cit)-specific T cells, predominantly of the memory T helper type 1 cell class.[51] Notably, the frequency of cit-specific T cells in RA patients is highest within the first 5 years of disease, and is decreased among patients on biologic therapies independent of disease duration. Autoreactive T cells in patients with RA recognize a combination of citrullinated epitopes carried on class II tetramers,[51] and demonstrate evidence of cellular immunity to citrullinated autoantigens using other techniques. For example, secretion of interleukin (IL)-6 and IL-17 and tumor necrosis factor (TNF)- α by CD4$^+$ cells was found to be present in normal controls and patients with RA, whereas interferon and IL-10 were specific for RA, with citrullinated aggrecan generating the most robust antigen-specific response.[52]

With regard to B cells, subjects with RA exhibit an increased number of peripheral blood plasmablasts and/or plasma cells, a substantial proportion of which produce

ACPAs.[53] Plasma cells producing ACPAs are also commonly found in the synovium.[54] B cells in patients with active RA also exhibit features of dysregulated control of anergy checkpoints during development,[55,56] as well as signaling alterations in the anergic population.[57]

In addition to antigen-specific lymphocytes, innate lymphoid cells, a novel family of effector cells that are reported to play important roles in the maintenance of lymphoid tissue, tissue repair, and response to infection, are also altered in patients with RA.[58] In this regard, there are several distinct subsets of innate lymphoid cells that secrete a variety of cytokines that are important in RA pathogenesis (IL-5, IL-13, IL-17, IL-22, TNF-α and interferon-γ).

Findings in at-risk populations

Although evidence of dysregulation of autoimmune B and T cells, as well as innate lymphoid cells, is anticipated to be present in the at-risk population, the studies necessary to assess this question are only just underway. In one sense, because antigen-specific T cells are more likely to be found earlier rather than later in disease,[51] systemic high titers of anti-CCP antibodies can also be present in FDRs,[42–44] and local production of anti-CCP antibodies has been described in the at-risk populations,[28] it is very likely that antigen-specific lymphocytes will be present and detectable. However, major questions include the epitope specificities of this early response, whether there a linked B- and T-cell response that is present, and if there are peptide specificities that can be targeted using antigen-specific immune tolerization approaches.

Cytokines and Chemokines

Findings in classified rheumatoid arthritis

Patients with classified RA exhibit a wide variety of elevated cytokines, with no single cytokine or pattern predominating (eg, see Hueber and colleagues[59]). There are patterns, however, that are associated with a highly inflammatory state, and IL-1, TNF-α, IL-12p40, and IL-13 have been found to be particularly elevated in early RA.[59]

Findings in at-risk populations

Using retrospective serum studies, it has been found that, shortly before the onset of clinically apparent arthritis, systemic levels of cytokines and chemokines increase in a heterogenous manner, both with regard to the number being elevated in an individual subject and the levels of each factor.[8,16,60,61] With regard to at-risk populations, elevated cytokines are associated with the presence of anti-CCP2 antibody,[62] as well as expanded in FDRs regardless of autoantibody status.[22] Thus, there is substantial evidence that immune dysregulation in at-risk populations is associated with systemic evidence of inflammation. Prospective analyses of this question in at-risk populations, however, have not been reported, and studies of other inflammation-related biomarkers including complement activation fragments are also now underway.

Genetics

Findings in classified rheumatoid arthritis

There are many genes that associate with RA, including high-risk HLA-DR alleles containing the SE[63] and PTPN22,[64] as well as more than 100 other linked genes with a modestly elevated relative risk.[65] Notably, a substantial number of these genes encode components of immune-related signaling pathways (reviewed in Bax and co-workers[66]) and/or also encompass genes expressed in memory effector T cells[67] and associated with CD40, TRAF1, TNFAIP3, and PRKCQ pathways.[68]

Differences in genetic relationships to disease are also present that are based on environmental exposures, such as a relationship between smoking, SE, and the presence of ACPA,[7,69] and the link between SE and the presence of antibodies to citrullinated enolase.[70]

Findings in at-risk populations

Despite the increasingly understood relationships between genetic risk and the presence of classified RA, little has been accomplished yet regarding the question of at what point during disease evolution these factors act. With regard to the major risks associated with the SE, in 1 study there was a trend between the presence of ACPA and the SE, but the size of the study apparently limited the ability to definitively answer this question.[45] Thus, this is another question that should be addressed and is indeed under active analysis.

Genomics

Findings in classified rheumatoid arthritis

In addition to the hardwired genetic contributions, there are genomic and epigenetic changes that are associated with RA and affect lymphocytes, fibroblastlike synoviocytes (FLS) and other cell populations.[65,71] Epigenetic modifications include DNA methylation, histone methylation, histone acetylation, histone phosphorylation, and expression of microRNAs, and changes are especially prominent in FLS, where they are chronically exposed to an environment rich in proinflammatory cytokines and mediators of oxidative stress.[71,72] These epigenetic changes represent key means by which environmental factors could influence gene expression and disease heterogeneity, and potentially heritability given that some epigenetic changes can be transmitted to offspring.[71,72] One important finding is that epigenetic changes in FLS seem to be "imprinted" and durable even after removal from the proinflammatory environment.[71]

Findings in at-risk populations

It is not yet known whether the same epigenetic findings in classified RA are also found in the preclinical disease state, or whether other stage-specific changes are found. One particularly important question is whether FLS exhibit changes that promote the transition from the presence of circulating autoimmunity to the development of local synovitis.

Imaging and Biopsy Studies

Findings in classified rheumatoid arthritis

Many types of imaging approaches have been applied to the study of patients with classified RA. Perhaps most relevant to the study of preclinical RA and at-risk populations, however, where the question of the presence or absence of changes consistent with inflammatory arthritis is most pressing, are ultrasound (US) and magnetic resonance imaging (reviewed by Tan and colleagues[73]). Using these techniques, one can detect by US synovitis by identifying within the images effusions, synovial expansion and a power Doppler signal. In addition, through US one can detect bony erosions and measure cartilage thickness. US is useful for tendon assessments and defining tenosynovitis and tendon rupture. Magnetic resonance imaging can also define the same structures, but in addition can visualize bone marrow pathologies not detectable by US, such as bone marrow edema.

Findings in at-risk populations
Studies in at-risk populations have focused on RA-related autoantibody-positive individuals as well as subjects who present to health care settings with arthralgia or early or unclassified inflammatory arthritis. Studies of anti-CCP positive arthralgia patients without clinically detectable arthritis have demonstrated histologic findings without inflammation but with a trend toward CD3 and CD8 T-cell infiltration.[74] Studies of FDR using magnetic resonance imaging of the hands and feet have not demonstrated evidence of synovial inflammation,[25] and analyses of arthralgia/IA populations demonstrate that a subset exhibit US abnormalities.[75] Thus, the situation remains uncertain, but is an important area for prospective investigation, as well as for the development of additional functional imaging approaches.

Dietary, Hormonal, and Environmental Exposures and Biomarkers
Findings in classified rheumatoid arthritis
With regard to environmental influences on RA susceptibility, there are several well-accepted exposures that increase or decrease the risk of developing RA, including smoke exposure, hormonal factors, dietary exposures, air pollutants, and silica dust[69,76]; however, the exact causal relationships are not understood beyond a potential relationship between smoke exposure and citrullination.[6] In this regard, autoreactivity to citrullinated α-enolase has demonstrated a linkage to both smoking and DR4 SE status.[70] Dietary factors have also been assessed, and particularly compelling findings have included an inverse relationship between omega-3 fatty acid intake and both the risk of developing and severity of RA (reviewed by James and colleagues[77]).

Findings in at-risk populations
Although limited in scope, studies have demonstrated an inverse relationship between birth control exposure and a direct relationship to smoking with the presence of RF in an FDR at-risk population.[78] In the same population, no association with vitamin D levels was found.[79] In addition, the relationship between air pollution exposure and RA-related autoantibodies in the FDR population has been studied, and demonstrated no relationship.[80] Ongoing studies are evaluating the relationships between omega-3 fatty acid intake and presence of RA-related autoantibodies.

Cardiovascular Disease Risk
Findings in classified rheumatoid arthritis
In addition to arthritis, other common and clinically significant manifestations of RA include an elevated risk for cardiovascular disease, although the exact time at which this elevated risk is manifest remains uncertain.[81]

Findings in at-risk populations
Reported studies of this important question are limited in nature, and many are ongoing in a number of at-risk populations. Importantly, identifying a risk of cardiovascular disease that precedes clinically apparent articular RA may drive interventions not only to prevent future RA, but cardiovascular disease as well.

Osteopenia and Erosions
Findings in classified rheumatoid arthritis
Loss of bone as manifest by osteopenia and local erosions commonly occurs along with the most severe forms of RA, likely through both local and systemic inflammatory and remodeling processes that alter relative rates of bone formation and degradation by osteoclasts and osteoblasts.[82,83] ACPA directed to citrullinated vimentin may be particularly important in inducing bone loss in patients with RA.[84]

Findings in at-risk populations

Studies in at-risk populations are limited; however, ACPA-positive individuals without detectable synovitis have been found to demonstrate diminished bone by the use of micro-computed tomography analyses.[85] Thus, it seems that in addition to evidence of systemic inflammation by cytokine elevations, local bone loss may also characterize the RA-related autoantibody at-risk status.

Pulmonary Disease

Findings in classified rheumatoid arthritis

Many links between RA and the lung have been made. For instance, cigarette smoke exposure is highly associated with risk for the development of RA, especially in the presence of HLA-expressing the DR4 SE.[6,69] In addition, through the use of sensitive high-resolution computed tomography, patients with early RA demonstrate a substantial number of pulmonary abnormalities.[86]

Findings in at-risk populations

Notably, at-risk individuals who do not have RA but exhibit high-risk RA-related autoantibodies demonstrate a high rate of inflammatory airway disease that is not associated with a smoking history or other similar exposures.[87] Local production of ACPA and other RA-related autoantibodies has been demonstrated through studies of induced sputa from FDR, where RF and anti-CCP antibodies can be readily demonstrated in the sputum but not in the peripheral blood of a subset of this population.[28] Because of these findings, the lung is now considered to be a primary site of the initiation of RA, although other mucosal sites may also be candidates for initiation of RA.

Microbiome Analyses

Findings in classified rheumatoid arthritis

Several lines of investigation suggest that dysbiosis occurs in patients with RA, which may be associated with risk, severity, or targets of injury. For example, an elevated occurrence of severe periodontitis is reproducibly found in patients with RA, and conversely patients with RA who exhibit severe periodontitis have higher disease activity scores.[88] Patients with severe periodontitis also manifest higher titers of IgG and IgM antibodies to *Porphyromonas gingivalis*, which is important because this organism exhibits enzymatic activity that can citrullinate fibrinogen and enolase in the presence of bacterial gingipains.[89] In addition, though, other studies have found that *Prevotella* and *Leptotrichia*, but not *P gingivalis*, are present in higher numbers in the subgingival microbiota in patients with recent onset untreated RA.[90]

Finally, studies of the gut, a mucosal site where microbes are well known to be able to influence immune responses and where experimental arthritis has been modulated by the exposure in the gut to a single organism,[91] have suggested that change in the microbiota are associated with concurrent RA,[92] especially an expansion of *Prevotella copri* species.[93]

Findings in at-risk populations

There is strong potential for the mucosa and/or mucosal dysbiosis to be an early driver of RA development. The rationale is based on recent studies strongly suggesting that mucosal inflammation,[87] production of RA-related autoantibodies,[28] and dysbiosis[93] can occur coincidently. In addition, in at-risk subjects, there is a specific elevation of antibodies to *P gingivalis* but not to related strains.[94] Therefore, substantial efforts are currently being made to further address these relationships in at-risk populations.

Metabolomics

Findings in classified rheumatoid arthritis

Measures of environmental and genetic influences include metabolic fingerprints that can be assessed through nuclear magnetic resonance spectroscopy-based metabolomics techniques.

With regard to patients with classified RA, the serum metabolic fingerprint was found to be clearly different than controls, with lactate and lipids as discriminators of the inflammatory burden in early RA; differences were also related to the level of C-reactive protein.[95]

Findings in at-risk populations

As a means by which one can assess a sum of many different endogenous and exogenous influences, metabolomics studies hold promise for helping to understand the biologic underpinnings of RA initiation and early evolution. Because of this, there are ongoing studies to evaluate this question.

INTEGRATION OF STUDIES OF AT-RISK INDIVIDUALS INTO STAGES OF DISEASE DEVELOPMENT

As is apparent from the status of many of the studies of at-risk populations described herein, this is a very active area of investigation. Notably, only a subset of environmental, and likely genetic, influences seem to be involved during the very early stages of development of RA. This is not surprising, given the complexity of this disease, and that stage-specific influences are found in other autoimmune diseases such as type 1 diabetes.[96] One way to portray the current state of understanding in RA is illustrated in **Fig. 2**. This figure also illustrates how much further the field needs to advance to understand, for instance, the stage-specific genetic influences and whether exposures early but not in later transitions. Nevertheless, the results of recently reported and ongoing studies do suggest that important insights into pathogenesis and treatment can be made in at-risk populations and that these can lead to novel population and individualized prevention and therapeutic strategies.

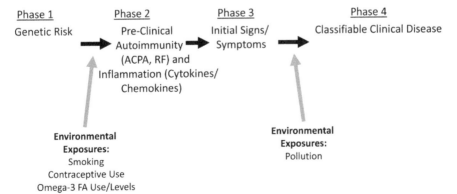

Fig. 2. Stage-specific environmental influences and biomarker alterations found during the evolution of seropositive RA. For earliest factors, current datasets do not allow conclusions regarding potential additional effects on later stages. Support for each is outlined in the text.

FUTURE CONSIDERATIONS

The results presented herein indicate that a subset of biomarkers commonly found in patients with classified RA is present in subjects who are at an increased future risk for developing clinically apparent RA. These results are consistent with a scenario wherein chronic mucosal inflammation related to genetic, environmental, microbial, and/or other local factors promoting immune dysregulation leads to the initial break in tolerance to self-antigens and systemic autoimmunity manifest by both IgG and IgA autoantibodies. Little is known regarding the precise mechanism that enables the transition from an autoimmune and inflammatory reaction at a mucosal site associated with circulating autoantibodies to an attack on the joints. Nevertheless, several potential mechanisms exist and have been explored either in patients or animal models (reviewed in Arend and colleagues[97] and Klarekog and colleagues[98]). One possibility, reflecting the presence of circulating immune complexes containing citrullinated fibrinogen in patients with RA,[99] which notably can more effectively activate macrophages through the synergistic engagement of Tool-like receptor-4 and Fc receptors,[100] is that immune complexes can enter the joint and deposit on cartilage and in synovial tissue. Another possibility is that transient expression of citrullinated antigens allows the ability of circulating autoantibodies[101,102] or T cells[103] to recognize and initiate or amplify inflammation. A third possibility, potentially explaining the link between the early involvement of the lung with later arthritis, may be shared expression of citrullinated vimentin that is recognized by pathogenic autoantibodies at both sites.[104] Further cross-sectional and especially prospective studies of at-risk subjects in this period will allow the definitive elucidation of causal mechanisms that will likely allow treatment with strategies that are unique to this early period of development.

REFERENCES

1. Fuchs HA, Sergent JS. Rheumatoid arthritis: the clinical picture. In: Koopman WJ, editor. Arthritis and allied conditions: a textbook of rheumatology. 13th edition. Baltimore (MD): Williams and Wilkins; 1997. p. 1041-70.
2. Lee DM, Weinblatt ME. Rheumatoid arthritis. Lancet 2001;359:903-11.
3. Schellekens GA, Visser H, de Jong BA, et al. The diagnostic properties of rheumatoid arthritis antibodies recognizing a cyclic citrullinated peptide. Arthritis Rheum 2000;43:155-63.
4. van Venrooij WJ, Pruijn GJ. Citrullination: a small change for a protein with great consequences for rheumatoid arthritis. Arthritis Res 2000;2:249-51.
5. Bas S, Genevay S, Meyer O, et al. Anti-cyclic citrullinated peptide antibodies, IgM and IgA rheumatoid factors in the diagnosis and prognosis of rheumatoid arthritis. Rheumatology 2003;42:677-80.
6. Klareskog L, Malmstrom V, Lundberg K, et al. Smoking, citrullination and genetic variability in the immunopathogenesis of rheumatoid arthritis. Semin Immunol 2011;23:92-8.
7. Padyukov L, Silva C, Stolt P, et al. A gene-environment interaction between smoking and shared epitope genes in HLA-DR provides a high risk of seropositive rheumatoid arthritis. Arthritis Rheum 2004;50:3085-92.
8. Deane KD, O'Donnell CI, Hueber W, et al. The number of elevated cytokines and chemokines in preclinical seropositive rheumatoid arthritis predicts time to diagnosis in an age-dependent manner. Arthritis Rheum 2010;62:3161-72.
9. Aho K, Heliovaara M, Maatela J, et al. Rheumatoid factors antedating clinical rheumatoid arthritis. J Rheumatol 1991;18:1282-4.

10. Aho K, Paluso T, Heliovaara M, et al. Antifilaggrin antibodies within "normal" range predict rheumatoid arthritis in a linear fashion. J Rheumatol 2000;27:2743–6.
11. Berglin E, Padyukov L, Sundin U, et al. A combination of autoantibodies to cyclic citrullinated peptide (CCP) and HLA-DRB1 locus antigens is strongly associated with the future onset of rheumatoid arthritis. Arthritis Res Ther 2004;6:R303–8.
12. del Puente A, Knowler WC, Pettitt DJ, et al. The incidence of rheumatoid arthritis is predicted by rheumatoid factor titer in a longitudinal population study. Arthritis Rheum 1988;31:1239–44.
13. Nielen MM, van Schaardenburg D, Reesink HW, et al. Increased levels of C-Reactive Protein in serum from blood donors before the onset of rheumatoid arthritis. Arthritis Rheum 2004;50:2423–7.
14. Nielen MM, van Schaardenburg D, Reesink HW, et al. Specific autoantibodies precede the symptoms of rheumatoid arthritis. Arthritis Rheum 2004;50:380–6.
15. Rantapaa Dahlqvist S, de Jong BA, Hallmans G, et al. Antibodies against citrullinated peptides (CCP) predict the development of rheumatoid arthritis. Arthritis Rheum 2003;48:2701–5.
16. Karlson EW, Chisnik LB, Tworoger SS, et al. Biomarkers of inflammation and development of rheumatoid arthritis in women from two prospective cohort studies. Arthritis Rheum 2009;60:641–52.
17. Deane KD, Norris JM, Holers VM. Pre-clinical rheumatoid arthritis: identification, evaluation and future directions for investigation. Rheum Dis Clin North Am 2010;13:236–41.
18. Gerlag DM, Raza K, van Baarsen LG, et al. EULAR recommendations for terminology and research in individuals at risk of rheumatoid arthritis: report from the Study Group for risk factors for rheumatoid arthritis. Ann Rheum Dis 2012;71: 638–41.
19. Raza K, Breese M, Nightingale P, et al. Predictive value of antibodies to cyclic citrullinated peptide in patients with very early inflammatory arthritis. J Rheumatol 2005;32:203–7.
20. Silman AJ, Ollier B, Mageed RA. Rheumatoid factor detection in the unaffected first degree relatives in families with multicase rheumatoid arthritis. J Rheumatol 1991;18:512–5.
21. Silman AJ. Epidemiology of rheumatoid arthritis. APMIS 1994;102:721–8.
22. El-Gabalawy HS, Robinson DB, Smolik I, et al. Familial clustering of the serum cytokine profile in the relatives of rheumatoid arthritis patients. Arthritis Rheum 2012;64:1720–9.
23. Kolfenbach JR, Deane KD, Derber LA, et al. A prospective approach to investigating the natural history of pre-clinical rheumatoid arthritis (RA) using first-degree relatives of probands with RA. Arthritis Care Res 2009;61:1735–41.
24. Bos WH, Dijkmans BA, Boers M, et al. Effect of dexamethasone on autoantibody levels and arthritis development in patients with arthralgia: a randomized trial. Ann Rheum Dis 2010;69:571–4.
25. van de Sande MG, de Hair MJ, van der Leij C, et al. Different stages of rheumatoid arthritis: features of the synovium in the preclinical phase. Ann Rheum Dis 2011;70:772–7.
26. van de Stadt LA, van der Horst AR, de Koning MH, et al. The extent of the anti-citrullinated protein antibody repertoire is associated with arthritis development in patients with seropositive arthralgia. Ann Rheum Dis 2011;70:128–33.
27. Deane KD, Striebich C, Goldstein BL, et al. Identification of undiagnosed inflammatory arthritis in a community health fair screen. Arthritis Care Res 2009;61: 1642–9.

28. Willis VC, Demoruelle MK, Derber LA, et al. Sputa autoantibodies in patients with established rheumatoid arthritis and subjects at-risk for future clinically apparent disease. Arthritis Rheum 2013;65:2545–54.

29. Aletaha D, Neogi T, Silman AJ, et al. 2010 Rheumatoid arthritis classification criteria: an American College of Rheumatology/European League against rheumatism collaborative initiative. Arthritis Rheum 2010;62:2569–81.

30. Arnett FC, Edworthy SM, Bloch DA, et al. The American Rheumatism Association 1987 revised criteria for the classification of rheumatoid arthritis. Arthritis Rheum 1998;31:314–24.

31. Coenen D, Verschueren P, Westhovens R, et al. Technical and diagnostic performance of 6 assays for the measurement of citrullinated protein/peptide antibodies in the diagnosis of rheumatoid arthritis. Clin Chem 2007;53:498–504.

32. Demoruelle MK, Deane KD. Antibodies to citrullinated protein antigens (ACPAs): clinical and pathophysiologic significance. Curr Rheumatol Rep 2011;13:421–30.

33. Goldbach-Mansky R, Lee J, McCoy A, et al. Rheumatoid arthritis associated autoantibodies in patients with synovitis of recent onset. Arthritis Res Ther 2000;2:236–43.

34. Demoruelle MK, Parish MC, Derber LA, et al. Performance of anti-cyclic citrullinated peptide assays differs in subjects at increased risk of rheumatoid arthritis and subjects with established disease. Arthritis Rheum 2013;65:2243–52.

35. Brink M, Hansson M, Mathsson L, et al. Multiplex analyses of antibodies against citrullinated peptides in individuals prior to the development of rheumatoid arthritis. Arthritis Rheum 2013;65:899–910.

36. Hueber W, Kidd BA, Tomooka BH, et al. Antigen microarray profiling of autoantibodies in rheumatoid arthritis. Arthritis Rheum 2005;52:2645–55.

37. Shi J, Knevel R, Suwannalai P, et al. Autoantibodies recognizing carbamylated proteins are present in sera of patients with rheumatoid arthritis and predict joint damage. Proc Natl Acad Sci U S A 2011;108:17372–7.

38. Vossenaar ER, Despres N, LaPointe E, et al. Rheumatoid arthritis specific anti-Sa antibodies target citrullinated vimentin. Arthritis Res Ther 2004;6:R142.

39. Hassfeld W, Steiner G, Graninger W, et al. Autoantibody to the nuclear antigen RA33: a marker for early rheumatoid arthritis. Br J Rheumatol 1993;32:199–203.

40. Harris ML, Darrah E, Lam GK, et al. Association of autoimmunity to peptidyl arginine deiminase type 4 with genotype and disease severity in rheumatoid arthritis. Arthritis Rheum 2008;58:1958–67.

41. Sokolove J, Bromberg R, Deane KD, et al. Autoantibody epitope spreading in the pre-clinical phase predicts progression to rheumatoid arthritis. PLoS One 2012;7:e35296.

42. El-Gabalawy HS, Robinson DB, Hart D, et al. Immunogenetic risks of anti-cyclical citrullinated peptide antibodies in a North American native population with rheumatoid arthritis and their first-degree relatives. J Rheumatol 2009;36:1130–5.

43. Arlestig L, Mullazehi M, Kokkonen H, et al. Antibodies against cyclic citrullinated peptides of IgG, IgA and IgM isotype and rheumatoid factor of IgM and IgA isotype are increased in unaffected members of multicase rheumatoid arthritis families from northern Sweden. Ann Rheum Dis 2012;71:825–9.

44. Young KA, Deane KD, Derber LA, et al. Relatives without rheumatoid arthritis show reactivity to anti-citrullinated protein/peptide antibodies that are associated with arthritis-related traits: studies of the etiology of rheumatoid arthritis. Arthritis Rheum 2013;65:1995–2004.

45. Barra L, Scinocca M, Saunders S, et al. Anti-citrullinated protein antibodies in unaffected first-degree relatives of rheumatoid arthritis patients. Arthritis Rheum 2013;65:1439–47.
46. Suwannalai P, van de Stadt LA, Radner H, et al. Avidity maturation of anti-citrullinated protein antibodies in rheumatoid arthritis. Arthritis Rheum 2012; 64:1323–8.
47. Trouw LA, Haisma EM, Levarht EW, et al. Anti-cyclic peptide antibodies from rheumatoid arthritis patients activate complement via both the classical and alternative pathways. Arthritis Rheum 2009;60:1923–31.
48. Ercan A, Cui J, Chatterton DE, et al. IgG galactosylation aberrancy precedes disease onset, correlates with disease activity and is prevalent in autoantibodies in rheumatoid arthritis. Arthritis Rheum 2010;62:2238–48.
49. Scherer HU, van der Woude D, Ioan-Facsinay A, et al. Glycan profiling of anti-citrullinated protein antibodies isolated from human serum and synovial fluid. Arthritis Rheum 2010;62:1620–9.
50. Barra L, Bykerk VP, Pope JE, et al. Anticitrullinated protein antibodies and rheumatoid factor fluctuate in early inflammatory arthritis and do not predict clinical outcomes. J Rheumatol 2013;40:1259–67.
51. James E, Rieck M, Pieper J, et al. Citrulline specific Th1 cells are increased in rheumatoid arthritis and their frequency is influenced by disease duration and therapy. Arthritis Rheum 2014;66(7):1712–22.
52. Law SC, Street S, Yu CH, et al. T-cell autoreactivity to citrullinated autoantigenic peptides in rheumatoid arthritis patients carrying HLA-DRB1 shared epitope alleles. Arthritis Res Ther 2012;14:R118.
53. Kerkaman PF, Rombouts Y, van der Voort E, et al. Circulating plasmablasts/plasma cells as a source of anticitrullinated protein antibodies in patients with rheumatoid arthritis. Ann Rheum Dis 2013;72:1259–63.
54. Amara K, Steen J, Murray F, et al. Monoclonal IgG antibodies generated from joint-derived B cells of RA patients have a strong bias toward citrullinated auto-antigen recognition. J Exp Med 2013;210:445–55.
55. Menard L, Samuels J, Meffre E. Inflammation-independent defective early B cell tolerance checkpoints in rheumatoid arthritis. Arthritis Rheum 2011;63:1237–45.
56. Samuels J, Ng YS, Coupillaud CP, et al. Impaired early B cell tolerance in patients with rheumatoid arthritis. J Exp Med 2005;210:1659–67.
57. Liubchenko GA, Appleberry HC, Striebich CC, et al. Rheumatoid arthritis is associated with signaling alterations in naturally occurring autoreactive B-lymphocytes. J Autoimmun 2013;40:111–21.
58. Spits H, Cupedo T. Innate lymphoid cells: emerging insights in development, lineage relationships, and function. Annu Rev Immunol 2012;30:647–75.
59. Hueber W, Tomooka BH, Zhao X, et al. Proteomic analysis of secreted proteins in early rheumatoid arthritis: anti-citrulline autoreactivity is associated with up regulation of proinflammatory cytokines. Ann Rheum Dis 2007;66:712–9.
60. Jorgensen KT, Wiik A, Pedersen M, et al. Cytokines, autoantibodies and viral antibodies in premorbid and postdiagnostic sera from patients with rheumatoid arthritis: case-control study nested in a cohort of Norwegian blood donors. Ann Rheum Dis 2008;67:860–6.
61. Kokkonen H, Soderstrom I, Rocklov J, et al. Up-regulation of cytokines and chemokines predates the onset of rheumatoid arthritis. Arthritis Rheum 2010;62:383–91.
62. Hughes-Austin J, Deane KD, Derber LA, et al. Multiple cytokines and chemokines are associated with rheumatoid arthritis-related autoimmunity in

first-degree relatives without rheumatoid arthritis: studies of the Aetiology of Rheumatoid Arthritis (SERA). Ann Rheum Dis 2012;72:901–7.

63. Nepom GT, Nepom BS. Prediction of susceptibility to rheumatoid arthritis by human leukocyte antigen phenotyping. Rheum Dis Clin North Am 1992;18:785–92.

64. Begovich AB, Carlton VE, Honigberg LA, et al. A missense single-nucleotide polymorphism in a gene encoding a protein tyrosine phosphatase (PTPN22) is associated with rheumatoid arthritis. Am J Hum Genet 2004;75:330–7.

65. Viatte S, Plant D, Raychaudhuri S. Genetics and epigenetics of rheumatoid arthritis. Nat Rev Rheumatol 2013;9:141–53.

66. Bax M, van Heemst J, Huizinga TW, et al. Genetics of rheumatoid arthritis: what have we learned? Immunogenetics 2011;63:459–66.

67. Hu X, Kim H, Stahl E, et al. Integrating autoimmune risk loci with gene-expression data identifies specific pathogenic immune cell subsets. Am J Hum Genet 2011;89:496–506.

68. Gregersen PK, Amos CI, Lee AT, et al. REL, encoding a member of the NF-kappaB family of transcription factors, is a newly defined risk locus for rheumatoid arthritis. Nat Genet 2009;41:820–3.

69. Klareskog L, Stolt P, Lundberg K, et al. A new model for an etiology of rheumatoid arthritis: smoking may trigger HLA-DR (shared epitope)-restricted immune reactions to autoantigens modified by citrullination. Arthritis Rheum 2006;54:38–46.

70. Mahdi H, Fisher BA, Kallberg H, et al. Specific interaction between genotype, smoking and autoimmunity to citrullinated alpha-enolase in the etiology of rheumatoid arthritis. Nat Genet 2009;41:1319–24.

71. Firestein GS. Evolving concepts of rheumatoid arthritis. Nature 2003;423:356–61.

72. Nakano K, Whitaker JW, Boyle DL, et al. DNA methylome signature in rheumatoid arthritis. Ann Rheum Dis 2013;72:110–7.

73. Tan YK, Ostergaard M, Conaghan PG. Imaging tools in rheumatoid arthritis: ultrasound vs magnetic resonance imaging. Rheumatology 2012;51(Suppl):vii36–42.

74. de Hair MJ, van de Sande MG, Ramwadhdoebe TH, et al. Features of the synovium of individuals at risk of developing rheumatoid arthritis: implications for understanding preclinical rheumatoid arthritis. Arthritis Rheum 2014;66:513–22.

75. Freeston JE, Wakefield RJ, Conaghan PG, et al. A diagnostic algorithm for persistence of very early inflammatory arthritis: the utility of power Doppler ultrasound when added to conventional assessment tools. Ann Rheum Dis 2010;69:417–9.

76. Karlson EW, Deane KD. Environmental and gene-environment interactions and risk of rheumatoid arthritis. Rheum Dis Clin North Am 2012;38:405–26.

77. James M, Proudman S, Cleland L. Fish oil and rheumatoid arthritis: past, present and future. Proc Nutr Soc 2010;69:316–23.

78. Bhatia SS, Majka DS, Kittelson JM, et al. Rheumatoid factor seropositivity is inversely associated with oral contraceptive use in women without arthritis. Ann Rheum Dis 2007;66:267–9.

79. Feser M, Derber LA, Deane KD, et al. Plasma 25,OH vitamin D levels are not associated with rheumatoid arthritis-related autoantibodies in individuals at elevated risk for rheumatoid arthritis. J Rheumatol 2009;36:943–6.

80. Gan RW, Deane KD, Zerbe GO, et al. Relationship between air pollution and positivity of RA-related autoantibodies in individuals without established RA: a report on SERA. Ann Rheum Dis 2013;72:2002–5.

81. Gabriel SE, Crowson CS, O'Fallon WM. Mortality in rheumatoid arthritis; have we made an impact in 4 decades. J Rheumatol 1999;26:2529–33.
82. Goldring SR. Periarticular bone changes in rheumatoid arthritis: pathophysiological implications and clinical utility. Ann Rheum Dis 2009;68:297–9.
83. Schett G, Gravallese EM. Bone erosion in rheumatoid arthritis: mechanisms, diagnosis and treatment. Nat Rev Rheumatol 2012;8:656–64.
84. Harre U, Georgess D, Bang H, et al. Induction of osteoclastogenesis and bone loss by human autoantibodies against citrullinated vimentin. J Clin Invest 2012; 122:1791–802.
85. Kleyer A, Finzel S, Rech J, et al. Bone loss before the clinical onset of rheumatoid arthritis in subjects with anticitrullinated protein antibodies. Ann Rheum Dis 2014;73:854–60.
86. Metafratzi ZM, Georgiadis AN, Ioannidou CV, et al. Pulmonary involvement in patients with early rheumatoid arthritis. Scand J Rheumatol 2007;38:338–44.
87. Demoruelle MK, Weisman MH, Simonian PL, et al. Airways abnormalities and rheumatoid arthritis-related autoantibodies in subjects without arthritis: early injury or initiating site of autoimmunity? Arthritis Rheum 2012;64:1756–61.
88. Smit MD, Westra J, Vissink A, et al. Periodontitis in established rheumatoid arthritis patients: a cross-sectional clinical, microbiological and serological study. Arthritis Res Ther 2012;14:R222.
89. Wegner N, Wait R, Sroka A, et al. Peptidylarginine deiminase from Porphyromonas gingivalis citrullinates human fibrinogen and a-enolase: implications for autoimmunity in rheumatoid arthritis. Arthritis Rheum 2010;62:2662–72.
90. Scher JU, Ubeda C, Equinda M, et al. Periodontal disease and the oral microbiota in new-onset rheumatoid arthritis. Arthritis Rheum 2012;64:3083–94.
91. Wu HJ, Ivanov I, Darce J, et al. Gut-residing segmented filamentous bacteria drive autoimmune arthritis via T helper 17 cells. Immunity 2010;32:815–27.
92. Vaahtovuo J, Munukka E, Korkeamaki M, et al. Fecal microbiota in early rheumatoid arthritis. J Rheumatol 2008;35:1500–5.
93. Scher JU, Sczesnak A, Longman RS, et al. Expansion of intestinal Prevotella copri correlates with enhanced susceptibility to arthritis. Elife (Cambridge) 2013;2: e01202. http://dx.doi.org/10.7554/eLife.01202.
94. Mikuls TR, Thiele GM, Deane KD, et al. Porphyromonas gingivalis and disease-related autoantibodies in individuals at increased risk of rheumatoid arthritis. Arthritis Rheum 2012;64:3522–30.
95. Young SP, Kapoor SR, Viant MR, et al. The impact of inflammation on metabolomic profiles in patients with arthritis. Arthritis Rheum 2013;65:2015–23.
96. Norris JM, Barriga K, Klingensmith G, et al. Timing of initial cereal exposure in infancy and risk of islet cell autoimmunity. JAMA 2003;290:1713–20.
97. Arend WP, Firestein GS. Pre-rheumatoid arthritis: predisposition and transition to clinical synovitis. Nat Rev Rheumatol 2012;8:573–6.
98. Klareskog L, Ronnelid J, Lundberg K, et al. Immunity to citrullinated proteins in rheumatoid arthritis. Annu Rev Immunol 2008;26:651–75.
99. Zhao X, Okeke NL, Sharpe O, et al. Circulating immune complexes contain citrullinated fibrinogen in rheumatoid arthritis. Arthritis Res Ther 2008;10: R94.
100. Sokolove J, Zhao X, Chandra PE, et al. Immune complexes containing citrullinated fibrinogen costimulate macrophages via Toll-like receptor 4 and Fc-gamma receptor. Arthritis Rheum 2011;63:53–62.
101. Kuhn KA, Kulik L, Tomooka B, et al. Antibodies to citrullinated proteins enhance tissue injury in experimental arthritis. J Clin Invest 2006;116:961–73.

102. Uysal H, Bockermann R, Nandakumar KS, et al. Structure and pathogenicity of antibodies specific for citrullinated collagen type II in experimental arthritis. J Exp Med 2009;206:449–62.

103. Cordova KN, Willis VC, Haskins K, et al. A citrullinated fibrinogen-specific T cell line enhances autoimmune arthritis in a mouse model of rheumatoid arthritis. J Immunol 2013;190:1457–65.

104. Ytterberg AJ, Reynisdottir G, Ossipova E, et al. Identification of shared citrullinated immunological targets in the lungs and joints of patients with rheumatoid arthritis. Ann Rheum Dis 2012;71:A19.

Preclinical Systemic Lupus Erythematosus

Julie M. Robertson, PhD[a], Judith A. James, MD, PhD[a,b,c,d],*

KEYWORDS

- SLE • Lupus • Autoantibodies • Preclinical autoimmunity • Incomplete lupus

KEY POINTS

- Autoantibodies are present and cytokine biomarkers are altered prior to systemic lupus erythematosus (SLE) diagnosis.
- Incomplete lupus erythematosus patients who transition to SLE classification often have mild SLE without major, life-threatening organ involvement.
- Undifferentiated connective tissue disease patients who have multiple autoreactivities, anti-nuclear antibody–homogeneous pattern, anti–double-stranded DNA, anti-samarium, and anti-cardiolipin responses are at higher risk for transitioning to SLE.
- New classification schemes are needed to adequately capture all phases of SLE.
- New preclinical lupus studies are warranted to elucidate mechanisms of disease progression without the confines of advance organ or tissue damage and immunosuppressive medication.

Conflict of Interest: The authors declare no conflict of interest.
This work was supported by the National Institute of Allergy and Infectious Diseases under award number U01AI101934, the National Institute of Allergy and Infectious Diseases and the Office of Research on Women's Health under award number U19AI082714, the National Institute of General Medical Sciences under award number P30GM103510, and the National Institute of Arthritis and Musculoskeletal and Skin Diseases under award number P30AR053483. The content of this article is the sole responsibility of the authors and does not necessarily represent the official views of the National Institutes of Health.

[a] Arthritis and Clinical Immunology Research Program, Oklahoma Medical Research Foundation, 825 Northeast 13th Street, Oklahoma City, OK 73104, USA; [b] Department of Medicine, University of Oklahoma Health Sciences Center, 1200 N. Phillips Avenue, Oklahoma City, OK 73104, USA; [c] Department of Pathology, University of Oklahoma Health Sciences Center, 1200 N. Phillips Avenue, Oklahoma City, OK 73104, USA; [d] Oklahoma Clinical and Translational Science Institute, University of Oklahoma Health Sciences Center, 1000 N. Lincoln Boulevard, Suite 2100, Oklahoma City, OK 73104, USA
* Corresponding author. Arthritis and Clinical Immunology Research Program, Oklahoma Medical Research Foundation, 825 Northeast 13th Street, Oklahoma City, OK 73104.
E-mail address: Judith-James@omrf.org

Rheum Dis Clin N Am 40 (2014) 621–635
http://dx.doi.org/10.1016/j.rdc.2014.07.004
0889-857X/14/$ – see front matter © 2014 Elsevier Inc. All rights reserved.

INTRODUCTION

Systemic lupus erythematosus (SLE) is a prototypical autoimmune disease featuring multiple organ system involvement and the presence of autoantibodies. The numerous variations of clinical symptom presentation often make diagnosis difficult. The current American College of Rheumatology (ACR) criteria for the classification (not diagnosis) of SLE requires that patients meet a minimum of 4 out of 11 defined clinical and/or serologic criteria.[1,2] In 2012, the Systemic Lupus International Collaborating Clinics (SLICC) group developed and proposed new classification criteria, which require at least one clinical and one serologic criterion to be met and allows disease classification based on the presence of 4 out of 17 criteria (**Fig. 1**).[3] However, clinical diagnosis of SLE is a distinct challenge from that of its classification for clinical studies and trials. Because SLE is a heterogeneous disorder, some individuals present with clinical symptoms of SLE but do not meet disease classification criteria. Due to the variety of possible clinical symptoms, individuals can wait years for a diagnosis while ongoing inflammatory processes cause irreversible organ damage.

Preclinical lupus thus encompasses a broad range of individuals, from individuals with enhanced genetic risk for SLE development without current clinical symptoms to individuals with autoantibodies and some clinical features of SLE that do not meet ACR disease classification criteria.[4] This period before SLE disease classification has, over the years, been categorized as latent lupus[5] or incomplete lupus.[6] Latent lupus identifies a group of individuals with features consistent with SLE that

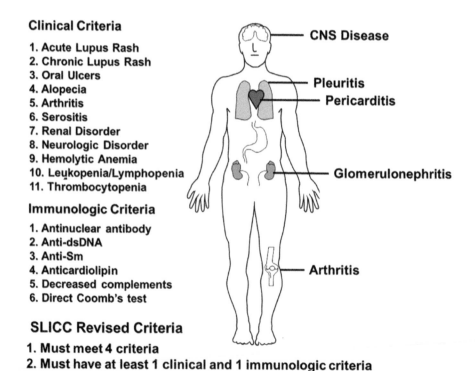

Clinical Criteria

1. Acute Lupus Rash
2. Chronic Lupus Rash
3. Oral Ulcers
4. Alopecia
5. Arthritis
6. Serositis
7. Renal Disorder
8. Neurologic Disorder
9. Hemolytic Anemia
10. Leukopenia/Lymphopenia
11. Thrombocytopenia

Immunologic Criteria

1. Antinuclear antibody
2. Anti-dsDNA
3. Anti-Sm
4. Anticardiolipin
5. Decreased complements
6. Direct Coomb's test

SLICC Revised Criteria

1. **Must meet 4 criteria**
2. **Must have at least 1 clinical and 1 immunologic criteria**
   OR Biopsy-proven lupus nephritis with anti-dsDNA or ANA

CNS Disease

Pleuritis
Pericarditis

Glomerulonephritis

Arthritis

Fig. 1. Systemic Lupus International Collaborating Clinics (SLICC) proposed new SLE classification criteria.

meet one or two of the ACR 1971 or 1982 classification criteria along with the presence of minor criteria such as fever, fatigue, low complement, or lymphadenopathy.[5] Incomplete lupus (ILE) refers to individuals with fewer than four of the ACR SLE classification criteria.[6] Additionally, undifferentiated connective tissue disease (UCTD) is a broader term referring to clinical symptom manifestations suggestive of a specific connective tissue disease without meeting disease classification criteria.[7] The UCTD group does contain a subset of individuals who may transition to SLE. This article examines preclinical lupus during the time before SLE classification, with particular attention to the time between serologic or cellular evidence of autoimmunity and SLE diagnosis (**Fig. 2**; see Refs.[5–10] for more information). Additionally, studies are discussed which examine individuals who transition to SLE from UCTD from ILE or from previously healthy mothers of neonatal lupus or congenital heart block children.

Significance of Autoantibodies in Preclinical Systemic Lupus Erythematosus

Autoantibodies are a hallmark SLE characteristic. Despite the variability of clinical symptoms, almost all newly diagnosed lupus patients have detectable autoantibodies. Through a partnership with US military rheumatologists and the US Department of Defense Serum Repository (DoDSR), a large sample repository comprised of longitudinal blood samples and basic laboratory evaluations were obtained on entry into the military and throughout military service. These samples span the time before clinical disease to at or after SLE diagnosis and provide a unique resource to examine serologic features of preclinical SLE. Using serial serum samples (n = 633) from 130 subjects who subsequently developed SLE while in the US military, 115 (88%) of the SLE subjects were found to have at least one autoantibody present in a prediagnosis serum sample. In some cases, this initial autoantibody was present up to 9.4 years

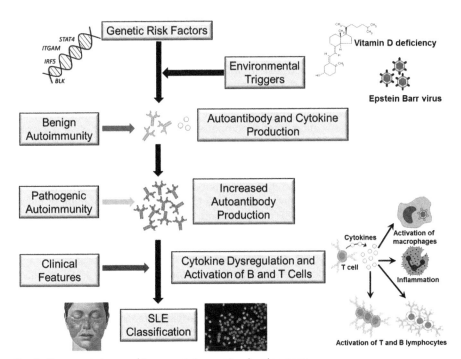

Fig. 2. Proposed stages of lupus autoimmunity development.

(mean 3.3 years) before SLE classification. Anti-phospholipid, anti-Ro, anti-La, and anti-nuclear antibodies (ANAs) were present significantly earlier (mean = 3.2 years) than anti-Sm and anti–nuclear ribonucleoprotein (anti-nRNP) antibodies (1.2 years) (P = .005). Anti–double stranded DNA (anti-dsDNA) antibodies appeared, on average, 2.2 years before diagnosis, whereas anti-ribosomal P and anti-C1q antibodies were detectable, on average, 1.1 and 1.4 years before classification, respectively.[11,12] Of the subjects who had at least two positive samples, one within 6 months of clinical SLE diagnosis and the second more than 6 months before diagnosis (N = 26), 73% (n = 19) had increases in their anti-dsDNA antibody levels as they moved toward diagnosis (mean = 227 units; SEM = 37 units vs mean = 743 units, SEM = 212 units, P = .018).[13] As such, autoantibodies are routinely observed to be present before SLE classification and display an increase in antibody specificity number and levels leading up to diagnosis.

Using a multiplexed, bead-based method to test for the presence of autoantibodies directed against the specific protein antigens 60kd Ro, 52kD Ro, La, Sm/nRNP, nRNP, nRNP 70K, nRNP A, histones, dsDNA, and ribosomal P, 33 of 114 subjects (25%) initially had a single, detectable autoantibody specificity and the others had multiple specificities in their first autoantibody-positive sample before SLE diagnosis.[14] The most common initial antibody recognized was anti-60kD Ro; anti-nRNP A, anti-dsDNA, and anti-La antibodies were the next most common single, initial autoantibodies.[12] Protein targets within linked autoantibody subsets were commonly targeted first, such as nRNP A before or with nRNP 70K or 60kD Ro before or with 52kd Ro. Other protein targets occurred with almost equal frequency, commonly simultaneous or closer together than could be assessed with DoDSR samples. Understanding these early autoantibody responses may provide keys to understanding the targets and mechanisms of initial breaks in tolerance in SLE that can, in turn, be developed into robust early diagnostic markers or tolerogens of early disease.

Some patients with antiphospholipid antibody syndrome subsequently develop clinical SLE.[15–17] Sera from the DoDSR were used to evaluate the temporal relationship between anti-phospholipid (aPL) antibodies and clinical SLE classification.[18] A total of 24 cases (18.5%) were positive for IgG and/or IgM aPL antibodies before SLE. Anti-cardiolipin (aCL) appeared, on average, 3.0 years before SLE classification. In addition, the presence of aCL before clinical classification was associated with a broader disease presentation. These subjects eventually met an average of 6.1 (of the 11) 1997 SLE classification criteria, compared with 4.9 criteria for other subjects (P<.001). The early aCL-positive population also had more frequent renal disease, central nervous system (CNS) disease, thrombocytopenia, and clotting events. In this population, aCL preceded initial thrombotic events by a mean of 3.1 years.[18]

Several studies have indicated that autoantibody specificities are associated with disease manifestations of SLE and may be able to predict the development of these clinical features. Within the DoDSR military cohort, one of the most common early clinical symptoms of SLE was arthritis. Stored samples from SLE subjects were analyzed for IgG rheumatoid factor (RF) to determine whether RF preceded arthritis onset. Of the 130 subjects in the DoDSR, 17 (13%) were found to have RF, present on average 2.1 years before the first documented arthritis symptom and 16 of the 17 RF-positive subjects eventually developed inflammatory arthritis. Anti-dsDNA responses have been associated with the presence of renal disease. Of the 80 subjects with anti-dsDNA positive samples, 38 (48%) developed ACR-defined renal disease with 35 having detectable antibodies against dsDNA before or concurrently with renal disease onset.[12] These data further support the associations between select lupus-specific autoantibodies and specific disease symptoms; however, how the concentration, specificity, and affinity of these autoantibodies change during the preclinical period is unknown. Taken together, these studies show that autoantibodies are detected years before SLE disease diagnosis.[4,11–13,18]

Serologic Markers Observed in a Swedish Systemic Lupus Erythematosus Cohort Before Diagnosis

Serologic biomarkers were examined in a Swedish retrospective cohort similar to the DoDSR. Both retrospective cohorts have samples before and at SLE diagnosis and have had extensive characterization along with medical record abstraction. However, the Swedish cohort contains only one sample collected before SLE diagnosis, whereas the DoDSR has, on average, 3.6 samples collected and studied before disease classification. Additionally, the Swedish cohort has 19 individuals enrolled from a pregnancy cohort and contains a mixture of serum and plasma samples that cannot be directly compared with each other for other serologic biomarkers, such as cytokines and chemokines. In contrast, the DoDSR only contains serum samples and has no pregnant individuals enrolled in the cohort.

SLE subjects seen at the Department of Rheumatology at the University Hospital in Umeå, Sweden were enrolled, examined, and donated a blood sample.[19] Thirty-eight of these individuals were found to have donated a sample before SLE disease classification. Despite the lack of numerous predisease samples, the Swedish cohort is still a rich source of preclinical SLE information. In the Eriksson[19] 2011 article, ANAs were detected in 63% of individuals who later transitioned to SLE, on average, 5.6 ± 4.7 years before onset of clinical symptoms. Anti-Ro antibodies were observed first 6.6 ± 2.5 years before clinical symptom presentation and 8.1 ± 2.3 years before SLE classification. Anti-RNP and anti-histone antibodies were also observed early at 5.9 ± 2.5 and 5.0 ± 1.5 years before clinical symptoms. Anti-Sm and anti-centromere antibodies were observed closer to disease classification at 1.4 ± 0.6 years before SLE classification.[19] The number of autoantibodies in preclinical SLE individuals increased after first clinical symptom from 1.4 to 3.1 ($P<.0005$). Similar to what was seen in the DoDSR cohort, autoantibodies were also associated with specific disease manifestations. For example, in preclinical individuals with serositis, the average number of autoantibodies was higher than individuals presenting with arthritis and skin manifestations (2.5 autoantibodies and 1.7 autoantibodies for arthritis, and 0.9 autoantibodies for skin manifestations of SLE).[19] Additionally, the autoantibodies observed in individuals with serositis appeared closer to diagnosis (1.9 years before diagnosis) than in individuals with arthritis (6.7 years before diagnosis) or skin manifestations (4.2 years before diagnosis).[19]

In another study by Eriksson and Rantapaa-Dahlqvist,[20] samples from the Swedish subject group were examined for alterations in cytokines and chemokines between predisease samples and samples collected following SLE diagnosis. Here, samples from 35 SLE subjects and 140 healthy controls were examined for chemokines and cytokines and their relationship to previously detected autoantibodies.[20] Increased levels of interferon gamma-induced protein (IP-10) were observed more frequently in predisease time points than in the healthy controls ($P = .02$). Concentrations of IFN-α (interferon-α) and IP-10 were significantly higher among autoantibody positive samples than autoantibody negative prediagnosis samples or controls. Specifically, IP-10 levels were increased in individuals positive for ANA, anti-Ro, and anti-Jo-1. IFN-α levels were increased in individuals positive for anti-La responses. IL-10 levels were higher in anti-RNP positive individuals. On the other hand, monocyte chemotactic protein 1 (MCP-1) levels were significantly decreased in anti-Ro and anti-La–positive individuals compared with samples from anti-Ro and anti-La–negative individuals and controls.[20] This study shows that, like autoantibodies, cytokines and chemokines are altered before SLE diagnosis.

Although this study provides valuable information on the alterations of cytokines before SLE diagnosis, it does have limitations. Half of the samples used for cytokine analysis were plasma whereas the samples obtained through the maternity cohort were sera. These two sample types are difficult to directly compare because biomarkers in serum often have a shorter half-life than the same biomarkers in plasma. Additionally, many studies have shown that during pregnancy the immune system of the mother is altered[21–30]; therefore, the cytokine alterations observed could be influenced by the pregnancy itself rather than the preclinical features of SLE. Further studies are required to elucidate alterations in soluble mediators during preclinical phases of SLE.

Although there is a lack of studies examining autoantibody and cytokine or chemokine biomarkers in preclinical periods of SLE, these studies suggest that altered biomarkers may also be critical during preclinical periods of SLE as well as in otherwise healthy ANA-positive individuals. Larger studies of ethnically diverse lupus subjects are needed to confirm and expand these initial findings and to elucidate the mechanisms responsible for the altered serologic biomarkers.

Transition from Incomplete to Classified Systemic Lupus Erythematosus

Incomplete lupus erythematosus (ILE) refers to individuals with clinical symptoms that indicate SLE but who have fewer than four 1997 ACR classification criteria. Several studies have followed groups of ILE subjects to evaluate and identify predictors of transition to SLE and to further elucidate preclinical features of SLE. In a 1989 paper, 38 ILE subjects (defined as meeting up to three ACR SLE classification criteria) were followed for an average of 1.6 years with only two individuals transitioning to SLE.[6] The Dallas Regional Autoimmune Disease Registry (DRADR) enrolls autoimmune disease subjects, first-degree relatives of autoimmune disease subjects, and healthy controls. In this retrospective study cohort, 15 individuals out of 124 were classified as ILE and 99 out of 124 were classified as SLE.[31] The ILE subjects were shown to have a significantly lower mean damage score than SLE subjects (0.67 ± 0.32 vs 1.67 ± 0.17; $P = .036$) and a significantly shorter disease duration (4.33 ± 0.94 years vs 10.24 ± 0.75 years; $P = .003$).[31] In another US-based study from the DRADR following 22 ILE subjects (<4 ACR criteria) for an average of 2.4 years, 14% (n = 3) transitioned to SLE classification.[32] All subjects who transitioned were female, of younger age, and showed increases in IgG autoreactivity. These transition individuals were more likely to have autoantibodies against proliferating cell nuclear antigen, β2-microglobulin, C1q, and hemocyanin at baseline compared with those who remained ILE. A quantitative risk score was generated to identify individuals who would transition to SLE. This risk score, comprised of female gender, baseline ANA ELISA greater than 200 units, baseline age less than 40, increase in overall IgG autoreactivity on an autoantigen array, and presence of IgG responses against seven baseline autoantigens, showed strong differentiation between ILE subjects who transitioned to SLE classification compared with those who remained ILE ($P = 1.38 \times 10^7$).[32]

In another study using SLE subjects (n = 73), ILE subjects (n = 43), unaffected first-degree relatives (n = 32), and healthy controls (n = 28) from the DRADR, ILE and SLE subjects had similar mean ANA levels ($P>.05$) that were significantly higher than first degree relatives ($P<.001$) and healthy controls ($P\leq.5$).[33] In examining differences in autoantibody response to autoantigens between ILE and SLE subjects, elevated levels of at least one IgG autoantibody were detected in 19% of ILE subjects compared with

26% of SLE. Additionally, the IgG to IgM autoantibody ratios showed a stepwise increase from healthy controls to ILE to SLE in this study.[34]

A study from Puerto Rico followed 87 subjects who met at least one ACR clinical SLE criterion for a mean of 2.2 years. Eight individuals transitioned to SLE in the follow-up period. Those subjects who evolved to SLE were more likely to have photosensitivity, malar rash, oral ulcerations, anti-dsDNA responses, and low levels of C3.[35] A collaborative study of 122 subjects with ILE (diagnosed less than 1 year) followed 100 subjects who did not transition to SLE for at least 3 years. These long-term ILE individuals had common baseline clinical symptoms of leukopenia, fatigue, arthritis, and mucocutaneous involvement.[36] In a Swedish study with 28 ILE subjects (<4 ACR criteria) followed an average of 5.3 years, malar rash, aCL, and thrombocytopenia were enriched in the 16 individuals who transitioned to SLE classification.[37]

When examining a small group of SLE subjects (n = 27), ILE subjects (n = 24), unaffected first-degree relatives (n = 22) and unaffected, unrelated healthy controls (n = 11), Li and colleagues[38] examined differences in interferon genes. A set of 63 interferon genes were upregulated in 83% of SLE subjects but only in 50% of ILE subjects, compared with no interferon-high individuals in the two control groups. Interferon-high status was shown to be associated with IgG autoantibody responses primarily targeted against DNA or RNA-binding proteins in both SLE subjects and ILE subjects. Additional longitudinal evaluation of ILE subjects, both in the interferon-high and interferon-low groups, are necessary to see if ILE patients with elevated interferon signatures are at higher risk of transition to SLE.

In the above studies, the ILE individuals who transitioned to SLE classification had relatively mild SLE without major organ involvement (**Table 1**). In total, approximately 10% of ILE patients will transition to SLE, often with a disease course that lacks nephritis, vasculitis, or major CNS involvement. As ILE may describe the time period with some SLE symptoms leading up to SLE diagnosis, many SLE patients may have a period of ILE; however, only individuals who do not transition to or have delayed transition to SLE are typically identified as having ILE. Further studies are needed to assess whether ILE is a different disease or a milder form of SLE, as well as to decipher mechanisms by which only approximately 10% of ILE patients may transition to SLE.

Transition from Undifferentiated Connective Tissue Disease to Systemic Lupus Erythematosus

Individuals with UCTD demonstrate clinical symptoms that indicate autoimmune connective tissue disease such as SLE, Sjögren syndrome (SS), or rheumatoid arthritis; however, these individuals do not meet clinical classification criteria. Although up to one-third of individuals with UCTD transition to a disease diagnosis,[39,40] the remaining individuals do not. Studies investigating clinical and serologic features of UCTD have begun to provide knowledge on preclinical features of disease.

A 1991 multi-institutional cohort study of 213 US-based early UCTD subjects (within 1 year of identification) investigated factors that were predictive of SLE onset. After 5 years of follow-up, 8.5% of the cohort (n = 18) transitioned to SLE.[41] A univariate analysis indicated that individuals more likely to transition to SLE were younger and African-American. The transition individuals also displayed alopecia, serositis, discoid lesions, anti-dsDNA, anti-Sm, positive ANA with a homogeneous pattern, Coombs positivity, or a false-positive syphilis test. After regression modeling, discoid lesions, serositis, anti-Sm (by precipitin), or ANA-homogenous patterns remained the best predictors of transition to SLE in these UCTD subjects.[41]

In a study from Italy, 84 subjects with early UCTD (symptoms onset within the past year) were followed for 5 years.[42] Baseline characteristics of these individuals included

Table 1
Summary table of studies with subjects who transitioned to systemic lupus erythematosus from incomplete lupus erythematosus

Reference, Year	Subject Population	Transitions to SLE	Predictors of Transition	Follow-up
Ganczarczyk et al,[5] 1989	Latent lupus (1–2 ARA criteria, 71 or 82), additional minor criteria	7 of 22 (31.8%)	No predictors	8 y (5–15 y)
Greer & Panush,[6] 1989	ILE	2 of 38 (5.3%)	No predictors	1.6 y
Vila et al,[35] 2000	ILE	8 of 87 (9.2%)	Photosensitivity, malar rash, oral ulcers, low C3 levels, and anti-dsDNA	2.2 y
Ståhl Hallengren et al,[37] 2004	ILE (positive ANA and at least one 1 ACR clinical criterion)	16 of 28 (57.1%)	Malar rash and anticardiolipin	5.3 y (1–10 y)
Laustrup et al,[58] 2010	ILE	7 of 26 (26.9%)	Mild disease, absence of renal and CNS involvement	8 y (1–8 y)
Olsen et al,[32] 2012	ILE	3 of 22 (14%)	Female, young age, increased levels of IgG, antibodies against β2 microglobulin, C1q, and hemocyanin	2.4 y

Raynaud (54%), arthralgia (51%), arthritis (23%), fever (23%), and weakness (16%). Thirty-three subjects (39%) developed a defined CTD, including seven subjects with SLE (8.3% of the cohort). Univariate analysis showed anti-dsDNA, aCL, and fever correlating with subsequent SLE disease classification. aCL responses were not significant in the multivariate analysis.[42] Another study of UCTD subjects (at least one clinical feature and autoantibody positive) were reported on 1 year[43] and 5 years[44] of follow-up. After 5 years, 18 of these subjects had transitioned to SLE (22%). The presence of aCL responses and multiple autoantibody specificities were associated with subsequent SLE classification. In another study from Milano, Italy, 148 subjects with UCTD were retrospectively evaluated. Of these, 36 developed a well-defined CTD after, on average, 4.5 years of follow-up. Anti-dsDNA responses were found to predict the evolution from UCTD to SLE classification.[45]

A large group of UCTD subjects (n = 665) were followed in Hungary between 1994 and 1999.[46] Of these 665 individuals, 230 developed a defined CTD, including 28 with SLE. Fever, serositis, photosensitivity, ANA homogenous pattern, and dsDNA antibodies were associated with the development of SLE. SLE subjects with a documented UCTD period were more likely to be older, have more serositis, less skin rash, less renal involvement, and less hemolytic anemia compared with SLE subjects without a documented UCTD period.[46] In a study from Portugal, 74 out of the 184 UCTD subjects presented with a lupus-like disease (based on clinical features and autoantibody profiles)[47]; however, longer-term follow-up of these individuals are not readily available. Nonetheless, in this cohort, arthralgia and arthritis were the most common symptoms, with 40% of the study participants showing lupus-like symptoms with a higher frequency of arthritis, cytopenia, oral ulcers, and dsDNA antibodies compared with other UCTD individuals in the cohort.[47] The presence of anti-dsDNA antibodies in the UCTD individuals with lupus-like disease was associated with decreased levels of C3 and C4, whereas aCL was associated with thrombocytopenia.[47] Finally, a study from the Netherlands followed 65 ANA-positive individuals (excluding anti-dsDNA antibody–positive individuals) referred for rheumatology evaluation. Of these 65 individuals, a specific rheumatic disease diagnosis could be established in 38 within the 2 years of follow-up, including six who transitioned to SLE after a median of 2.2 years.[48]

Several studies have examined cellular and serologic differences in individuals with UCTD in hopes of further identifying UCTD individuals who transition to a defined connective tissue disease. In examining the cellular differences between UCTD individuals who do and do not transition to defined disease along with healthy controls, individuals with UCTD have elevated numbers and percentages of activated T cells, memory T cells, and natural killer T cells compared with healthy, unaffected controls.[49] In UCTD individuals who transition to defined disease, the percentages of CD4+ IFN-γ+ T-helper 1 cells here higher than controls and UCTD individuals who do not transition to disease. Additionally, the percentage and number of CD4+ CD25+ Foxp3+ natural regulatory T cells were diminished in UCTD individuals compared with healthy controls.[49] When vitamin D levels were examined in a collection of 161 UCTD individuals, so UCTD subjects demonstrated significantly lower levels of vitamin D in both summer and winter compared with controls ($P = .01$ and $P = .0001$, respectively). Clinical symptoms of photosensitivity, erythema, and discoid rash were associated with low vitamin D levels in the UCTD subjects. Additionally, autoantibodies against RNP, Ro, and CCP were associated with low vitamin D levels in UCTD subjects.[50] Importantly, Zold and colleagues[50] showed that the UCTD subjects with the lowest vitamin D levels were the ones who tended to transition to a defined connective tissue disease and that low vitamin D levels in UCTD subjects impaired regulatory T-cell homeostasis.[51]

Although most UCTD patients remain within the UCTD category, preclinical lupus information can be gleaned from the cumulative transition across these studies of 93 individuals to SLE diagnosis. UCTD individuals with multiple autoreactivities, ANA-homogeneous pattern, dsDNA antibodies, Sm antibodies, and aCL responses are at higher risk for transitioning to SLE, as are individuals with multiple lupus-like clinical features (**Table 2**). Patients who remain in the UCTD group tend to have a mild clinical picture with little to no major organ involvement, arthralgia, arthritis, Raynaud phenomenon, and leucopenia.[40,52] See Refs.[40,53,54] for more detailed information.

Transition of Neonatal Lupus Erythematosus or Congenital Heart Block Patient Mothers to Systemic Lupus Erythematosus

The Research Registry for Neonatal Lupus was created to help study the disease evolution of the mothers of and the neonates with neonatal lupus erythematosus (NLE). This rich resource, started in 1994, collects diagnostic information on enrolled mothers and their children affected with congenital heart block or NLE. Importantly, in terms of evolution of SLE, a study using this resource examined rheumatic disease progression in mothers of neonates with NLE; 387 NLE children and 321 anti-Ro antibody positive mothers were assessed.[55] Among the mothers of neonates with NLE, 51 were

Table 2
Summary table of studies with subjects who transitioned to systemic lupus erythematosus from undifferentiated connective tissue disease

Reference, Year	Subject Population	Transitions to SLE	Predictors of Transition	Follow-up
Calvo-Alen et al,[41] 1996	Started with 213 eUCTD (symptoms <1 y); complete 5 y data on 143	18 of 143 (12.6%)	Predictors: discoid lupus, serositis, ANA homogeneous, and anti-Sm by precipitation	5 y (1–5 y)
Danieli et al,[42] 1998	eUCTD, 84 subjects	7 of 33 (21.2%)	Fever and anti-DNA antibodies	5 y (1–5 y)
Mosca et al,[43] 1998	UCTD (1 autoantibody and 1 clinical feature)	12 of 91 (13.2%)	Multiple autoantibodies; less sicca Raynaud and photosensitivity	3 y (1–8 y)
Belfiore et al,[59] 2000	UCTD	5 of 57 (8.77%)	Anti-60kD alone associated with transition	5 y (1–23 y)
Cavazzana et al,[45] 2001	UCTD (retrospective study)	45 of 148 (30.4%)	Anti-dsDNA antibodies	5 y (1–9 y)
Bodolay et al,[46] 2003	UCTD	28 of 665 (4.2%)	Fever, serositis, photosensitivity, ANA homogenous pattern, anti-dsDNA antibodies	5 y

Abbreviation: eUCTD, early undifferentiated connective tissue disease.

asymptomatic (no clinical symptoms of rheumatic disease), 20 pauci–undifferentiated autoimmune syndrome (UAS; with up to two of arthralgias, oral or nasal ulcers, photosensitivity, lymphopenia, Raynaud phenomenon, dry eyes or dry mouth, or parotid enlargement), 12 poly-UAS (present with more than two of the pauci-UAS symptoms), 12 probable SS (at least two of dry eyes, dry mouth, or parotid enlargement), 6 SS (met the revised European classification of SS), 10 SLE (met four or more ACR SLE classification criteria), and 11 with SLE and SS. In mothers that were asymptomatic at enrollment (n = 51), 49% remained asymptomatic up to a mean 4.1 years of follow-up. Thus, the presence of NLE in the neonate does not directly associate with the development of SLE in the mothers.[55] Additionally, mothers with only anti-Ro antibodies were more likely to remain asymptomatic, whereas mothers with both anti-Ro and anti-La antibodies were 1.8 times more likely to develop a rheumatic disease.[55]

Future Considerations

Preclinical lupus is a broad concept that seeks to categorize a wide range of individuals, including those with increased genetic risk of developing SLE but no clinical symptoms or positive standard lupus serology tests as well as individuals with autoantibodies and clinical features consistent with SLE who do not meet the current ACR SLE classification criteria. In addition, there is some debate over what time frame preclinical lupus encompasses. Some investigators argue that preclinical lupus should focus on the period between evidence of immune dysregulation to before the first clinical feature in an individual who eventually will be diagnosed with SLE. On the other hand, others have identified the preclinical SLE phase as the entire clinically asymptomatic period leading up to SLE classification. Due to the variation between these two definitions, several terms have been proposed to describe this preclinical period, including latent lupus,[5] incomplete lupus,[6] and lupus-like or probable lupus.[56] Additionally, the broader term of UCTD, which identifies individuals with clinical symptoms suggestive of a connective tissue disease, has also been used to identify preclinical SLE patients. However, UCTD also encompasses individuals who develop non-SLE connective tissue disease such as SS or systemic sclerosis. Clearly more studies are needed to better classify individuals with preclinical lupus. These studies can be used to create a consensus on preclinical lupus terminology as well as to help understand and investigate early SLE natural history.

Studying preclinical lupus may also lead to several potential benefits. **Box 1** provides a partial list. Individuals in the preclinical phase of disease are often not on immunosuppressive medications. This allows a clearer picture of early disease events without the confounding effects of medications, irreversible or severe organ damage, or ongoing aggressive inflammation. In addition, studying subjects during preclinical or early clinical stages can identify individuals at increased risk for full SLE development or for severe SLE complications that can lead to the potential of early intervention. These studies can also lead to improved understandings of specific etiologic factors of SLE, such as environmental or epigenetic triggers of disease development, as well as the earliest events in lupus autoimmunity, allowing for improved diagnostic tools, identification of biomarkers of early disease activity, and elucidating novel pathways for therapeutic development.

Early identification of individuals at high-risk for development of clinically apparent disease or who have early mild clinical disease will allow for closer monitoring and early treatment to reduce or inhibit major organ involvement in SLE. Early intervention would also allow for the modulation of the dysregulated immune and inflammatory responses, thus reducing morbidity and early mortality. Therefore, the preclinical study of SLE along with additional longitudinal cohorts is poised to develop prospective studies to assess immune parameters and other serologic responses of disease onset and to understand mechanisms of disease to drive directed therapeutic development and create potential prevention trials. A retrospective analysis of individuals in the DoDSR suggested that early intervention with hydroxychloroquine (HCQ) and/or prednisone may delay disease onset and slow accrual of autoantibody specificities.[57] In this study, individuals treated with HCQ before diagnosis had a longer time between the onset of the first clinical symptom and SLE classification than matched, HCQ-untreated SLE subjects (median times of 1.08 vs 0.29 years, respectively; $P = .018$). Subjects treated with prednisone before SLE classification progressed more slowly

---

Box 1
Reasons for studying preclinical systemic lupus erythematosus

1. Understand disease pathogenesis without confounding effects of concurrent medication or extensive, irreversible disease damage

2. Identify at-risk individuals to allow for close monitoring and implementation early interventions to delay disease progression and damage

3. Characterize biomarkers of early disease for the development of early screening tests and improved diagnostic tools

4. Create prevention studies to assess effectiveness of preventative treatment in high-risk individuals

to ACR classification criteria than matched prednisone-untreated SLE subjects (P = .011). Additionally, individuals receiving both HCQ and prednisone (n = 13) had a significantly longer time between initial clinical symptoms and SLE classification than individuals treated with only prednisone (n = 14) before diagnosis (P = .03). Importantly, subjects treated with HCQ had a lower rate of autoantibody accumulation and decreased numbers of autoantibody specificities at and after SLE diagnosis.[57] These findings indicate that preventative treatment in individuals at increased risk of SLE development may be beneficial and a preclinical study of HCQ in high-risk individuals for subsequent disease development is warranted.

REFERENCES

1. Tan EM, Cohen AS, Fries JF, et al. The 1982 revised criteria for the classification of systemic lupus erythematosus. Arthritis Rheum 1982;25(11):1271–7.
2. Hochberg MC. Updating the American College of Rheumatology revised criteria for the classification of systemic lupus erythematosus. Arthritis Rheum 1997; 40(9):1725.
3. Petri M, Orbai AM, Alarcon GS, et al. Derivation and validation of the Systemic Lupus International Collaborating Clinics classification criteria for systemic lupus erythematosus. Arthritis Rheum 2012;64(8):2677–86.
4. Deane KD, El-Gabalawy H. Pathogenesis and prevention of rheumatic disease: focus on preclinical RA and SLE. Nat Rev Rheumatol 2014;10(4):212–28.
5. Ganczarczyk L, Urowitz MB, Gladman DD. Latent lupus. J Rheumatol 1989; 16(4):475–8.
6. Greer JM, Panush RS. Incomplete lupus erythematosus. Arch Intern Med 1989; 149(11):2473–6.
7. Alarcon GS, Williams GV, Singer JZ, et al. Early undifferentiated connective tissue disease. I. Early clinical manifestation in a large cohort of patients with undifferentiated connective tissue diseases compared with cohorts of well established connective tissue disease. J Rheumatol 1991;18(9):1332–9.
8. Cooper GS. Unraveling the etiology of systemic autoimmune diseases: peering into the preclinical phase of disease. J Rheumatol 2009;36(9):1853–5.
9. Klareskog L, Gregersen PK, Huizinga TW. Prevention of autoimmune rheumatic disease: state of the art and future perspectives. Ann Rheum Dis 2010;69(12):2062–6.
10. Doria A, Zen M, Canova M, et al. SLE diagnosis and treatment: when early is early. Autoimmun Rev 2010;10(1):55–60.
11. Heinlen LD, Ritterhouse LL, McClain MT, et al. Ribosomal P autoantibodies are present before SLE onset and are directed against non-C-terminal peptides. J Mol Med (Berl) 2010;88(7):719–27.
12. Heinlen LD, McClain MT, Merrill J, et al. Clinical criteria for systemic lupus erythematosus precede diagnosis, and associated autoantibodies are present before clinical symptoms. Arthritis Rheum 2007;56(7):2344–51.
13. Arbuckle MR, James JA, Kohlhase KF, et al. Development of anti-dsDNA autoantibodies before clinical diagnosis of systemic lupus erythematosus. Scand J Immunol 2001;54(1–2):211–9.
14. Bruner BF, Guthridge JM, Lu R, et al. Comparison of autoantibody specificities between traditional and bead-based assays in a large, diverse collection of patients with systemic lupus erythematosus and family members. Arthritis Rheum 2012;64(11):3677–86.
15. Andrews PA, Frampton G, Cameron JS. Antiphospholipid syndrome and systemic lupus erythematosus. Lancet 1993;342(8877):988–9.

16. Derksen RH, Gmelig-Meijling FH, de Groot PG. Primary antiphospholipid syndrome evolving into systemic lupus erythematosus. Lupus 1996;5(1):77–80.

17. Mujic F, Cuadrado MJ, Lloyd M, et al. Primary antiphospholipid syndrome evolving into systemic lupus erythematosus. J Rheumatol 1995;22(8):1589–92.

18. McClain MT, Arbuckle MR, Heinlen LD, et al. The prevalence, onset, and clinical significance of antiphospholipid antibodies before diagnosis of systemic lupus erythematosus. Arthritis Rheum 2004;50(4):1226–32.

19. Eriksson C, Kokkonen H, Johansson M, et al. Autoantibodies predate the onset of systemic lupus erythematosus in northern Sweden. Arthritis Res Ther 2011; 13(1):R30.

20. Eriksson C, Rantapaa-Dahlqvist S. Cytokines in relation to autoantibodies before onset of symptoms for systemic lupus erythematosus. Lupus 2014. [Epub ahead of print].

21. Aluvihare VR, Kallikourdis M, Betz AG. Regulatory T cells mediate maternal tolerance to the fetus. Nat Immunol 2004;5(3):266–71.

22. Davis D, Kaufmann R, Moticka EJ. Nonspecific immunity in pregnancy: monocyte surface Fcgamma receptor expression and function. J Reprod Immunol 1998;40(2):119–28.

23. Faas MM, Donker RB, van Pampus MG, et al. Plasma of pregnant and preeclamptic women activates monocytes in vitro. Am J Obstet Gynecol 2008; 199(1):84.e1–8.

24. Luppi P, Haluszczak C, Betters D, et al. Monocytes are progressively activated in the circulation of pregnant women. J Leukoc Biol 2002;72(5):874–84.

25. Luppi P, Haluszczak C, Trucco M, et al. Normal pregnancy is associated with peripheral leukocyte activation. Am J Reprod Immunol 2002;47(2):72–81.

26. Naccasha N, Gervasi MT, Chaiworapongsa T, et al. Phenotypic and metabolic characteristics of monocytes and granulocytes in normal pregnancy and maternal infection. Am J Obstet Gynecol 2001;185(5):1118–23.

27. Sacks GP, Studena K, Sargent K, et al. Normal pregnancy and preeclampsia both produce inflammatory changes in peripheral blood leukocytes akin to those of sepsis. Am J Obstet Gynecol 1998;179(1):80–6.

28. Saito S, Nakashima A, Shima T, et al. Th1/Th2/Th17 and regulatory T-cell paradigm in pregnancy. Am J Reprod Immunol 2010;63(6):601–10.

29. Somerset DA, Zheng Y, Kilby MD, et al. Normal human pregnancy is associated with an elevation in the immune suppressive CD25+ CD4+ regulatory T-cell subset. Immunology 2004;112(1):38–43.

30. Ueda Y, Hagihara M, Okamoto A, et al. Frequencies of dendritic cells (myeloid DC and plasmacytoid DC) and their ratio reduced in pregnant women: comparison with umbilical cord blood and normal healthy adults. Hum Immunol 2003; 64(12):1144–51.

31. Olsen NJ, Yousif M, Mutwally A, et al. Organ damage in high-risk patients with systemic and incomplete lupus syndromes. Rheumatol Int 2013;33(10): 2585–90.

32. Olsen NJ, Li QZ, Quan J, et al. Autoantibody profiling to follow evolution of lupus syndromes. Arthritis Res Ther 2012;14(4):R174.

33. Wandstrat AE, Carr-Johnson F, Branch V, et al. Autoantibody profiling to identify individuals at risk for systemic lupus erythematosus. J Autoimmun 2006;27(3): 153–60.

34. Li QZ, Zhou J, Wandstrat AE, et al. Protein array autoantibody profiles for insights into systemic lupus erythematosus and incomplete lupus syndromes. Clin Exp Immunol 2007;147(1):60–70.

35. Vila LM, Mayor AM, Valentin AH, et al. Clinical outcome and predictors of disease evolution in patients with incomplete lupus erythematosus. Lupus 2000; 9(2):110–5.

36. Swaak AJ, van de Brink H, Smeenk RJ, et al. Incomplete lupus erythematosus: results of a multicentre study under the supervision of the EULAR Standing Committee on international clinical studies including therapeutic trials (ESCISIT). Rheumatology (Oxford) 2001;40(1):89–94.

37. Ståhl Hallengren C, Nived O, Sturfelt G. Outcome of incomplete systemic lupus erythematosus after 10 years. Lupus 2004;13(2):85–8.

38. Li QZ, Zhou J, Lian Y, et al. Interferon signature gene expression is correlated with autoantibody profiles in patients with incomplete lupus syndromes. Clin Exp Immunol 2010;159(3):281–91.

39. Osnes LT, Nakken B, Bodolay E, et al. Assessment of intracellular cytokines and regulatory cells in patients with autoimmune diseases and primary immunodeficiencies - novel tool for diagnostics and patient follow-up. Autoimmun Rev 2013; 12(10):967–71.

40. Mosca M, Tani C, Carli L, et al. Undifferentiated CTD: a wide spectrum of autoimmune diseases. Best Pract Res Clin Rheumatol 2012;26(1):73–7.

41. Calvo-Alen J, Alarcon GS, Burgard SL, et al. Systemic lupus erythematosus: predictors of its occurrence among a cohort of patients with early undifferentiated connective tissue disease: multivariate analyses and identification of risk factors. J Rheumatol 1996;23(3):469–75.

42. Danieli MG, Fraticelli P, Salvi A, et al. Undifferentiated connective tissue disease: natural history and evolution into definite CTD assessed in 84 patients initially diagnosed as early UCTD. Clin Rheumatol 1998;17(3):195–201.

43. Mosca M, Tavoni A, Neri R, et al. Undifferentiated connective tissue diseases: the clinical and serological profiles of 91 patients followed for at least 1 year. Lupus 1998;7(2):95–100.

44. Mosca M, Neri R, Bencivelli W, et al. Undifferentiated connective tissue disease: analysis of 83 patients with a minimum followup of 5 years. J Rheumatol 2002; 29(11):2345–9.

45. Cavazzana I, Franceschini F, Belfiore N, et al. Undifferentiated connective tissue disease with antibodies to Ro/SSa: clinical features and follow-up of 148 patients. Clin Exp Rheumatol 2001;19(4):403–9.

46. Bodolay E, Csiki Z, Szekanecz Z, et al. Five-year follow-up of 665 Hungarian patients with undifferentiated connective tissue disease (UCTD). Clin Exp Rheumatol 2003;21(3):313–20.

47. Vaz CC, Couto M, Medeiros D, et al. Undifferentiated connective tissue disease: a seven-center cross-sectional study of 184 patients. Clin Rheumatol 2009; 28(8):915–21.

48. Dijkstra S, Nieuwenhuys EJ, Swaak AJ. The prognosis and outcome of patients referred to an outpatient clinic for rheumatic diseases characterized by the presence of antinuclear antibodies (ANA). Scand J Rheumatol 1999;28(1):33–7.

49. Szodoray P, Nakken B, Barath S, et al. Progressive divergent shifts in natural and induced T-regulatory cells signify the transition from undifferentiated to definitive connective tissue disease. Int Immunol 2008;20(8):971–9.

50. Zold E, Szodoray P, Gaal J, et al. Vitamin D deficiency in undifferentiated connective tissue disease. Arthritis Res Ther 2008;10(5):R123.

51. Zold E, Szodoray P, Kappelmayer J, et al. Impaired regulatory T-cell homeostasis due to vitamin D deficiency in undifferentiated connective tissue disease. Scand J Rheumatol 2010;39(6):490–7.

52. Mosca M, Tani C, Carli L, et al. Analysis of the evolution of UCTD to defined CTD after a long term follow-up. Clin Exp Rheumatol 2013;31(3):471.
53. Mosca M, Neri R, Bombardieri S. Undifferentiated connective tissue diseases (UCTD): a review of the literature and a proposal for preliminary classification criteria. Clin Exp Rheumatol 1999;17(5):615–20.
54. Mosca M, Tani C, Bombardieri S. Defining undifferentiated connective tissue diseases: a challenge for rheumatologists. Lupus 2008;17(4):278–80.
55. Rivera TL, Izmirly PM, Birnbaum BK, et al. Disease progression in mothers of children enrolled in the research registry for neonatal lupus. Ann Rheum Dis 2009;68(6):828–35.
56. Asherson RA, Cervera R, Lahita RG. Latent, incomplete or lupus at all? J Rheumatol 1991;18(12):1783–6.
57. James JA, Kim-Howard XR, Bruner BF, et al. Hydroxychloroquine sulfate treatment is associated with later onset of systemic lupus erythematosus. Lupus 2007;16(6):401–9.
58. Laustrup H, Voss A, Green A, et al. SLE disease patterns in a Danish population-based lupus cohort: an 8-year prospective study. Lupus 2010;19(3):239–46.
59. Belfiore N, Rossi S, Bobbio-Pallavicini F, et al. Anti-Ro(SS-A) 52 kDa and 60 kDa specificities in undifferentiated connective tissue disease. Joint Bone Spine 2000;67(3):183–7.

Genetics, Environment, and Gene-Environment Interactions in the Development of Systemic Rheumatic Diseases

CrossMark

Jeffrey A. Sparks, MD, MMSc*, Karen H. Costenbader, MD, MPH

KEYWORDS

- Rheumatoid arthritis • Systemic lupus erythematosus • Ankylosing spondylitis
- Environment • Genetics • Interaction • Smoking

KEY POINTS

- Genetic and environmental risk factors have been identified for rheumatic diseases using case-control, cohort, and genome-wide association studies.
- The identification of gene-environment interactions (GEIs) may elucidate biological mechanisms for rheumatic diseases by causally linking established genetic and environmental risk factors.
- The most well studied example of GEIs in rheumatic disease susceptibility is for cigarette smoking and the *HLA-DRB1* for seropositive rheumatoid arthritis (RA); the presence of both risk factors greatly increases the risk for RA development.
- Owing to the relative rarity of systemic lupus erythematosus (SLE), comprehensive studies of GEIs have not yet been performed for SLE. However, there is some evidence that genes may interact with smoking and ultraviolet-B radiation exposure in increasing the risk for SLE.
- *HLA-B27* is the most potent genetic risk factor for ankylosing spondylitis, and there are suggestions that molecular mimicry by gut microbes might stimulate autoimmunity through GEIs with *HLA-B27*.
- Emerging research frontiers such as epigenetics, metabolomics, and the study of the oral, respiratory, and gastrointestinal microbiome may provide new biological mechanisms to link genetic and environmental risk factors in the pathogenesis of rheumatic diseases.

Funding: This work was supported by the National Institute of Arthritis and Musculoskeletal and Skin Diseases (grants AR057327 and AR059073, AR066109 to Dr K.H. Costenbader). Dr J.A. Sparks was supported by the Rheumatology Research Foundation Scientist Development Award. The funders had no role in the preparation of the article.
Division of Rheumatology, Immunology and Allergy, Department of Medicine, Brigham and Women's Hospital, Harvard Medical School, 75 Francis Street, Boston, MA 02115, USA
* Corresponding author.
E-mail address: jasparks@partners.org

INTRODUCTION

The current paradigm for the etiology of autoimmune rheumatic disease is that several preclinical stages precede the onset of clinically apparent disease. When individuals at increased genetic risk are exposed to environmental or lifestyle factors, early alterations in the immune system and the breakdown of self-tolerance ensue, eventually leading to the presentation of overt disease (**Fig. 1**).[1,2] Indeed, several genetic and environmental risk factors have been strongly associated with the risk of incident rheumatic diseases, and many more are weakly associated or hypothesized to be related.[3,4] However, the pathogenesis and biological mechanisms for the development of autoimmune rheumatic diseases remain poorly understood.

Interactions between genetic and environmental factors may elucidate biological mechanisms for rheumatic disease susceptibility and bridge findings in several fields of research. Greater understanding of the etiology of rheumatic disease may provide important insights into prevention, screening, and treatment options. Therefore, researchers in rheumatic disease are motivated to explore the intersection of genetic and environmental risk factors. However, rheumatic diseases present distinct challenges for the identification of gene-environment interactions (GEIs). These challenges include heterogeneous phenotypes, low disease incidence and prevalence, geographic variation in epidemiology, and the difficulty in identifying individuals at elevated risk for disease before clinical diagnosis.

This article serves as an overview to contextualize genetic and environmental risk factors in the development of rheumatic diseases, and highlights future research directions according to study designs and molecular approaches. Specific successes and challenges concerning rheumatoid arthritis (RA), systemic lupus erythematosus (SLE), and ankylosing spondylitis (AS) are addressed.

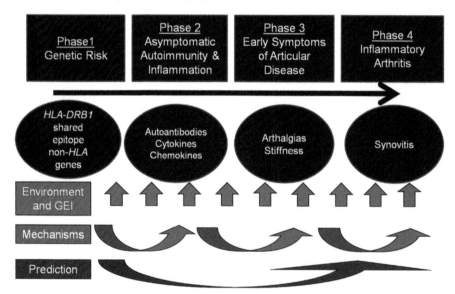

Fig. 1. The preclinical phases of rheumatoid arthritis. Other rheumatic diseases likely follow similar phases of progression from genetic susceptibility, immune dysregulation, and subclinical disease to classifiable disease. Environmental factors and gene-environment interactions likely occur throughout this process of disease pathogenesis. (*From* Karlson EW, Deane K. Environmental and gene-environment interactions and risk of rheumatoid arthritis. Rheum Dis Clin North Am 2012;38(2):406; with permission.)

CURRENT RESEARCH STRATEGIES FOR ENVIRONMENTAL AND GENETIC RISK FACTORS

As in other areas of research, bias, confounding, chance, and generalizability are major threats to validity that must be considered in study designs and analyses investigating genetic and environmental risk factors (**Table 1**). Investigators studying environmental and lifestyle risk factors for rheumatic disease risk have primarily used traditional epidemiologic techniques: the case-control and prospective cohort study designs.

Case-Control Studies

Case-control studies identify incident disease cases and match them to controls. Advantages of case-control studies are relative efficiency, especially when cases are rare and difficult to identify prospectively. Disadvantages are inherent biases based on the retrospective nature of these studies: selection and recall bias. In particular, the selection of inappropriate controls may introduce biases that lead to erroneous conclusions. Preclinical disease changes, such as dietary intake, physical activity, or weight changes, might also truly influence factors, introducing the potential for reverse causation bias. Important environmental exposures may occur early in life and may be difficult to assess. In addition, when genes are associated with established disease, it is unclear whether the effect of these genes is for disease etiology or disease propagation. Given these nuances, multiple case-control studies in diverse populations are usually warranted to establish an association between an environmental factor and disease susceptibility. Population-based case-control studies whereby inclusion is compulsory, as in national registries, may overcome some of these challenges.

Cohort Studies

Cohort studies offer solutions to some of the biases inherent in case-control studies. This study design follows populations prospectively based on a common exposure or demographic factor before individuals might develop incident disease. The major advantage of cohort studies is that data are collected without bias for all individuals before disease onset. Design issues such as selection or recall bias are therefore less problematic, although subtle subclinical manifestations might still introduce the

Table 1
Threats to validity in study designs

	Case-Control Study	Cohort Study	Genome-Wide Association Study
Bias	Selection bias Recall bias Inappropriate matching Reverse causation	Selection bias Misclassification Length-time bias Reverse causation Loss to follow-up	Phenotype misclassification Inappropriate controls Genomic inflation
Confounding	Unmeasured confounders	Unmeasured confounders	Population stratification
Chance	Multiple testing Power	Multiple testing Power	Multiple testing False discovery rate Rare variants Power
Generalizability	Study-specific	Cohort-specific	Race/region-specific Phenotype-specific

potential for reverse causation bias.[5] Inclusion criteria, however, might affect generalizability. Nested case-control studies on stored samples performed within cohort studies can evaluate biomarkers in the preclinical period. Confirmation of incident cases is often a limiting factor in cohort studies, because most rheumatic diseases have a low incidence and require either extremely large cohorts, long follow-up, or specific populations at increased risk, such as first-degree relatives or those with preclinical symptoms (such as arthralgias). Meta-analyses of multiple large cohorts may overcome some of these limitations; however, heterogeneity in study designs and populations may also be limiting. These different cohort designs (general population, unaffected relative, and symptomatic but nonclassifiable individuals) may correspond to particular phases in the development of autoimmune diseases (see **Fig. 1**).[1,6]

Early studies seeking to identify genetic risk factors often focused on heritability, usually in the context of familial disease. Heritability was estimated by evaluating rates of disease within homozygote and heterozygote twins. Linkage analyses used entire families, with affected and unaffected family members. These methods were able to establish the familial heritability of a disease, although shared environmental factors might still contribute to this heritability. Linkage analyses were most useful in identifying highly penetrant genes with large effect sizes. In addition, candidate gene studies genotyped a few loci at a time, a slow process focusing on known mechanisms of cellular pathways.[7]

Genome-Wide Association Studies

The advent of high-throughput genotyping brought about the era of genome-wide association studies (GWAS), which evaluate initially thousands (and more recently, hundreds of thousands) of different genetic loci at once for association with disease.[8] This hypothesis-free method is capable of evaluating the entire genome for potential disease-susceptibility genes.[9] However, GWAS depend on the performance and composition of specific platforms of single-nucleotide polymorphisms (SNPs) across the genome, which might vary widely according to race, ethnicity, and geography. Potentially associated loci may not necessarily be included on each platform, and therefore would not be tested. The ability of GWAS to detect true associations depends on a homogeneous disease phenotype with similar disease pathogenesis. Appropriate control selection, with similar race and genetic structure, is therefore important. For example, most early GWAS in RA were performed for seropositive RA cases among whites with European heritage.[10–12] Findings from these studies may not be generalizable to seronegative RA or nonwhite European populations. This concept presents major challenges for diseases such as SLE with heterogeneous subtypes and variation by race, ethnicity, and geography. The genetic components of rheumatic diseases might also be more pronounced in early-onset than in older-onset disease, in which environmental or age-related factors may be more important.[13,14]

GWAS usually offer only statistical associations with probabilities of disease development. Disease susceptibility loci detected through this method are not necessarily causal for rheumatic diseases, but may be proxies for causal loci because of linkage disequilibrium. GWAS are most successful at discovering common variants, as opposed to rare variants. The latter, however, often have higher effect sizes, and therefore may provide important pathogenic information in comparison with common variants with lower effect sizes. For example, single mutations of genes involved in the complement cascade (C1q, C2, and C4) occur rarely but are very strongly associated with an increased risk for SLE.[15] Methodological issues such as genomic inflation, population stratification, false discovery rates, linkage disequilibria, and multiple comparisons are major design and computational obstacles for GWAS, requiring advanced statistical expertise.[16] Despite these caveats, GWAS have rapidly and efficiently detected numerous loci with rheumatic disease susceptibility.[17] To date, however, findings from GWAS for rheumatic diseases have had little clinical impact, as significant SNPs may not be causal and have low effect size estimates, and thus offer little ability to classify individuals according to risk for disease development.

Genetic Risk Scores

Genetic risk scores (GRS) have been developed to combine many validated genetic loci into a single summary variable, improving statistical power to detect potential associations.[18] GRS can be calculated simply by counts of risk alleles. However, if effect sizes of individual genetic components vary appreciably, weighted GRS (wGRS) should be used.[19] Typically, wGRS are weighted using the natural logarithm of odds ratios found in large GWAS or meta-analyses.[19] Because human leukocyte antigen (HLA) loci are often more strongly associated with the risk of rheumatic disease in comparison with non-*HLA* SNPs, wGRS have been used in rheumatic disease research.[14,19–22]

GENE-ENVIRONMENT INTERACTIONS

The rapid emergence of genetic susceptibility loci and the identification and replication of specific environmental risk factors provide the opportunity to evaluate specific GEIs that may offer new biological mechanisms in disease pathogenesis, and potentially provide personalized medicine approaches whereby an individual's risk for disease can be calculated using a combination of genetic and environmental factors.[23] However, study design, statistical power, and expertise are major challenges in the identification of potential GEIs.[24] Because GWAS require very large samples sizes to detect associations of genetic factors with disease, often with modest effect sizes, studies with statistical power to detect GEIs may not be feasible using current techniques. Although GEIs may suggest biological mechanisms for disease development, it is not clear that they will be able to provide robust predictive abilities for rheumatic diseases, at least in the foreseeable future.[25,26]

GEIs can be identified statistically through additive or multiplicative interactions (**Table 2**). An additive interaction is an effect beyond the sum of the risks associated with individual factors, and can be measured by the relative excess risk due to

Table 2
Statistical measures of interaction

Type of Interaction		Statistical Measure	Interpretation	Null Hypothesis
Additive	RERI	Relative excess risk due to interaction	Additional risk compared with the expected risk from adding the risks for each exposure	RERI = 0
	AP	Attributable proportion due to interaction	Proportion due to interaction of overall risk among those with both exposures	AP = 0
	S	Synergy index	Excess risk from combined exposures relative to the risks from each exposure	S = 1
Multiplicative	ROR	Ratio of odds ratios	Additional risk compared with the expected risk from multiplying risks of each exposure	ROR = 1

interaction (RERI), attributable proportion due to interaction (AP), or synergy index (S).[27] A multiplicative interaction is an effect greater than the multiplied effects of the individual factors, and is measured by the ratio of odds ratios (ROR).[27] The interpretation and suitability of interaction terms depend on the scale of the statistical model used. Logistic regression models are on a multiplicative scale, whereas linear regression models are on an additive scale. Therefore, in a logistic regression model (eg, with an outcome of development of disease or not), a statistically significant interaction term implies a multiplicative interaction between the 2 factors. Additive interactions have been considered to represent biological interaction of 2 factors within the same pathway.[24] However, a statistical interaction does not necessarily imply a biological interaction. In studies of disease pathogenesis, a statistically significant additive GEI should be ideally replicated in independent studies and animal models to validate biological plausibility. GEIs usually have statistically significant main effects for both genetic and environmental factors in predicting disease onset, although this may not be a requirement if factors work exclusively in synergy.

Recent advancements in fine mapping of genetic regions of interest and high-throughput next-generation sequencing will result in yet more genetic loci associated with the risk of rheumatic diseases, so these issues are timely. Specific examples of genetic factors, environment factors, and GEIs in RA, SLE, and AS susceptibility are provided here.

Rheumatoid Arthritis

The study of genetic and environmental risk factors for RA is the most developed among the rheumatic diseases, owing to a relatively homogeneous disease phenotype and high disease prevalence.[28] Despite these advantages, differences in the risk-factor assessment for RA are appreciated based on serologic status.[29] Early studies of RA risk factors were stratified by the presence of absence of rheumatoid factor (RF). However, RF positivity may be seen in other diseases or as a consequence of aging.[30] Recent studies have used anticitrullinated peptide antibody (ACPA) to classify RA, which is more specific for RA and thus has less potential for misclassification.[31] Despite validated classification criteria for RA, atypical presentations of other systemic rheumatic diseases have the potential to be misclassified as seronegative RA.[32,33]

Genetic risk factors for rheumatoid arthritis: the shared epitope and beyond

Genetic variants in the major histocompatibility complex (MHC) region on chromosome 6 were identified to be potently associated with RA susceptibility and were deemed the "shared epitope."[34] Polymorphisms in 3 HLA genes (*HLA-DRB1*, *HLA-DPB1*, *HLA-B*) in the MHC region are highly associated with RA.[35] Polymorphisms in *HLA-DRB1*, in particular, the classic shared epitope genotypes of *04:01* and *04:04* are strongly associated with RA (odds ratios of approximately 4 for risk variants).[36] Specific amino acid positions (11, 71, and 74) that correspond to the *HLA-DRB1* shared epitope classic genotypes are located in the peptide-binding groove of the protein HLA-DRβ1, offering a potential biological mechanism for this potent RA genetic risk factor.[35]

Large genetic consortia have identified many non-*HLA* SNPs associated with RA using GWAS.[4,11,37,38] Most recently, a large transethnic GWAS associated 101 genetic loci with RA across European and Asian populations.[4] However, most of the non-*HLA* SNPs are only modestly associated with RA.[37] An exception is an SNP near the gene *PTPN22* (encoding a tyrosine-phosphatase protein expressed in lymphoid tissue), which is strongly associated with RA (odds ratio 1.78).[37] SNPs near the genes *TNFAIP3* and *TYK2* also have relatively large effect sizes for RA risk.[17]

Most early genetic studies focused on seropositive RA among Caucasian or Japanese populations.[4] In a recent large genetic consortium study, Han and colleagues[39] made special efforts to correctly classify ACPA-positive and APCA-negative RA cases by using a highly specific ACPA assay. This study identified new genetic risk factors associated with ACPA-negative RA: serine or leucine at amino acid position 11 in *HLA-DRB1* and aspartate in position 9 in *HLA-B*.[39] These findings provide further evidence that ACPA-positive and ACPA-negative RA are genetically distinct, and thus may have separate pathogeneses.[4,17,39,40]

Despite the significance of the *HLA* shared epitope to RA risk and the growing number of non-*HLA* SNPs associated with RA, most genetic heritability remains unexplained. The *HLA* shared epitope explains only 12% of the genetic variance for RA while only about 4% is explained by all other non-*HLA* SNPs.[37] Gene-gene interactions for RA may also be present, in particular an association between the *HLA* shared epitope and *PTPN22,* specifically based on the presence of the R620W allele, for the development of seropositive RA.[41,42] Studies among familial RA and twins suggest that environmental factors have an important role in the development of RA and RA-related antibodies, so GEIs may be important in linking these discoveries.[20,43]

Environmental risk factors for rheumatoid arthritis: cigarette smoking and more

Strong epidemiologic evidence supports cigarette smoking as an environmental risk factor for RA development. Multiple studies have shown an increased RA risk from smoking among men and women in various populations.[44-53] Furthermore, there is a dose-dependent effect between smoking pack-years and RA development.[46,54] After 20 years of smoking cessation, RA risk of former smokers returns to the RA risk of the general population.[46] Murine models evaluating exposure to cigarette smoke have induced inflammatory arthritis, providing further biological evidence.[55] This association is particularly strong for the development of seropositive RA.[44] Smoking may contribute up to 25% of RA risk, and up to 35% of risk for ACPA-positive RA.[56] However, studies of smoking and seronegative RA have revealed less powerful associations.[44,47]

Other environmental factors have been associated with the development of RA. It is beyond the scope of this article to review these factors extensively, but they include occupational exposures such as silica, reproductive factors in women, and excess body mass.[57-59] Dietary factors that might be protective for RA include intake of alcohol and fish.[60-65]

Given the knowledge of a period of preclinical RA autoimmunity during which autoantibodies are present in the absence of clinically apparent joint inflammation, there is growing interest that the induction of RA may occur at extra-articular sites. The induction of autoimmunity in RA may specifically occur at mucosal surfaces in the respiratory tract, mouth, or gut.[66] Mucosal involvement in the lung has been posited as a possible site for RA initiation because of the increased risk seen in both smoking and particulate silica exposure.[44,62] Citrullination of peptides occurs in the lung because of inflammation, and this is most pronounced in smokers.[66,67] Interstitial lung disease is a well-known nonarticular manifestation of RA, and may occur even without articular involvement. Periodontitis has also been associated with both prevalent and incident RA, although smoking and secondary Sjögren syndrome may confound these associations.[68,69] *Porphyromonas gingivalis*, a causative bacterium for periodontitis, expresses the enzyme peptidylarginine deiminase, which can citrullinate both enolase and fibrinogen, self-antigens thought to be involved in the joint specificity of RA.[70] A study composed of RA first-degree relatives reported higher concentrations of *P gingivalis* antibodies in RA relatives who had developed RA-related antibodies, arguing that preclinical infection, or its immune response, may be important in the development of altered immunity in RA.[71]

Rheumatoid arthritis gene-environment interaction: HLA-DRB1–cigarette smoking interaction

The strong association of smoking with RA risk and evidence for induction of autoimmunity and citrullination in mucosa led to a hypothesized biological mechanism for the role of smoking in the development of RA. Studies initially performed by Klareskog and colleagues[72,73] demonstrated a strong GEI between cigarette smoking and HLA-DRB1 in determining RA risk.[42,74–76] This association was strongest for seropositive RA and has been replicated in several populations, including United States women, and Swedish and Malaysian populations.[72,74,75] The presence of heavy smoking and 2 HLA-DRB1 genes increased the odds for RA by 23-fold compared with those with neither risk factor.[42,75]

Transgenic mouse models have demonstrated a strong immune response between HLA-DRβ1 and citrullinated self-antigens implicated in smoking, offering more evidence of biological plausibility for this GEI.[77] Smoking in particular, but also other inflammatory exposures, are now thought to cause citrullination of a large array of peptides. The specific responses to these citrullinated peptides are likely genetically determined, generating a diversity of ACPAs to different citrullinated antigens, which arise before onset of clinical disease and have varying pathogenicity. The HLA-smoking interaction may contribute to citrullination processes and autoimmunity and might explain the seroconversion noted in preclinical RA (**Fig. 2**).[78,79] This GEI seems to apply only to seropositive RA, and possibly in particular to those with antibodies to citrullinated α-enolase and vimentin.[80] Other genes (GSTT1 and HMOX1) in which polymorphisms might interfere with the metabolism of cigarette smoke are hypothesized to also enhance RA susceptibility.[81]

Although HLA-smoking GEIs have led to robust findings about the pathogenesis of ACPA-positive RA among those with both risk factors, they confer little ability to discriminate between RA cases and controls in risk modeling, emphasizing the need for continued research of other biological pathways involved in RA pathogenesis.[20,21]

Systemic Lupus Erythematosus

Because of its elevated morbidity and mortality, there is interest in identifying risk factors for the development of SLE.[82] SLE has a heterogeneous clinical phenotype,

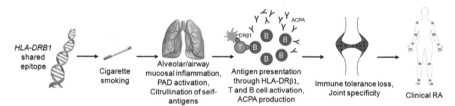

Fig. 2. HLA-DRB1–cigarette smoking interaction in the development of seropositive rheumatoid arthritis (RA). Individuals with 1 or more HLA-DRB1 shared epitope alleles smoke cigarettes, which induces inflammation in the airways and alveolar mucosa. Peptidylarginine deiminase (PAD) is activated, which citrullinates self-antigens. Antigen-presenting cells stimulate T cells through aberrant HLA-DRβ1 interactions and stimulate B cells to produce anticitrullinated peptide antibodies (ACPA). Immune tolerance is lost specifically in joints, which manifests clinically as synovitis with signs and symptoms compatible with RA. (From Klareskog L, Ronnelid J, Lundberg K, et al. Immunity to citrullinated proteins in rheumatoid arthritis. Annu Rev Immunol 2008;26:651–75; with permission. Modified from Figures on Pages 660–2.)

ranging from mild mucocutaneous or musculoskeletal involvement to severe, life-threatening neurologic or renal manifestations.[83] The American College of Rheumatology (ACR) classification criteria for SLE considers these varied manifestations as a single disease entity.[84,85] This singularity presents methodological challenges, as different SLE subtypes may have separate pathogeneses and, therefore, different genetic and environmental risk factors. This aspect further partitions an already rare disease, decreasing the statistical power of even large studies with long follow-up periods. Despite these challenges, specific autoantibody and biomarker profiles offer insight into defining distinct SLE subtypes.

Genetic risk factors for systemic lupus erythematosus

As in RA and other autoimmune diseases, HLA genes are thought to have a central role in SLE susceptibility. The haplotypes HLA-DRB1*03:01 and *15:01 are strong genetic risk factors for SLE in European populations.[36] GWAS have associated more than 40 genetic loci with SLE susceptibility.[86] Several genes, such as PTPN22, are implicated in SLE and other autoimmune diseases, RA in particular.[87] However, many other genes are specifically associated with SLE susceptibility.[88]

SLE-associated genetic loci have been categorized according to putative functionality.[86] These categories include DNA degradation and cellular debris, immune complex clearance, toll-like receptors, interferon regulation, nuclear factor κB, and regulation of B cells, T cells, monocytes, and neutrophils.[86] The role of DNA repair genes, in particular ATG5, TREX1, and DNASE1, may be of particular interest given the nearly ubiquitous presence of antinuclear antibodies in SLE.[86] A wGRS for SLE, composed of 22 SNPs including HLA-DRB1, has been developed and used to calculate GRS of particular SLE subtypes based on validated SNPs for SLE and ACR criteria (such as renal involvement and presence of anti-dsDNA antibodies).[22] This wGRS is associated with earlier-onset SLE, consistent with the notion that increased genetic burden may correspond to earlier disease onset.[22] Gene-gene interactions may also be present in SLE, specifically between CTLA4, IRF5, and ITGAM with HLA-DRB1 as well as between PDCD1 and IL21, among others.[89]

Environmental risk factors for systemic lupus erythematosus

Smoking and exposure to ultraviolet radiation have been implicated as possible environmental factors for SLE susceptibility.[90–93] Ultraviolet-B radiation is well known to cause SLE exacerbations, and its potential pathogenic mechanism in aberrant apoptosis and the removal of cellular debris make this a key candidate in the etiology of SLE, particularly for cutaneous manifestations.[94] Epstein-Barr virus (EBV) has been suggested to be involved in the pathogenesis of SLE, based on high EBV viral loads in pediatric SLE patients compared with controls, with posited molecular mimicry of EBV antigens and autoantigens targeted by lupus autoantibodies.[95,96] However, the association between EBV and risk of SLE remains controversial. The female predominance in SLE argues strongly for hormonal and reproductive influences. Oral contraceptives and postmenopausal hormones have both been related to an increased risk for SLE, in particular among women taking higher doses of ethinyl estradiol.[97–100]

Systemic lupus erythematosus gene-environment interactions

Unlike RA, there is not yet strong evidence associating particular genetic and environmental factors to SLE susceptibility, which makes GEIs for SLE challenging to identify. However, GEIs for both smoking and ultraviolet-B exposure have been reported.[101,102] In the Carolina Lupus Study, women with null homozygous genotypes for GSTM1 and more than 2 years of occupational sun exposure had 3-fold increased odds for SLE, with a trend toward statistical significance.[102] Other genes involved in DNA repair (such as *ATG5, TREX1,* and *DNASE1*) have not been specifically studied for a GEI with ultraviolet-B light for SLE development. A Japanese case-control study found that women who were smokers and had the slow acetylator *N*-acetyltransferase-2 (*NAT2*) genotype had 6-fold increased odds of SLE, compared with never smokers with the rapid acetylator form of *NAT2*. This interaction bore a significant additive interaction, an AP of 50%, suggesting that metabolism of oxidants from cigarette smoke may play a role in SLE pathogenesis.[101] In addition, genes for toll-like receptors (such as *IRF5* and *TLR7*) may engage microbes, inappropriately resulting in SLE autoimmunity. Infections with several potential organisms may trigger immune responses that go awry in genetically predisposed individuals and leading to SLE autoimmunity, although particular pathogens and interactions have not yet been identified.

Ankylosing Spondylitis

The incidence and prevalence of AS varies markedly by geography, perhaps owing to the prevalence of *HLA-B27* in these populations.[103] The identification of individuals at risk therefore may be comparably easier for AS than for other rheumatic diseases based on geography, *HLA-B27*-positivity, or AS relatives. However, AS classification criteria are still evolving, which makes consistent phenotyping challenging.[104,105] There is considerable clinical overlap between AS and other *HLA-B27*–associated diseases, such as reactive arthritis, psoriatic arthritis, and inflammatory bowel disease. Inconsistent phenotyping could hinder the identification of genetic and environmental associations in AS. Because AS patients often present in adolescence or go undiagnosed for many years, identifying exposure windows before disease onset is challenging. Cohort studies used in rheumatic diseases comparing exposed with unexposed subjects are typically not large enough to detect AS and most do not follow children or adolescents, who might go on to develop AS in early adulthood.

Genetic risk factors for ankylosing spondylitis: HLA-B27 dominates

Unlike other rheumatic diseases, AS has long been associated with a gene with very large effect size.[106] *HLA-B27* positivity confers an odds ratio of approximately 90 for developing AS compared with *HLA-B27*–negative individuals.[107] *HLA-B27* is present in about 90% of patients with AS, but only about 5% of *HLA-B27*–positive individuals develop AS or another form of spondyloarthritis.[107] This finding illustrates the difficulty in the clinical implementation of genetic testing for rheumatic disease susceptibility. A recent large GWAS associated 31 genetic loci with AS.[108] However, these non-*HLA* loci are overwhelmed by the influence of *HLA-B27*. The overall contribution of *HLA-B27* to AS heritability is estimated to be 20%, with about 4% being due to other loci.[108] Other genes implicated in AS risk include *IL23R* and *IL1R2* in addition to the intergenic region at 2p15.[107] These associations offer insight into the role of cytokines interleukin (IL)-17/IL-23 and IL-1 in the pathogenesis of AS.

Several possible explanations might explain the striking association of *HLA-B27* with AS development. The arthritogenic peptide hypothesis states that similarity between microbial peptides and HLA-B27–specific CD8-positive lymphocytes could induce autoimmunity.[109] The heavy-chain homodimer hypothesis states that HLA-B27 dimers are resistant to normal degradation and engage natural killer receptors inappropriately, resulting in autoimmunity.[110] The protein misfolding hypothesis, which states that unfolded HLA-B27 accumulates in the endoplasmic reticulum and stimulates the release of proinflammatory cytokines, is the most widely accepted.[111,112]

Environmental risk factors for ankylosing spondylitis: microbial and gut influences?
Microbes have been postulated to trigger altered immunity in AS through molecular mimicry. Some suggest that this might specifically occur in the gut through the microbiome. The etiologic role of *Chlamydia* species and enterobacteria in reactive arthritis has been posited to also apply to AS pathogenesis.[113,114] Transgenic HLA-B27 murine models have also demonstrated that the introduction of bacteria is necessary for the development of spondyloarthropathy.[115] Inflammation in the gut has been consistently observed in spondyloarthritis.[116] Cigarette smoking has also been implicated in AS susceptibility, underscoring its role in multiple inflammatory and autoimmune diseases.[117] Unlike in most other rheumatic diseases, men are more likely than women to develop AS, so male-specific factors such as testosterone may also be involved in the pathogenesis of AS.[118]

Ankylosing spondylitis gene-environment interactions: engaging HLA-B27
Given the large influence of *HLA-B27* on AS susceptibility, any GEI will need to have biological plausibility with *HLA-B27* functionality.[112] In this sense, finding significant GEIs may be more straightforward in AS than in RA and SLE (**Table 3**). A proteomic analysis of *Chlamydia trachomatis* identified peptides that interact with *HLA-B27* in mouse models and also stimulate T cells from patients with spondyloarthritis.[119] The role of environmental factors in AS pathogenesis, and the reason why many *HLA-B27*–positive individuals never develop AS or other forms of spondyloarthritis, are as yet unsolved.[120,121]

Table 3					
Selected genetic, environment, and gene-environment interactions in RA, SLE, and AS					
Phenotype	MHC Genes (Variance Explained)	No. of Non-HLA SNPs Associated[Ref.]	Selected Non-*HLA* Genes/Loci	Key Environmental Factors	Proposed Gene-Environment Interactions
RA	HLA-DRB1 HLA-DPB1 HLA-B (12%)	101[4]	PTPN22 TNAIF3 TYK2	Cigarette smoking Reproductive factors and hormonal exposures Silica Periodontitis Excess body mass Alcohol intake Fish intake	HLA-DRB1– smoking PTPN22- smoking
SLE	HLA-DRB1 HLA-DPB1 HLA-G	>40[86]	ATG5 TREX1 DNASE1 IRF5 TLR7 FCGR2A	Ultraviolet-B radiation Current cigarette smoking Silica Reproductive factors and hormonal exposures Alcohol intake Epstein-Barr virus	DNA repair genes–UV-B radiation and smoking TLR gene– infections
AS	HLA-B27 (20%)	30[108]	IL23R IL1R2 2p15	Gut microbiome Cigarette smoking Testosterone	HLA-B27– infections

Abbreviations: AS, ankylosing spondylitis; HLA, human leukocyte antigen; MHC, major histocompatibility complex; RA, rheumatoid arthritis; SLE, systemic lupus erythematosus; SNPs, single nucleotide polymorphisms; TLR, toll-like receptor; UV-B, ultraviolet-B.

EMERGING RESEARCH STRATEGIES
Epigenetics

Epigenetic regulation is thought to be largely responsible for the cell-specific expression of genes. Epigenetic changes are heritable from one cell cycle to the next, are potentially reversible, and do not alter nucleotide sequences.[122] Biochemical modifications involved in epigenetics include acetylation, histone modifications, methylation, phosphorylation, sumoylation, and microRNA.[123]

Epigenetic modifications provide an important potential link between genes and the environment, because environmental factors influence epigenetic processes, such as methylation and acetylation, whereas other epigenetic factors are inherited.[124] It also adds many layers of complexity to the notions of inheritance of complex disease phenotypes. Epigenetic responses to environmental exposures are likely in part genetically determined themselves, and can be inherited as stable traits and act as bona fide epigenetic quantitative trait loci, perhaps responsible for a great deal of unexplained heritability. This notion leads to added complexity in understanding the interplay between genetic factors and environmental exposures, and epigenetic control and modification with subsequent genetic expression, in determining disease susceptibility.[125]

Studies performed in rheumatic diseases have mostly focused on inflammatory pathways in distinct immune cell types.[126] Demethylation has been linked to drug-induced lupus in humans and murine models.[127,128] Sophisticated techniques are required to systematically identify and isolate cells of the same immunophenotype. The differential expression of epigenetic markers between cell types and innumerable immunophenotypes make population-based epigenetic studies difficult to implement. At present, specific hypotheses, radiation based on known genetic findings and immune function, are often needed for epigenetic investigations. As the technological aspects of high-throughput epigenetic screening evolve, population-based studies using epigenetics are likely to become increasingly feasible. For example, a study examined epigenetic patterns in more than 200 neonates to investigate the roles of genetic and maternal factors.[129] Another study performed a genome-wide methylation analysis of peripheral blood mononuclear cells in a cohort of African American women to find and identify more than 900 statistically significant loci potentially related to cigarette smoking.[130] Methylation patterns have also been implicated as an intermediary of genetic risk seen in ACPA-positive RA.[131] Methods for epigenome-wide association studies are currently being refined, and may be ready for large-scale use in the near future.[132]

Microbiome

The microbiome refers to the symbiosis and interaction of individuals and their bacterial flora. It has long been recognized that bacteria occupy the mucosal surfaces in the gut, mouth, respiratory system, and skin. Recent findings implicating autoimmunity at these sites have heightened the search for imbalances of the microbiome and rheumatic disease susceptibility. The relationship of microbiota to diseases such as acute rheumatic fever and reactive arthritis provide a precedent for the potential importance of microbes to other rheumatic diseases.

Scher and colleagues[133] examined stools from RA cases and healthy controls, and found a potential role for the bacteria *Prevotella copri* in RA disease susceptibility. Though provocative, this study requires replication, as factors related to having RA (such as socioeconomic status, health care utilization, and medications) might explain this association. Studies are currently exploring mechanisms to link specific bacteria in the microbiome and disease susceptibility. Comparisons between high-risk, asymptomatic individuals, the general population, and patients with established disease could elucidate the microbiome's role in the etiology of rheumatic disease. Exploration of the microbiome of other mucosal surfaces, such as the mouth and lung, are ongoing in RA and other diseases. High-throughput methods to assess microbiota need to be developed so that large population-based studies can be performed in diverse populations and geographic areas, incorporating knowledge of other environmental factors and host genetics.

Metabolomics

Metabolomics is the study of metabolites and their relationship to disease. Metabolomics may serve as the bridge between host genetics and environmental exposures. Unlike epigenetics and the microbiome, high-throughput methods involving mass spectrometry already exist for metabolomics.[134] However, metabolite levels may depend on many factors such as sleep, fasting status, comorbidities, and medication use, making study design challenging and sensitive to many variables. Metabolomic studies require sophisticated statistical support to allow for multiple comparisons, mutual adjustments, and principal-components analysis.

Despite these qualifications, studies have been performed to investigate metabolomic profiles in rheumatic diseases. Serum metabolite profiles related to lipids and lactate were related to the inflammatory burden in RA patients.[135] Urine metabolite profiles in RA patients distinguished responders to tumor necrosis factor inhibitors from nonresponders.[136] Though provocative, it is unclear whether these methods provide clinically meaningful data beyond currently available biomarkers or whether metabolite dysregulation occurs in the preclinical disease period. Identification of novel metabolite biomarkers in the preclinical phase may prove to be helpful in identifying individuals at risk for autoimmune rheumatic disease, and contribute to the understanding of pathophysiology. Thus, metabolomics may be a powerful tool in identifying biomarker patterns associated with drug response, and could influence treatment decisions.

FUTURE CONSIDERATIONS AND SUMMARY

Genetic and environmental factors, and the interactions between them, some of which may be mediated by epigenetic modification followed by posttranslational effects, are associated with the development of rheumatic diseases. The discovery and validation of the *HLA-DRB1*–smoking interaction in RA is a model among rheumatic diseases for GEI studies. For SLE, genetics have elucidated pathways that may lead to the differentiation of disease subtypes and form hypotheses that integrate environmental risk factors. *HLA-B27* must be considered a potential etiologic mechanism in AS. Despite these advances, the etiology of rheumatic disease remains enigmatic. GEIs have provided, and could continue to provide, insights into biological mechanisms that link genetic and environmental risk factors. However, much of the risk for rheumatic disease susceptibility remains unexplained. Future research will investigate whether this risk can be explained by rare genetic variants, epigenetic controls and modifications, novel environmental factors, gene-gene interactions, or GEIs. In addition, understanding which genes may be involved in the development of autoimmunity and those that lead to progression of disease will be important in evaluating longitudinal studies. Emerging research strategies, including epigenetics, metabolomics, and the microbiome, will likely further elucidate susceptibility to rheumatic disease.

REFERENCES

1. van Steenbergen HW, Huizinga TW, van der Helm-van Mil AH. The preclinical phase of rheumatoid arthritis: what is acknowledged and what needs to be assessed? Arthritis Rheum 2013;65(9):2219–32.
2. Klareskog L, Alfredsson L, Rantapaa-Dahlqvist S, et al. What precedes development of rheumatoid arthritis? Ann Rheum Dis 2004;63(Suppl 2):ii28–31.
3. Lahiri M, Morgan C, Symmons DP, et al. Modifiable risk factors for RA: prevention, better than cure? Rheumatology (Oxford) 2012;51(3):499–512.
4. Okada Y, Wu D, Trynka G, et al. Genetics of rheumatoid arthritis contributes to biology and drug discovery. Nature 2014;506(7488):376–81.
5. Choi HK, Nguyen US, Niu J, et al. Selection bias in rheumatic disease research. Nat Rev Rheumatol 2014;10:403–12.
6. Karlson EW, Deane K. Environmental and gene-environment interactions and risk of rheumatoid arthritis. Rheum Dis Clin North Am 2012;38(2):405–26.
7. Chernajovsky Y, Winyard PG, Kabouridis PS. Advances in understanding the genetic basis of rheumatoid arthritis and osteoarthritis: implications for therapy. Am J Pharmacogenomics 2002;2(4):223–34.
8. Neale BM, Purcell S. The positives, protocols, and perils of genome-wide association. Am J Med Genet B Neuropsychiatr Genet 2008;147B(7):1288–94.
9. Brookes AJ. Rethinking genetic strategies to study complex diseases. Trends Mol Med 2001;7(11):512–6.
10. Raychaudhuri S, Remmers EF, Lee AT, et al. Common variants at CD40 and other loci confer risk of rheumatoid arthritis. Nat Genet 2008;40(10):1216–23.
11. Stahl EA, Raychaudhuri S, Remmers EF, et al. Genome-wide association study meta-analysis identifies seven new rheumatoid arthritis risk loci. Nat Genet 2010;42(6):508–14.
12. Plenge RM, Seielstad M, Padyukov L, et al. TRAF1-C5 as a risk locus for rheumatoid arthritis–a genomewide study. N Engl J Med 2007;357(12):1199–209.
13. Webb R, Kelly JA, Somers EC, et al. Early disease onset is predicted by a higher genetic risk for lupus and is associated with a more severe phenotype in lupus patients. Ann Rheum Dis 2011;70(1):151–6.
14. Scott IC, Seegobin SD, Steer S, et al. Predicting the risk of rheumatoid arthritis and its age of onset through modelling genetic risk variants with smoking. PLoS Genet 2013;9(9):e1003808.
15. Tsokos GC. Systemic lupus erythematosus. N Engl J Med 2011;365(22):2110–21.
16. Hayes B. Overview of statistical methods for genome-wide association studies (GWAS). Methods Mol Biol 2013;1019:149–69.
17. Viatte S, Plant D, Raychaudhuri S. Genetics and epigenetics of rheumatoid arthritis. Nat Rev Rheumatol 2013;9(3):141–53.
18. Horne BD, Anderson JL, Carlquist JF, et al. Generating genetic risk scores from intermediate phenotypes for use in association studies of clinically significant endpoints. Ann Hum Genet 2005;69(Pt 2):176–86.
19. Karlson EW, Chibnik LB, Kraft P, et al. Cumulative association of 22 genetic variants with seropositive rheumatoid arthritis risk. Ann Rheum Dis 2010;69(6):1077–85.
20. Sparks JA, Chen C, Jiang X, et al. Improved performance of epidemiologic and genetic risk models for rheumatoid arthritis serologic phenotypes using family history. Ann Rheum Dis 2014. [Epub ahead of print].
21. Karlson EW, Ding B, Keenan BT, et al. Association of environmental and genetic factors and gene-environment interactions with risk of developing rheumatoid arthritis. Arthritis Care Res (Hoboken) 2013;65(7):1147–56.

22. Taylor KE, Chung SA, Graham RR, et al. Risk alleles for systemic lupus erythematosus in a large case-control collection and associations with clinical subphenotypes. PLoS Genet 2011;7(2):e1001311.

23. Kraft P, Hunter D. Integrating epidemiology and genetic association: the challenge of gene-environment interaction. Philos Trans R Soc Lond B Biol Sci 2005;360(1460):1609–16.

24. Karlson EW, Costenbader KH. Epidemiology: interpreting studies of interactions between RA risk factors. Nat Rev Rheumatol 2010;6(2):72–3.

25. Aschard H, Chen J, Cornelis MC, et al. Inclusion of gene-gene and gene-environment interactions unlikely to dramatically improve risk prediction for complex diseases. Am J Hum Genet 2012;90(6):962–72.

26. Milne RL, Gaudet MM, Spurdle AB, et al. Assessing interactions between the associations of common genetic susceptibility variants, reproductive history and body mass index with breast cancer risk in the breast cancer association consortium: a combined case-control study. Breast Cancer Res 2010;12(6): R110.

27. Knol MJ, van der Tweel I, Grobbee DE, et al. Estimating interaction on an additive scale between continuous determinants in a logistic regression model. Int J Epidemiol 2007;36(5):1111–8.

28. Crowson CS, Matteson EL, Myasoedova E, et al. The lifetime risk of adult-onset rheumatoid arthritis and other inflammatory autoimmune rheumatic diseases. Arthritis Rheum 2011;63(3):633–9.

29. Gabriel SE, Crowson CS, O'Fallon WM. The epidemiology of rheumatoid arthritis in Rochester, Minnesota, 1955-1985. Arthritis Rheum 1999;42(3):415–20.

30. Tighe H, Carson DA. Rheumatoid factor. In: Ruddy S, Harris ED, Sledge C, editors. Kelley's textbook of rheumatology. Philadelphia: WB Saunders Company; 2001. p. 151–61.

31. Schellekens GA, Visser H, de Jong BA, et al. The diagnostic properties of rheumatoid arthritis antibodies recognizing a cyclic citrullinated peptide. Arthritis Rheum 2000;43(1):155–63.

32. Aletaha D, Neogi T, Silman AJ, et al. 2010 Rheumatoid arthritis classification criteria: an American College of Rheumatology/European League Against Rheumatism collaborative initiative. Arthritis Rheum 2010;62(9):2569–81.

33. Arnett FC, Edworthy SM, Bloch DA, et al. The American Rheumatism Association 1987 revised criteria for the classification of rheumatoid arthritis. Arthritis Rheum 1988;31(3):315–24.

34. Gregersen PK, Silver J, Winchester RJ. The shared epitope hypothesis. An approach to understanding the molecular genetics of susceptibility to rheumatoid arthritis. Arthritis Rheum 1987;30(11):1205–13.

35. Raychaudhuri S, Sandor C, Stahl EA, et al. Five amino acids in three HLA proteins explain most of the association between MHC and seropositive rheumatoid arthritis. Nat Genet 2012;44(3):291–6.

36. Fernando MM, Stevens CR, Walsh EC, et al. Defining the role of the MHC in autoimmunity: a review and pooled analysis. PLoS Genet 2008;4(4):e1000024.

37. Eyre S, Bowes J, Diogo D, et al. High-density genetic mapping identifies new susceptibility loci for rheumatoid arthritis. Nat Genet 2012;44(12):1336–40.

38. Plenge RM, Cotsapas C, Davies L, et al. Two independent alleles at 6q23 associated with risk of rheumatoid arthritis. Nat Genet 2007;39(12):1477–82.

39. Han B, Diogo D, Eyre S, et al. Fine mapping seronegative and seropositive rheumatoid arthritis to shared and distinct HLA alleles by adjusting for the effects of heterogeneity. Am J Hum Genet 2014;94(4):522–32.

40. Kurreeman F, Liao K, Chibnik L, et al. Genetic basis of autoantibody positive and negative rheumatoid arthritis risk in a multi-ethnic cohort derived from electronic health records. Am J Hum Genet 2011;88(1):57–69.
41. Morgan AW, Thomson W, Martin SG, et al. Reevaluation of the interaction between HLA-DRB1 shared epitope alleles, PTPN22, and smoking in determining susceptibility to autoantibody-positive and autoantibody-negative rheumatoid arthritis in a large UK Caucasian population. Arthritis Rheum 2009;60(9):2565–76.
42. Kallberg H, Padyukov L, Plenge RM, et al. Gene-gene and gene-environment interactions involving HLA-DRB1, PTPN22, and smoking in two subsets of rheumatoid arthritis. Am J Hum Genet 2007;80(5):867–75.
43. Haj Hensvold A, Magnusson PK, Joshua V, et al. Environmental and genetic factors in the development of anticitrullinated protein antibodies (ACPAs) and ACPA-positive rheumatoid arthritis: an epidemiological investigation in twins. Ann Rheum Dis 2013. [Epub ahead of print].
44. Sugiyama D, Nishimura K, Tamaki K, et al. Impact of smoking as a risk factor for developing rheumatoid arthritis: a meta-analysis of observational studies. Ann Rheum Dis 2010;69(1):70–81.
45. Criswell LA, Merlino LA, Cerhan JR, et al. Cigarette smoking and the risk of rheumatoid arthritis among postmenopausal women: results from the Iowa Women's Health Study. Am J Med 2002;112(6):465–71.
46. Costenbader KH, Feskanich D, Mandl LA, et al. Smoking intensity, duration, and cessation, and the risk of rheumatoid arthritis in women. Am J Med 2006;119(6): 503.e1–9.
47. Yahya A, Bengtsson C, Lai TC, et al. Smoking is associated with an increased risk of developing ACPA-positive but not ACPA-negative rheumatoid arthritis in Asian populations: evidence from the Malaysian MyEIRA case-control study. Mod Rheumatol 2012;22(4):524–31.
48. Vessey MP, Villard-Mackintosh L, Yeates D. Oral contraceptives, cigarette smoking and other factors in relation to arthritis. Contraception 1987;35(5):457–64.
49. Hernandez Avila M, Liang MH, Willett WC, et al. Reproductive factors, smoking, and the risk for rheumatoid arthritis. Epidemiology 1990;1(4):285–91.
50. Hazes JM, Dijkmans BA, Vandenbroucke JP, et al. Lifestyle and the risk of rheumatoid arthritis: cigarette smoking and alcohol consumption. Ann Rheum Dis 1990;49(12):980–2.
51. Heliovaara M, Aho K, Aromaa A, et al. Smoking and risk of rheumatoid arthritis. J Rheumatol 1993;20(11):1830–5.
52. Karlson EW, Lee IM, Cook NR, et al. A retrospective cohort study of cigarette smoking and risk of rheumatoid arthritis in female health professionals. Arthritis Rheum 1999;42(5):910–7.
53. Uhlig T, Hagen KB, Kvien TK. Current tobacco smoking, formal education, and the risk of rheumatoid arthritis. J Rheumatol 1999;26(1):47–54.
54. Di Giuseppe D, Orsini N, Alfredsson L, et al. Cigarette smoking and smoking cessation in relation to risk of rheumatoid arthritis in women. Arthritis Res Ther 2013;15(2):R56.
55. Okamoto S, Adachi M, Chujo S, et al. Etiological role of cigarette smoking in rheumatoid arthritis: nasal exposure to cigarette smoke condensate extracts augments the development of collagen-induced arthritis in mice. Biochem Biophys Res Commun 2011;404(4):1088–92.
56. Kallberg H, Ding B, Padyukov L, et al. Smoking is a major preventable risk factor for rheumatoid arthritis: estimations of risks after various exposures to cigarette smoke. Ann Rheum Dis 2011;70(3):508–11.

57. Wesley A, Bengtsson C, Elkan AC, et al. Association between body mass index and anti-citrullinated protein antibody-positive and anti-citrullinated protein antibody-negative rheumatoid arthritis: results from a population-based case-control study. Arthritis Care Res (Hoboken) 2013;65(1):107–12.

58. Shapiro JA, Koepsell TD, Voigt LF, et al. Diet and rheumatoid arthritis in women: a possible protective effect of fish consumption. Epidemiology 1996;7(3): 256–63.

59. Symmons DP, Bankhead CR, Harrison BJ, et al. Blood transfusion, smoking, and obesity as risk factors for the development of rheumatoid arthritis: results from a primary care-based incident case-control study in Norfolk, England. Arthritis Rheum 1997;40(11):1955–61.

60. Karlson EW, Mandl LA, Hankinson SE, et al. Do breast-feeding and other reproductive factors influence future risk of rheumatoid arthritis? Results from the Nurses' Health Study. Arthritis Rheum 2004;50(11):3458–67.

61. Orellana C, Wedren S, Kallberg H, et al. Parity and the risk of developing rheumatoid arthritis: results from the Swedish Epidemiological Investigation of Rheumatoid Arthritis study. Ann Rheum Dis 2013;73:752–5.

62. Stolt P, Kallberg H, Lundberg I, et al. Silica exposure is associated with increased risk of developing rheumatoid arthritis: results from the Swedish EIRA study. Ann Rheum Dis 2005;64(4):582–6.

63. Stolt P, Yahya A, Bengtsson C, et al. Silica exposure among male current smokers is associated with a high risk of developing ACPA-positive rheumatoid arthritis. Ann Rheum Dis 2010;69(6):1072–6.

64. Rosell M, Wesley AM, Rydin K, et al. Dietary fish and fish oil and the risk of rheumatoid arthritis. Epidemiology 2009;20(6):896–901.

65. Di Giuseppe D, Wallin A, Bottai M, et al. Long-term intake of dietary long-chain n-3 polyunsaturated fatty acids and risk of rheumatoid arthritis: a prospective cohort study of women. Ann Rheum Dis 2013. [Epub ahead of print].

66. Demoruelle MK, Deane KD, Holers VM. When and where does inflammation begin in rheumatoid arthritis? Curr Opin Rheumatol 2014;26(1):64–71.

67. Makrygiannakis D, Hermansson M, Ulfgren AK, et al. Smoking increases peptidylarginine deiminase 2 enzyme expression in human lungs and increases citrullination in BAL cells. Ann Rheum Dis 2008;67(10):1488–92.

68. de Pablo P, Dietrich T, McAlindon TE. Association of periodontal disease and tooth loss with rheumatoid arthritis in the US population. J Rheumatol 2008; 35(1):70–6.

69. Chen HH, Huang N, Chen YM, et al. Association between a history of periodontitis and the risk of rheumatoid arthritis: a nationwide, population-based, case-control study. Ann Rheum Dis 2013;72(7):1206–11.

70. Mangat P, Wegner N, Venables PJ, et al. Bacterial and human peptidylarginine deiminases: targets for inhibiting the autoimmune response in rheumatoid arthritis? Arthritis Res Ther 2010;12(3):209.

71. Mikuls TR, Thiele GM, Deane KD, et al. *Porphyromonas gingivalis* and disease-related autoantibodies in individuals at increased risk of rheumatoid arthritis. Arthritis Rheum 2012;64(11):3522–30.

72. Klareskog L, Stolt P, Lundberg K, et al. A new model for an etiology of rheumatoid arthritis: smoking may trigger HLA-DR (shared epitope)-restricted immune reactions to autoantigens modified by citrullination. Arthritis Rheum 2006;54(1): 38–46.

73. Klareskog L, Padyukov L, Ronnelid J, et al. Genes, environment and immunity in the development of rheumatoid arthritis. Curr Opin Immunol 2006;18(6):650–5.

74. Too CL, Yahya A, Murad S, et al. Smoking interacts with HLA-DRB1 shared epitope in the development of anti-citrullinated protein antibody-positive rheumatoid arthritis: results from the Malaysian Epidemiological Investigation of Rheumatoid Arthritis (MyEIRA). Arthritis Res Ther 2012;14(2):R89.

75. Karlson EW, Chang SC, Cui J, et al. Gene-environment interaction between HLA-DRB1 shared epitope and heavy cigarette smoking in predicting incident rheumatoid arthritis. Ann Rheum Dis 2010;69(1):54–60.

76. Lundstrom E, Kallberg H, Alfredsson L, et al. Gene-environment interaction between the DRB1 shared epitope and smoking in the risk of anti-citrullinated protein antibody-positive rheumatoid arthritis: all alleles are important. Arthritis Rheum 2009;60(6):1597–603.

77. Hill JA, Southwood S, Sette A, et al. Cutting edge: the conversion of arginine to citrulline allows for a high-affinity peptide interaction with the rheumatoid arthritis-associated HLA-DRB1*0401 MHC class II molecule. J Immunol 2003; 171(2):538–41.

78. Klareskog L, Malmstrom V, Lundberg K, et al. Smoking, citrullination and genetic variability in the immunopathogenesis of rheumatoid arthritis. Semin Immunol 2011;23(2):92–8.

79. Mahdi H, Fisher BA, Kallberg H, et al. Specific interaction between genotype, smoking and autoimmunity to citrullinated alpha-enolase in the etiology of rheumatoid arthritis. Nat Genet 2009;41(12):1319–24.

80. Lundberg K, Bengtsson C, Kharlamova N, et al. Genetic and environmental determinants for disease risk in subsets of rheumatoid arthritis defined by the anticitrullinated protein/peptide antibody fine specificity profile. Ann Rheum Dis 2013;72(5):652–8.

81. Keenan BT, Chibnik LB, Cui J, et al. Effect of interactions of glutathione S-transferase T1, M1, and P1 and HMOX1 gene promoter polymorphisms with heavy smoking on the risk of rheumatoid arthritis. Arthritis Rheum 2010;62(11): 3196–210.

82. Urowitz MB, Gladman DD, Tom BD, et al. Changing patterns in mortality and disease outcomes for patients with systemic lupus erythematosus. J Rheumatol 2008;35(11):2152–8.

83. Von Feldt JM. Systemic lupus erythematosus. Recognizing its various presentations. Postgrad Med 1995;97(4):79, 83, 86 passim.

84. Hochberg MC. Updating the American College of Rheumatology revised criteria for the classification of systemic lupus erythematosus. Arthritis Rheum 1997; 40(9):1725.

85. Tan EM, Cohen AS, Fries JF, et al. The 1982 revised criteria for the classification of systemic lupus erythematosus. Arthritis Rheum 1982;25(11):1271–7.

86. Rullo OJ, Tsao BP. Recent insights into the genetic basis of systemic lupus erythematosus. Ann Rheum Dis 2013;72(Suppl 2):ii56–61.

87. Chung SA, Criswell LA. PTPN22: its role in SLE and autoimmunity. Autoimmunity 2007;40(8):582–90.

88. Suarez-Gestal M, Calaza M, Dieguez-Gonzalez R, et al. Rheumatoid arthritis does not share most of the newly identified systemic lupus erythematosus genetic factors. Arthritis Rheum 2009;60(9):2558–64.

89. Hughes T, Adler A, Kelly JA, et al. Evidence for gene-gene epistatic interactions among susceptibility loci for systemic lupus erythematosus. Arthritis Rheum 2012;64(2):485–92.

90. Borchers AT, Naguwa SM, Shoenfeld Y, et al. The geoepidemiology of systemic lupus erythematosus. Autoimmun Rev 2010;9(5):A277–87.

91. Costenbader KH, Kim DJ, Peerzada J, et al. Cigarette smoking and the risk of systemic lupus erythematosus: a meta-analysis. Arthritis Rheum 2004;50(3): 849–57.
92. Bengtsson AA, Rylander L, Hagmar L, et al. Risk factors for developing systemic lupus erythematosus: a case-control study in southern Sweden. Rheumatology (Oxford) 2002;41(5):563–71.
93. Cooper GS, Wither J, Bernatsky S, et al. Occupational and environmental exposures and risk of systemic lupus erythematosus: silica, sunlight, solvents. Rheumatology (Oxford) 2010;49(11):2172–80.
94. Barbhaiya M, Costenbader KH. Ultraviolet radiation and systemic lupus erythematosus. Lupus 2014;23:588–95.
95. Kang I, Quan T, Nolasco H, et al. Defective control of latent Epstein-Barr virus infection in systemic lupus erythematosus. J Immunol 2004;172(2): 1287–94.
96. Poole BD, Scofield RH, Harley JB, et al. Epstein-Barr virus and molecular mimicry in systemic lupus erythematosus. Autoimmunity 2006;39(1):63–70.
97. Cooper GS, Dooley MA, Treadwell EL, et al. Hormonal and reproductive risk factors for development of systemic lupus erythematosus: results of a population-based, case-control study. Arthritis Rheum 2002;46(7):1830–9.
98. Simard JF, Costenbader KH. What can epidemiology tell us about systemic lupus erythematosus? Int J Clin Pract 2007;61(7):1170–80.
99. Costenbader KH, Feskanich D, Stampfer MJ, et al. Reproductive and menopausal factors and risk of systemic lupus erythematosus in women. Arthritis Rheum 2007;56(4):1251–62.
100. Bernier MO, Mikaeloff Y, Hudson M, et al. Combined oral contraceptive use and the risk of systemic lupus erythematosus. Arthritis Rheum 2009;61(4):476–81.
101. Kiyohara C, Washio M, Horiuchi T, et al. Cigarette smoking, N-acetyltransferase 2 polymorphisms and systemic lupus erythematosus in a Japanese population. Lupus 2009;18(7):630–8.
102. Fraser PA, Ding WZ, Mohseni M, et al. Glutathione S-transferase M null homozygosity and risk of systemic lupus erythematosus associated with sun exposure: a possible gene-environment interaction for autoimmunity. J Rheumatol 2003; 30(2):276–82.
103. Shapira Y, Agmon-Levin N, Shoenfeld Y. Geoepidemiology of autoimmune rheumatic diseases. Nat Rev Rheumatol 2010;6(8):468–76.
104. van der Linden S, Valkenburg HA, Cats A. Evaluation of diagnostic criteria for ankylosing spondylitis. A proposal for modification of the New York criteria. Arthritis Rheum 1984;27(4):361–8.
105. Sieper J, Rudwaleit M, Baraliakos X, et al. The Assessment of SpondyloArthritis international Society (ASAS) handbook: a guide to assess spondyloarthritis. Ann Rheum Dis 2009;68(Suppl 2):ii1–44.
106. Schlosstein L, Terasaki PI, Bluestone R, et al. High association of an HL-A antigen, W27, with ankylosing spondylitis. N Engl J Med 1973;288(14):704–6.
107. Reveille JD. Genetics of spondyloarthritis–beyond the MHC. Nat Rev Rheumatol 2012;8(5):296–304.
108. Cortes A, Hadler J, Pointon JP, et al. Identification of multiple risk variants for ankylosing spondylitis through high-density genotyping of immune-related loci. Nat Genet 2013;45(7):730–8.
109. Sorrentino R, Bockmann RA, Fiorillo MT. HLA-B27 and antigen presentation: at the crossroads between immune defense and autoimmunity. Mol Immunol 2014;57(1):22–7.

110. Payeli SK, Kollnberger S, Marroquin Belaunzaran O, et al. Inhibiting HLA-B27 homodimer-driven immune cell inflammation in spondylarthritis. Arthritis Rheum 2012;64(10):3139–49.
111. Mear JP, Schreiber KL, Munz C, et al. Misfolding of HLA-B27 as a result of its B pocket suggests a novel mechanism for its role in susceptibility to spondyloarthropathies. J Immunol 1999;163(12):6665–70.
112. Colbert RA, DeLay ML, Klenk EI, et al. From HLA-B27 to spondyloarthritis: a journey through the ER. Immunol Rev 2010;233(1):181–202.
113. Carter JD, Gerard HC, Espinoza LR, et al. Chlamydiae as etiologic agents in chronic undifferentiated spondylarthritis. Arthritis Rheum 2009;60(5):1311–6.
114. Nickerson CL, Luthra HS, David CS. Role of enterobacteria and HLA-B27 in spondyloarthropathies: studies with transgenic mice. Ann Rheum Dis 1990; 49(Suppl 1):426–33.
115. Berthelot JM, Glemarec J, Guillot P, et al. New pathogenic hypotheses for spondyloarthropathies. Joint Bone Spine 2002;69(2):114–22.
116. Van Praet L, Van den Bosch F, Mielants H, et al. Mucosal inflammation in spondylarthritides: past, present, and future. Curr Rheumatol Rep 2011;13(5): 409–15.
117. Wendling D, Prati C. Spondyloarthritis and smoking: towards a new insight into the disease. Expert Rev Clin Immunol 2013;9(6):511–6.
118. Gooren LJ, Giltay EJ, van Schaardenburg D, et al. Gonadal and adrenal sex steroids in ankylosing spondylitis. Rheum Dis Clin North Am 2000;26(4):969–87.
119. Kuon W, Holzhutter HG, Appel H, et al. Identification of HLA-B27-restricted peptides from the *Chlamydia trachomatis* proteome with possible relevance to HLA-B27-associated diseases. J Immunol 2001;167(8):4738–46.
120. Hjelholt A, Carlsen T, Deleuran B, et al. Increased levels of IgG antibodies against human HSP60 in patients with spondyloarthritis. PLoS One 2013;8(2): e56210.
121. Feng XG, Xu XJ, Ye S, et al. Recent *Chlamydia pneumoniae* infection is highly associated with active ankylosing spondylitis in a Chinese cohort. Scand J Rheumatol 2011;40(4):289–91.
122. Costenbader KH, Gay S, Alarcon-Riquelme ME, et al. Genes, epigenetic regulation and environmental factors: which is the most relevant in developing autoimmune diseases? Autoimmun Rev 2012;11(8):604–9.
123. Brooks WH, Le Dantec C, Pers JO, et al. Epigenetics and autoimmunity. J Autoimmun 2010;34(3):J207–19.
124. Ballestar E, Esteller M, Richardson BC. The epigenetic face of systemic lupus erythematosus. J Immunol 2006;176(12):7143–7.
125. Cortijo S, Wardenaar R, Colome-Tatche M, et al. Mapping the epigenetic basis of complex traits. Science 2014;343(6175):1145–8.
126. Garaud S, Le Dantec C, Jousse-Joulin S, et al. IL-6 modulates CD5 expression in B cells from patients with lupus by regulating DNA methylation. J Immunol 2009;182(9):5623–32.
127. Lu Q, Wu A, Richardson BC. Demethylation of the same promoter sequence increases CD70 expression in lupus T cells and T cells treated with lupus-inducing drugs. J Immunol 2005;174(10):6212–9.
128. Lu Q, Kaplan M, Ray D, et al. Demethylation of ITGAL (CD11a) regulatory sequences in systemic lupus erythematosus. Arthritis Rheum 2002;46(5):1282–91.
129. Teh AL, Pan H, Chen L, et al. The effect of genotype and in utero environment on inter-individual variation in neonate DNA methylomes. Genome Res 2014;24: 1064–74.

130. Dogan MV, Shields B, Cutrona C, et al. The effect of smoking on DNA methylation of peripheral blood mononuclear cells from African American women. BMC Genomics 2014;15:151.

131. Liu Y, Aryee MJ, Padyukov L, et al. Epigenome-wide association data implicate DNA methylation as an intermediary of genetic risk in rheumatoid arthritis. Nat Biotechnol 2013;31(2):142–7.

132. Liu Y, Li X, Aryee MJ, et al. GeMes, clusters of DNA methylation under genetic control, can inform genetic and epigenetic analysis of disease. Am J Hum Genet 2014;94(4):485–95.

133. Scher JU, Sczesnak A, Longman RS, et al. Expansion of intestinal *Prevotella copri* correlates with enhanced susceptibility to arthritis. Elife (Cambridge) 2013;2: e01202.

134. Scrivo R, Casadei L, Valerio M, et al. Metabolomics approach in allergic and rheumatic diseases. Curr Allergy Asthma Rep 2014;14(6):445.

135. Young SP, Kapoor SR, Viant MR, et al. The impact of inflammation on metabolomic profiles in patients with arthritis. Arthritis Rheum 2013;65(8):2015–23.

136. Kapoor SR, Filer A, Fitzpatrick MA, et al. Metabolic profiling predicts response to anti-tumor necrosis factor alpha therapy in patients with rheumatoid arthritis. Arthritis Rheum 2013;65(6):1448–56.

Is Preclinical Autoimmunity Benign?

The Case of Cardiovascular Disease

 CrossMark

Darcy S. Majka, MD, MS[a,b],*, Rowland W. Chang, MD, MPH[a,b]

KEYWORDS

- Autoantibodies • Autoimmunity • Preclinical • Cardiovascular disease
- Coronary artery calcification • Intima media thickness

KEY POINTS

- Preclinical rheumatic disease–related autoantibodies have been identified in stored samples before development of systemic lupus erythematosus and rheumatoid arthritis (RA).
- Autoreactive B cells can drive RA pathogenesis through generation of autoantibody-secreting plasma cells, presentation of autoantigens such as citrullinated peptides to T cells, production of proinflammatory cytokines, and formation of ectopic tertiary lymphoid structures, as are found in the RA synovium.
- It has been hypothesized that atherosclerosis might have autoimmune features because of the involvement of autoantigens and their autoantibodies in atherogenesis in both humans and animal models.
- Antiphospholipid antibodies, antinuclear antibodies, and RA–related autoantibodies have been associated with atherosclerosis in clinically active rheumatic diseases as well as in general population study samples.

INTRODUCTION

Preclinical autoimmunity, or the presence of autoantibodies before disease symptoms, has been well described for several autoimmune rheumatic diseases, such as rheumatoid arthritis (RA), systemic lupus erythematosus (SLE), Sjögren syndrome,

Funding Sources: R01 HL104047, P60AR064464 (Dr D.S. Majka); R21 AR062317, P60 AR064464, R01 AR054155, R01 HL104047 (Dr R.W. Chang).
Disclosures/Conflict of Interest: None.
[a] Division of Rheumatology, Northwestern University Feinberg School of Medicine, 240 East Huron, M300, Chicago, IL 60611, USA; [b] Department of Preventive Medicine, Northwestern University Feinberg School of Medicine, 680 North Lake Shore Drive, Suite 1400, Chicago, IL 60611, USA
* Corresponding author. Northwestern University Feinberg School of Medicine, 240 East Huron, M300, Chicago, IL 60611.
E-mail address: d-majka@northwestern.edu

Rheum Dis Clin N Am 40 (2014) 659–668
http://dx.doi.org/10.1016/j.rdc.2014.07.006
0889-857X/14/$ – see front matter © 2014 Elsevier Inc. All rights reserved.

rheumatic.theclinics.com

and antiphospholipid antibody syndrome (APS).[1–7] In studies of preclinical autoanti-bodies before SLE development, Arbuckle and colleagues[2] noted that autoantibodies less commonly associated with clinical sequelae of SLE such as antinuclear anti-bodies (ANA), anti-Ro, and antiphospholipid antibodies (APA) were present in the preclinical period more remote to clinical illness, whereas antibodies more specific for pathogenic features of SLE such as anti-Smith, antibodies against double-stranded DNA (dsDNA), and ribonucleoprotein (RNP) developed later, simultaneous to the onset of clinical features of SLE. Thus, benign autoimmunity was used to describe the earlier phase of autoantibody appearance during the preclinical period (**Fig. 1**). Certainly, there are many examples of autoantibodies occurring in disease-free individuals: RA-related autoantibodies and ANA occur in increased number and titer with age-related loss of tolerance[8–11]; healthy relatives of individuals with autoimmune rheumatic diseases also have increased rates of autoantibody positi-vity.[9,12,13] However, although ANA, rheumatoid factor, and APA may occur in the general population, individuals with such autoantibodies are also at increased risk for development of autoimmune rheumatic disease, with odds estimated as high as 10-fold to 30-fold.[6,7]

Autoantibodies are markers for autoreactive B-cell activation, which can drive dis-ease pathogenesis through a variety of mechanisms. Autoreactive B cells lead to the generation of autoantibody-secreting plasma cells, formation of immune complexes, presentation of autoantigens to T cells and costimulation, as well as the production of proinflammatory cytokines, chemokines, and lymphangiogenic growth factors. But when does benign become pathogenic autoimmunity during disease develop-ment? Early on, autoantigens activate self-reactive B cells, leading to the formation of short-lived plasma cells secreting autoantibodies. However, if self-reactive B cells enter germinal centers, they may undergo somatic hypermutation and affinity maturation of B-cell receptors, immunoglobulin class switching, generation of long-lived self-reactive B cells, and differentiation into long-lived plasma cells secreting high-affinity Fc receptor-binding autoantibodies.[14,15] An example of such a transition

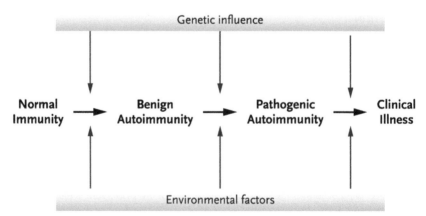

Fig. 1. Phases in the development of pathogenic autoimmunity. Normal immunity pro-gresses to benign autoimmunity through the influence of genetic composition and environ-ment. Later, benign autoimmunity progresses to pathogenic autoimmunity. Symptoms of clinical illness appear soon after pathogenic autoimmunity develops. (*From* Arbuckle MR, McClain MT, Rubertone MV, et al. Development of autoantibodies before the clinical onset of systemic lupus erythematosus. N Engl J Med 2003;349:1532; with permission.)

is the formation of the ectopic tertiary lymphoid structures in the RA synovium, which clearly leads to the pathogenic autoimmune features of RA.[16,17]

As described in detail elsewhere in this issue of *Rheumatic Disease Clinics*, the identification of preclinical autoimmunity before rheumatic disease development has led to substantial efforts to accurately describe autoimmune rheumatic disease pathogenesis such that individuals might be identified and targeted for primary prevention strategies, or secondary prevention strategies in the case of early disease features not yet meeting disease classification criteria. Recent data suggest that autoantibodies might be risk factors for development of cardiovascular disease (CVD) as well.

ANTIPHOSPHOLIPID ANTIBODIES, RHEUMATOID ARTHRITIS-RELATED AUTOANTIBODIES, AND CARDIOVASCULAR DISEASE, AS WELL AS SUBCLINICAL ATHEROSCLEROSIS, IN PATIENTS WITH AUTOIMMUNE RHEUMATIC DISEASE

Patients with RA have an increased risk for CVD of 1.5-fold to 2-fold, comparable with the risk in type II diabetes mellitus.[18,19] Moreover, the presence of traditional risk factors does not fully account for this degree of excess risk. Therefore, it has been proposed that autoimmune-mediated inflammation may contribute to increased CVD risk in RA.[20] RA-related autoantibody positivity has been associated with increased risk of CVD events among patients with RA.[21-23] There is an increased prevalence of subclinical measures of atherosclerosis in RA,[24] and antibodies to modified citrullinated vimentin and anticyclic citrullinated peptide antibodies (anti-CCP) have been correlated with carotid intima media thickness (IMT) in early RA.[25,26]

CVD is a leading cause for mortality in SLE,[27] and given that APA are present in greater abundance in SLE compared with the general population, they have been evaluated as potential risk factors for CVD in SLE. In a large US prospective cohort of patients with SLE evaluated for myocardial infarction (MI) and subclinical atherosclerosis, patients with history of positivity for the lupus anticoagulant had a higher prevalence of history of MI (22% vs 9%, $P = .04$).[28] In a unique prospective study for hard clinical cardiovascular end points in 182 Swedish patients with SLE free from CVD at baseline, Gustafsson and colleagues[29] found that presence of any anti-cardiolipin autoantibodies (aCL) or anti-β2 glycoprotein (anti-β2GPI) autoantibodies were strongly associated with an increased risk of first CVD events over a mean of 8.3 years (hazard ratio [HR] 4.9, 95% confidence interval [CI] 1.76, 17.72). In contrast, anti-Smith, anti-dsDNA, and RNP had lower point estimates for this association, but these did not reach statistical significance. In a follow-up of 208 patients with SLE in the same inclusion cohort over 12 years, presence of any APA was predictive of cardiovascular mortality (HR 2.8, 95% CI 1.1–1.7) and again, whereas specific anti-dsDNA antibodies were associated with noncardiovascular mortality, they were not associated with cardiovascular mortality.[30] Moreover, levels of aCL and anti-β2GPI autoantibodies were also associated with myocardial perfusion defects detected by single-photon emission computed tomography, but not in the distribution of major coronary arteries, suggesting that APA may also cause small, undetected thrombi in the coronary microcirculation.[31]

Previously, there was no known association in patients with SLE between APA and coronary artery calcification (CAC), a marker of overall atherosclerotic burden.[28] However, in a small group of patients with SLE (N = 60), Plazak and colleagues[32] recently reported an increased risk of CAC in patients with both increased aCL and anti-β2GPI IgG levels, and among 139 patients with SLE, Romero-Diaz and colleagues[33] reported increased levels of aCL in those with CAC.

ANTIPHOSPHOLIPID ANTIBODIES, ANTINUCLEAR ANTIBODIES, AND RHEUMATOID ARTHRITIS-RELATED AUTOANTIBODIES AND CARDIOVASCULAR DISEASE, AS WELL AS SUBCLINICAL ATHEROSCLEROSIS, IN PATIENTS WITHOUT AUTOIMMUNE RHEUMATIC DISEASE

The increased prevalence of CVD in autoimmune rheumatic diseases such as RA and lupus, and the increased risk of CVD in patients with rheumatic disease with auto-antibodies suggest that CVD may have autoimmune features. Studies identifying relationships between autoantibodies and cardiovascular outcomes in individuals without clinically active autoimmune diseases certainly support the role of autoimmunity in the pathogenesis of CVD. In 3 general population samples,[34–36] RF positivity has been associated with ischemic heart disease. Tomasson and colleagues[36] reported an increased risk of cardiovascular mortality in RF-positive patients followed prospectively over 23 years in their Icelandic Reykjavik population-based cohort, even after excluding participants with any joint symptoms (HR 1.60, 95% CI 1.08–2.37). Also, in a recent nested case-control study within a cohort of middle-aged healthy UK men followed for CVD,[37] participants with anti-CCP2 positivity had more ischemic heart disease (odds ratio [OR] 4.23, 95% CI 1.22–14.61). We measured the association of RA-related autoantibodies with CAC, using data from a community-based sample of 6814 men and women enrolled in the MESA (Multi-Ethnic Study of Atherosclerosis) trial.[38] Although we found that RA-related autoantibodies were associated with CAC in African American and white women, these data need to be verified in other general population cohorts without clinically active RA, and associations between RA-related autoantibodies and IMT need to be investigated.

Although there is a paucity of studies identifying clear-cut associations between specific ANA and cardiovascular outcomes in patients with SLE, one study evaluating patients without SLE presenting with chest pain[39] found that patients with triple vessel coronary artery disease had higher odds of positive ANA (OR 11.67, 95% CI 3.91–17.82) compared with controls with negative angiograms. In addition, in a population-based cohort study of 7852 patients who had ANA testing, Liang and colleagues[35] found that a positive ANA was associated with risk of MI, independent of the presence of SLE diagnosis (HR 1.29, 95% CI 1.03–1.61). Furthermore, there are numerous studies reporting associations between APA and cardiovascular outcomes in individuals without autoimmune rheumatic diseases. In particular, in several studies,[40–49] APA have been found in the sera and plaques of individuals with clinical cardiovascular events. A few studies have reported positive correlations between APA and IMT, and in a case-control study of 50 male patients with acute MI, Dropinski and colleagues[42] found APA level to be higher in MI cases, and APA level correlated with IMT as well.[50,51] Although previous studies in individuals without SLE did not identify associations between APA and CAC,[45,52] we did find associations when we tested the hypothesis that circulating APA are associated with subsequent subclinical atherosclerosis, measured as CAC in a cohort of community-based African American and white young adults followed prospectively for subclinical and clinical cardiovascular outcomes in the CARDIA (Coronary Artery Risk Development in Young Adults) study.[53] After adjustment for traditional cardiovascular risk factors, APA were associated with subclinical atherosclerosis measured as CAC greater than 0 after 15 years of follow-up. IgG and IgA anti-β2GPI antibodies were associated with CAC greater than 0 measured after 15 years of follow-up (anti-β2GPI IgG: OR 6.4, 95% CI 2.4–16.8; IgA: OR 5.6, 95% CI 2.3–13.2). Anti-β2GPI IgM was marginally associated with CAC greater than 0 (IgM: OR 1.7, 95% CI 1.0–3.1), and aCL IgG were also associated with CAC greater than 0 (OR 5.1, 95% CI 1.4–18.6).

Associations between rheumatic disease autoantibodies and subclinical and clinical atherosclerosis in individuals without rheumatic disease have led us to propose a possible model in which preclinical autoantibodies are not only risk factors for connective tissue disease development but also for subclinical and clinical CVD (**Fig. 2**), and their association with CVD development might occur in parallel with, or even independent of the presence of autoimmune rheumatic diseases.

POSSIBLE MECHANISMS FOR ASSOCIATIONS BETWEEN AUTOANTIBODIES AND ATHEROSCLEROSIS

As reported elsewhere in this issue, there is abundant evidence that autoimmune processes occur before clinical diagnosis of RA and SLE. Work by Maradit-Kremers and colleagues[54] furthermore reported that in the preclinical period of RA development, pre-RA cases already had increased risk for coronary heart disease. In their landmark retrospective longitudinal RA incidence cohort study within the Rochester Epidemiology Project, during the preclinical period 2 years before RA diagnosis, cases had increased odds of acute MI (OR 3.17, 95% CI 1.16–8.68), sudden death (HR 1.94, 95% CI 1.06–3.55), and unrecognized MI (OR 5.86, 95% CI 1.29–26.64) compared with controls. Therefore, autoimmune-mediated processes occurring during the preclinical period may lead to coronary artery disease development. Sokolove and colleagues[55] reported citrullinated proteins within atherosclerotic aorta segments from men without autoimmune rheumatic diseases. These citrullinated proteins were also recognized by anti-citrullinated peptide antibodies (ACPAs) derived from patients with RA, indicating that ACPAs might propagate the progression of atherosclerosis. In addition, the previous findings of associations between APA and subclinical atherosclerosis suggest that the role of APA in the pathogenesis of atherosclerosis is not merely prothrombotic. This theory has been explored in animal models. Both monoclonal aCL bound to β2GPI and anti-β2GPI IgG derived from an APS mouse model

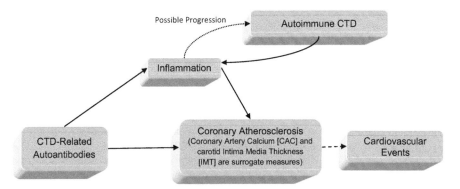

Conceptual Model for the Relationship between Autoimmunity and
Cardiovascular Disease Development

Fig. 2. Connective tissue disease (CTD)-related autoimmunity might lead to inflammation and epitope spreading, which can progress to clinically active autoimmune CTD. It is hypothesized that the increased prevalence of atherosclerosis and subsequent cardiovascular events in autoimmune CTD is mediated by inflammation from disease activity. CTD-related autoimmunity might be independently associated with the development of atherosclerosis, which can be measured by the surrogate CAC or IMT. Subclinical atherosclerosis might then progress to clinical cardiovascular events.

enhanced oxidized low-density lipoprotein (LDL)/β2GPI complex binding to macrophages, and oxidized LDL uptake by macrophages promotes foam cell formation.[56,57] Moreover, APA increased atherosclerotic lesions in a mouse model of atherosclerosis, the LDL-receptor knockout mouse (LDL-RKO): mouse aCL, induced by immunization of LDL-RKO mice with human aCL, led to increased fatty streak formation,[58] and immunization of LDL-RKO mice with β2GPI also led to accelerated atherosclerotic lesions.[59] These mechanistic studies lend biological plausibility to the theory that autoantibodies are direct risk factors for atherosclerosis.

FUTURE CONSIDERATIONS

These collective data indicate that preclinical autoimmunity or autoimmunity in individuals without clinically apparent disease are decidedly not benign. Numerous studies indicate autoantibodies might be markers for humoral and cell-mediated immune mechanisms driving CVD not only in individuals with but also in those without autoimmune rheumatic diseases. For patients with active RA, the European League Against Rheumatism[60] recently recommended annual cardiovascular risk assessment and management. Moreover, evidence is increasing for risk reduction from pharmaceutical interventions in active RA, such as anti–tumor necrosis factor α, hydroxychloroquine, statins, and possibly, methotrexate.[19,20] Because it has recently been shown that both rheumatologists and primary care physicians identify and manage cardiovascular risk factors less often in patients with RA compared with controls from the general population, interventions may be needed to improve CVD risk in patients with RA.[19,60–62] Potential preventive interventions for CVD development in SLE are of course being proposed as well.[63] It seems that the presence of autoantibodies might also be a pertinent risk marker for subclinical atherosclerosis and clinical CVD in the general population as well. Although further studies are needed to confirm the relevance of autoantibodies as CVD risk markers, we propose that preclinical autoimmunity might one day enable clinicians to identify individuals in the general population who might benefit from traditional risk factor assessment and measures targeted at CVD prevention, perhaps even measures targeting the process of autoimmunity.

REFERENCES

1. Arbuckle MR, James JA, Kohlhase KF, et al. Development of anti-dsDNA autoantibodies prior to clinical diagnosis of systemic lupus erythematosus. Scand J Immunol 2001;54(1–2):211–9.
2. Arbuckle MR, McClain MT, Rubertone MV, et al. Development of autoantibodies before the clinical onset of systemic lupus erythematosus. N Engl J Med 2003; 349(16):1526–33.
3. Arslan S, Erkut B, Ates A, et al. Pseudoaneurysm of left ventricular following left ventricular apical venting. Clin Res Cardiol 2009;98(4):280–2.
4. Majka DS, Deane KD, Parrish LA, et al. Duration of preclinical rheumatoid arthritis-related autoantibody positivity increases in subjects with older age at time of disease diagnosis. Ann Rheum Dis 2008;67(6):801–7.
5. Majka DS, Holers VM. Can we accurately predict the development of rheumatoid arthritis in the preclinical phase? Arthritis Rheum 2003;48(10): 2701–5.
6. Rantapaa-Dahlqvist S, de Jong BA, Berglin E, et al. Antibodies against cyclic citrullinated peptide and IgA rheumatoid factor predict the development of rheumatoid arthritis. Arthritis Rheum 2003;48(10):2741–9.

7. Eriksson C, Kokkonen H, Johansson M, et al. Autoantibodies predate the onset of systemic lupus erythematosus in northern Sweden. Arthritis Res Ther 2011; 13(1):R30.

8. Gerli R, Monti D, Bistoni O, et al. Chemokines, sTNF-Rs and sCD30 serum levels in healthy aged people and centenarians. Mech Ageing Dev 2000;121(1–3): 37–46.

9. Kim SK, Bae J, Lee H, et al. Greater prevalence of seropositivity for anti-cyclic citrullinated peptide antibody in unaffected first-degree relatives in multicase rheumatoid arthritis-affected families. Korean J Intern Med 2013;28(1):45–53.

10. Satoh M, Chan EK, Ho LA, et al. Prevalence and sociodemographic correlates of antinuclear antibodies in the United States. Arthritis Rheum 2012;64(7): 2319–27.

11. van Schaardenburg D, Lagaay AM, Otten HG, et al. The relation between class-specific serum rheumatoid factors and age in the general population. Br J Rheumatol 1993;32(7):546–9.

12. Arlestig L, Mullazehi M, Kokkonen H, et al. Antibodies against cyclic citrullinated peptides of IgG, IgA and IgM isotype and rheumatoid factor of IgM and IgA isotype are increased in unaffected members of multicase rheumatoid arthritis families from northern Sweden. Ann Rheum Dis 2012;71(6):825–9.

13. Ramos PS, Kelly JA, Gray-McGuire C, et al. Familial aggregation and linkage analysis of autoantibody traits in pedigrees multiplex for systemic lupus erythematosus. Genes Immun 2006;7(5):417–32.

14. Anolik JH. B cell biology and dysfunction in SLE. Bull NYU Hosp Jt Dis 2007; 65(3):182–6.

15. Townsend MJ, Monroe JG, Chan AC. B-cell targeted therapies in human autoimmune diseases: an updated perspective. Immunol Rev 2010;237(1):264–83.

16. Canete JD, Celis R, Moll C, et al. Clinical significance of synovial lymphoid neogenesis and its reversal after anti-tumour necrosis factor alpha therapy in rheumatoid arthritis. Ann Rheum Dis 2009;68(5):751–6.

17. Weyand CM, Goronzy JJ. Ectopic germinal center formation in rheumatoid synovitis. Ann N Y Acad Sci 2003;987:140–9.

18. Avina-Zubieta JA, Thomas J, Sadatsafavi M, et al. Risk of incident cardiovascular events in patients with rheumatoid arthritis: a meta-analysis of observational studies. Ann Rheum Dis 2012;71(9):1524–9.

19. Barbhaiya M, Solomon DH. Rheumatoid arthritis and cardiovascular disease: an update on treatment issues. Curr Opin Rheumatol 2013;25(3):317–24.

20. van Breukelen-van der Stoep DF, Klop B, van Zeben D, et al. Cardiovascular risk in rheumatoid arthritis: how to lower the risk? Atherosclerosis 2013;231(1): 163–72.

21. Ajeganova S, Andersson ML, Frostegard J, et al. Disease factors in early rheumatoid arthritis are associated with differential risks for cardiovascular events and mortality depending on age at onset: a 10-year observational cohort study. J Rheumatol 2013;40(12):1958–66.

22. Goodson NJ, Wiles NJ, Lunt M, et al. Mortality in early inflammatory polyarthritis: cardiovascular mortality is increased in seropositive patients. Arthritis Rheum 2002;46(8):2010–9.

23. Lopez-Longo FJ, Oliver-Minarro D, de la Torre I, et al. Association between anti-cyclic citrullinated peptide antibodies and ischemic heart disease in patients with rheumatoid arthritis. Arthritis Rheum 2009;61(4):419–24.

24. Kramer HR, Giles JT. Cardiovascular disease risk in rheumatoid arthritis: progress, debate, and opportunity. Arthritis Care Res (Hoboken) 2011;63(4):484–99.

25. El-Barbary AM, Kassem EM, El-Sergany MA, et al. Association of anti-modified citrullinated vimentin with subclinical atherosclerosis in early rheumatoid arthritis compared with anti-cyclic citrullinated peptide. J Rheumatol 2011; 38(5):828–34.

26. Gerli R, Sherer Y, Bocci EB, et al. Precocious atherosclerosis in rheumatoid arthritis: role of traditional and disease-related cardiovascular risk factors. Ann N Y Acad Sci 2007;1108:372–81.

27. Yurkovich M, Vostretsova K, Chen W, et al. Overall and cause-specific mortality in patients with systemic lupus erythematosus: a meta-analysis of observational studies. Arthritis Care Res (Hoboken) 2014;66(4):608–16.

28. Petri M. The lupus anticoagulant is a risk factor for myocardial infarction (but not atherosclerosis): Hopkins Lupus Cohort. Thromb Res 2004;114(5–6):593–5.

29. Gustafsson J, Gunnarsson I, Borjesson O, et al. Predictors of the first cardiovascular event in patients with systemic lupus erythematosus–a prospective cohort study. Arthritis Res Ther 2009;11(6):R186.

30. Gustafsson JT, Simard JF, Gunnarsson I, et al. Risk factors for cardiovascular mortality in patients with systemic lupus erythematosus, a prospective cohort study. Arthritis Res Ther 2012;14(2):R46.

31. Plazak W, Gryga K, Milewski M, et al. Association of heart structure and function abnormalities with laboratory findings in patients with systemic lupus erythematosus. Lupus 2011;20(9):936–44.

32. Plazak W, Pasowicz M, Kostkiewicz M, et al. Influence of chronic inflammation and autoimmunity on coronary calcifications and myocardial perfusion defects in systemic lupus erythematosus patients. Inflamm Res 2011;60(10):973–80.

33. Romero-Diaz J, Vargas-Vorackova F, Kimura-Hayama E, et al. Systemic lupus erythematosus risk factors for coronary artery calcifications. Rheumatology (Oxford) 2012;51(1):110–9.

34. Edwards CJ, Syddall H, Goswami R, et al. The autoantibody rheumatoid factor may be an independent risk factor for ischaemic heart disease in men. Heart 2007;93(10):1263–7.

35. Liang KP, Kremers HM, Crowson CS, et al. Autoantibodies and the risk of cardiovascular events. J Rheumatol 2009;36(11):2462–9.

36. Tomasson G, Aspelund T, Jonsson T, et al. Effect of rheumatoid factor on mortality and coronary heart disease. Ann Rheum Dis 2010;69(9):1649–54.

37. Cambridge G, Acharya J, Cooper JA, et al. Antibodies to citrullinated peptides and risk of coronary heart disease. Atherosclerosis 2013;228(1):243–6.

38. Majka DS, Chang RW, Pope RM, et al. Autoantibodies are associated with subclinical atherosclerosis and cardiovascular endpoints in Caucasian and African American women in a prospective study: the Multi-Ethnic Study of Atherosclerosis (MESA) [abstract]. Arthritis Rheum 2012;64(10):S711.

39. Grainger DJ, Bethell HW. High titres of serum antinuclear antibodies, mostly directed against nucleolar antigens, are associated with the presence of coronary atherosclerosis. Ann Rheum Dis 2002;61(2):110–4.

40. Adler Y, Finkelstein Y, Zandeman-Goddard G, et al. The presence of antiphospholipid antibodies in acute myocardial infarction. Lupus 1995;4(4):309–13.

41. Brey RL, Abbott RD, Curb JD, et al. Beta(2)-Glycoprotein 1-dependent anticardiolipin antibodies and risk of ischemic stroke and myocardial infarction: the Honolulu heart program. Stroke 2001;32(8):1701–6.

42. Dropinski J, Szczeklik W, Rubis P, et al. Anti-phospholipid antibodies and carotid-artery intima-media thickness in young survivors of myocardial infarction. Med Sci Monit 2003;9(4):BR105–9.

43. Hughes JR, Davies JA. Anticardiolipin antibodies in clinical conditions associated with a risk of thrombotic events. Thromb Res 1998;89(3):101–6.
44. Meroni PL, Peyvandi F, Foco L, et al. Anti-beta 2 glycoprotein I antibodies and the risk of myocardial infarction in young premenopausal women. J Thromb Haemost 2007;5(12):2421–8.
45. Sherer Y, Tenenbaum A, Praprotnik S, et al. Coronary artery disease but not coronary calcification is associated with elevated levels of cardiolipin, beta-2-glycoprotein-I, and oxidized LDL antibodies. Cardiology 2001;95(1):20–4.
46. Veres K, Lakos G, Kerenyi A, et al. Antiphospholipid antibodies in acute coronary syndrome. Lupus 2004;13(6):423–7.
47. Zuckerman E, Toubi E, Shiran A, et al. Anticardiolipin antibodies and acute myocardial infarction in non-systemic lupus erythematosus patients: a controlled prospective study. Am J Med 1996;101(4):381–6.
48. George J, Harats D, Gilburd B, et al. Immunolocalization of beta2-glycoprotein I (apolipoprotein H) to human atherosclerotic plaques: potential implications for lesion progression. Circulation 1999;99(17):2227–30.
49. Doria A, Sherer Y, Meroni PL, et al. Inflammation and accelerated atherosclerosis: basic mechanisms. Rheum Dis Clin North Am 2005;31(2):355–62, viii.
50. Ames PR, Margarita A, Delgado Alves J, et al. Anticardiolipin antibody titre and plasma homocysteine level independently predict intima media thickness of carotid arteries in subjects with idiopathic antiphospholipid antibodies. Lupus 2002;11(4):208–14.
51. Margarita A, Batuca J, Scenna G, et al. Subclinical atherosclerosis in primary antiphospholipid syndrome. Ann N Y Acad Sci 2007;1108:475–80.
52. Asanuma Y, Oeser A, Shintani AK, et al. Premature coronary-artery atherosclerosis in systemic lupus erythematosus. N Engl J Med 2003;349(25):2407–15.
53. Majka DS, Liu K, Pope RM, et al. Antiphospholipid antibodies and sub-clinical atherosclerosis in the Coronary Artery Risk Development in Young Adults (CARDIA) cohort. Inflamm Res 2013;62(10):919–27.
54. Maradit-Kremers H, Crowson CS, Nicola PJ, et al. Increased unrecognized coronary heart disease and sudden deaths in rheumatoid arthritis: a population-based cohort study. Arthritis Rheum 2005;52(2):402–11.
55. Sokolove J, Brennan MJ, Sharpe O, et al. Brief report: citrullination within the atherosclerotic plaque: a potential target for the anti-citrullinated protein antibody response in rheumatoid arthritis. Arthritis Rheum 2013;65(7):1719–24.
56. Kobayashi K, Lopez LR, Matsuura E. Atherogenic antiphospholipid antibodies in antiphospholipid syndrome. Ann N Y Acad Sci 2007;1108:489–96.
57. Hasunuma Y, Matsuura E, Makita Z, et al. Involvement of beta 2-glycoprotein I and anticardiolipin antibodies in oxidatively modified low-density lipoprotein uptake by macrophages. Clin Exp Immunol 1997;107(3):569–73.
58. George J, Harats D, Gilburd B, et al. Adoptive transfer of beta(2)-glycoprotein I-reactive lymphocytes enhances early atherosclerosis in LDL receptor-deficient mice. Circulation 2000;102(15):1822–7.
59. George J, Afek A, Gilburd B, et al. Induction of early atherosclerosis in LDL-receptor-deficient mice immunized with beta2-glycoprotein I. Circulation 1998;98(11):1108–15.
60. Peters MJ, Symmons DP, McCarey D, et al. EULAR evidence-based recommendations for cardiovascular risk management in patients with rheumatoid arthritis and other forms of inflammatory arthritis. Ann Rheum Dis 2010;69(2):325–31.

61. Desai SS, Myles JD, Kaplan MJ. Suboptimal cardiovascular risk factor identification and management in patients with rheumatoid arthritis: a cohort analysis. Arthritis Res Ther 2012;14(6):R270.
62. Toms TE, Panoulas VF, Douglas KM, et al. Statin use in rheumatoid arthritis in relation to actual cardiovascular risk: evidence for substantial undertreatment of lipid-associated cardiovascular risk? Ann Rheum Dis 2010;69(4):683–8.
63. Iaccarino L, Bettio S, Zen M, et al. Premature coronary heart disease in SLE: can we prevent progression? Lupus 2013;22(12):1232–42.

Detecting the Earliest Signs of Rheumatoid Arthritis: Symptoms and Examination

 CrossMark

Tabitha N. Kung, MD, MPH, FRCPC[a], Vivian P. Bykerk, MD, FRCPC[b],*

KEYWORDS

- Preclinical disease • Symptoms • Clinical features • Examination

KEY POINTS

- The understanding of signs and symptoms associated with the development of rheumatoid arthritis (RA) is emerging.
- No definitive screening tool or a tool solely incorporating signs and symptoms has yet been validated as having sufficient predictive ability for RA.
- Studies of individuals at risk for RA need to include symptoms and signs that are not necessarily derived from classification criteria to provide new insights and novel detection tools.
- Qualitative methods applied to cohorts of individuals at risk of developing arthritis are integral to identify and validate novel symptom complexes important in preclinical disease.

INTRODUCTION

The concept of preclinical disease has gained increasing attention over the past decade as researchers and providers aspired to prevent and cure chronic disease. In seropositive autoimmune diseases, autoantibodies have been identified well before the onset of disease or even symptoms not only in type 1 diabetes[1] and celiac disease,[2] but also in rheumatic diseases, including rheumatoid arthritis (RA), antiphospholipid syndrome, and systemic lupus erythematosis.[3] Of the rheumatic diseases, prediagnosis and preclinical RA clinics are becoming more prevalent because RA is the most common of the inflammatory arthritides, affecting approximately 1% of the general population. These clinics follow those individuals at risk for RA in whom

Disclosures: Postgraduate fellowships from UCB and Janssen Canada (T.N. Kung).
[a] Department of Medicine, Mount Sinai Hospital, University of Toronto, Toronto, Ontario M5T3L9, Canada; [b] Division of Rheumatology, Hospital for Special Surgery, Weill Cornell Medical College, New York, NY 10021, USA
* Corresponding author.
E-mail address: bykerkv@hss.edu

risk may include the presence of autoantibodies without symptoms, symptoms without signs of synovitis, a first-degree relative (FDR) with RA, and/or a propensity to RA based on belonging to a specific at-risk population (eg, first nations). These clinics are generally aimed at identifying predictors of developing arthritis. Moreover, as the importance of the preclinical phase of inflammatory arthritis has gained prominence, the terminology describing persons in this preclinical phase has evolved. In a recent publication, the European League Against Rheumatism (EULAR) propose that prospective studies should use the following terminology to describe individuals at risk of RA having genetic risk factors for RA, having environmental risk factors for RA, having systemic autoimmunity associated with RA, having symptoms without clinical arthritis, and having unclassified arthritis.[4] These recommendations further suggest that "pre-RA" should refer to the period of time or phase, assessed retrospectively, before RA can be classified. Studies examining the pre-RA phase usually compare patients who were recently classified as RA and those not classified as RA but followed over a similar period of time. These studies compare risk factors in each group. The term "individuals at risk" implies a longitudinal study design in which individuals with risk factors for RA are followed to determine the probability of, or time course to, developing classifiable RA given a set of risk factors. This article focuses on individuals at risk who have symptoms and/or one or more other risk factors for RA but who have not developed clinical arthritis it also looks at studies that examined patients in the pre-RA phase.

Despite an increased interest in the preclinical phases of RA, there are few studies designed to examine the symptoms in this period. This article therefore extrapolates findings about symptoms in the preclinical phase from existing studies and summarizes these from studies that included information about clinical symptoms. Included are studies examining (1) screening tools to detect RA, and (2) physical features examined in cohorts of people with undifferentiated arthritis to predict who developed classifiable RA or persistent arthritis. This article also highlights the signs and symptoms being captured prospectively among patients followed in cohort studies of people at risk for RA, including cohorts of people who screened positively for increased risk of RA (eg, FDRs of individuals with RA, or those who carry antibodies associated with RA, or have symptoms without clinical arthritis [eg, arthralgia without synovitis]). Underscoring the need to understand symptoms in the presynovitis phase, a study by van de Stadt and colleagues[5] identified that joint symptoms are important components of predicting future RA in autoantibody-positive individuals initially without arthritis.

SCREENING AND TRIAGE TOOLS

Screening tools have been developed to screen populations with varying degrees of risk to detect people with RA. These tools may identify people with musculoskeletal (MSK) symptoms, or may be used to help triage those with symptoms or signs to either general practitioner or rheumatologist care in an attempt to improve early identification of inflammatory arthritis and RA. Because MSK symptoms are common, these tools are designed to identify only those people with true inflammatory disease. A recent systematic review of strategies to promote early diagnosis identified available screening tools to increase detection of individuals with inflammatory arthritis.[6] The symptoms queried by these self-report tools included questions about the presence of joint pain, stiffness, swelling, symmetry, duration of disease, and functional limitation (**Tables 1** and **2**). Some tools (such as the Connective Screening Questionnaire [CSQ]) were less specific for RA and queried an extensive list of extra-articular features

Table 1
Screening tools for detection of RA

Name	P and O	Questions Pertaining to Symptoms	Performance
CSQ[7]	P: general P O: any connective tissue disease 30-Item self-report questionnaire	Presence of: 1. Joint stiffness 2. Nodules or bumps around the elbow or ankle 3. Swelling in upper extremities or knees 4. Extra-articular features	Sensitivity: 85% Specificity: 87%–93%
ERASE[36]	7-Item self-report questionnaire	Presence of: 1. MCP involvement 2. Wrist involvement 3. Duration of symptoms weeks/months 4. Absence of fibromyalgia symptoms (any 2 of IBS, jaw pain, chronic fatigue, or daily headaches)	Not reported
RASQ[37]	P: patients referred from GPs for MSK symptoms O: ACR 1987 RA diagnosis	Presence of: 1. Pain in joints (indicate on diagram) 2. Swelling in joints (indicate on diagram) 3. ACR1987 diagnostic criteria	Sensitivity: 67.2% Specificity: 60.4%
EIA Detection Tool[38]	P: patients referred to early arthritis clinic O: inflammatory arthritis	Presence of: 1. Pain in joints; wrists, hands (make a fist) 2. Morning stiffness (>60 min) 3. Disease duration (>6 wk; <1 y) 4. Symmetry 5. Functional limitation	Sensitivity: 91.5% Specificity: 85.5%[39]
P-VAS/D-ADL ratio[40]	P: patients referred to rheumatology clinic O: RA	Ratio of P-VAS/-ADL score 1. P-VAS 2. D-ADL (includes the first 8 questions from the MDHAQ)	Cutoff ≥3 Sensitivity: 72% Specificity: 67%

Abbreviations: ACR 1987, American College of Rheumatology 1987 RA criteria; CSQ, Clinical Screening Questionnaire; D-ADL, Difficulty in Activities of Daily Living; ERASE, E-triage RA Study in Early Arthritis; GP, general practitioner; IBS, irritable bowel syndrome; MCP, metacarpophalangeal; MDHAQ, MD Health Assessment Questionnaire; O, outcome; P, population; P-VAS, Pain Visual Analogue Scale; RASQ, RA Screening Questionnaire.

associated with autoimmune diseases in general (eg, mucositis, rash, nodules). Ascertainment of these might identify not only RA but also a variety of connective tissue diseases.[7] The questions that pertain to symptoms, the populations examined with these tools, and their performance characteristics are listed in **Table 1**. The clinical signs and symptoms incorporated into these screening tools were selected by a variety of

Table 2
Early symptoms predictive of arthritis (X indicates that the symptoms or lack of symptoms were found)

Tool or Study	Joint Stiffness	Joint Pain		Joint Swelling		Symmetry	Functional Limitation	Duration of Symptoms	Extra-Articular Features	Absence of Symptoms
		Upper Extremities	Lower Extremities	Upper Extremities	Lower Extremities					
Screening Tools										
CSQ[7]	X (>1 h)	—	—	X (wrists, MCPs, PIPs, elbows)	X (knees)	—	—	X (>3 mo)	X	—
ERASE[36]	—	X (wrists, MCPs)	—	—	—	—	—	X (weeks/months)	—	X (absence of fibromyalgia symptoms)
RASQ[37]	X (ACR1987)	X	—	X	—	X (ACR1987)	—	X (ACR1987)	X (ACR1987)	—
EIA Detection Tool[38]	X (morning, >1 h)	X (wrists, hands)	X	X (wrists, hands)	—	X	X (making a fist, other ADL/IADL)	X (>6 wk, <1 y)	—	—
P-VAS: D-ADL[40]	—	X	—	—	—	—	X	—	—	—
Undifferentiated Arthritis Studies										
Leiden Prediction Rule[8]	X (VAS)	X	X	X	X	X	—	—	—	—
Systematic Review by Kuriya et al[11]	X[41,42]	—	X (on examination, MTP pain)[29]	X[30] (wrist[43], small joints)[44]	—	—	—	X[30,41] (>12 wk, >6 mo)	—	—

Abbreviations: ACR1987, based on American College of Rheumatology 1987 RA criteria; IADL, instrumental activities of daily living; MTP, metatarsophalangeal joint; PIP, proximal interphalangeal.

methods, including qualitative studies of patients, and Delphi consensus with input from patients and providers. These tools most often reflect domains that are part of existing classification criteria either for autoimmune diseases in general or for specific diseases. Although these features may be important to help clinicians to identify eventual persistent and classifiable RA, earlier detection of inflammatory arthritis may need to systematically study symptoms or signs not necessarily included in classification criteria because they may have important predictive value. This approach is the basis of many of the newer cohort studies examining individuals at risk of RA, the goals of which include identifying incident inflammatory arthritis in addition to classifiable RA.

UNDIFFERENTIATED ARTHRITIS COHORTS

Undifferentiated arthritis cohort studies were developed to detect and treat arthritis early in the disease course to improve outcomes. These cohorts identify individuals who already have clinically detectable inflammatory arthritis (eg, swollen joints) within a specified duration of symptoms (eg, within 1 year) and follow them over time.

Because the wish is to identify the clinical signs and symptoms that manifest in people who ultimately develop persistent disease, one approach is to identify the signs and symptoms used in cohorts of undifferentiated arthritis followed prospectively to derive prediction rules for the development of classifiable RA. The Leiden Prediction Rule is one such rule in which a score including clinical symptoms and signs could predict people who go on to develop classifiable RA by 1987 criteria. This tool was created for use in patients with undifferentiated arthritis.[8] The rule weighted involvement of upper and lower extremities, small joint involvement, symmetry, numbers of tender and swollen joints, and morning stiffness greater than 60 minutes as predictive signs and symptoms for the development of RA. Combining the weights from the clinical variables with other demographic and laboratory variables (age, sex, C-reactive protein level, rheumatoid factor [RF] and anti–cyclic citrullinated protein [anti-CCP] positivity), a threshold of greater than or equal to 9 points was 31% and 99% specific for RA by 1987 criteria.[9] A threshold of greater than or equal to 6 points was 81% sensitive and 79% specific predictive of the development of classifiable RA by American College of Rheumatology (ACR/EULAR) 2010 criteria in later studies performed after the development of the newer classification criteria (see **Table 2**).[10]

Examining undifferentiated arthritis cohorts for clinical features that predicted the development of persistent arthritis can also provide an understanding of the clinical features that occur before the development of classifiable arthritis. A systematic review by Kuriya and colleagues[11] examined the diagnostic and prognostic value of elements of history and physical examination with respect to persistent arthritis published in observational studies of undifferentiated peripheral inflammatory arthritis. The clinical elements in histories that predicted the development of persistent arthritis included symptom duration greater than 12 weeks, early morning stiffness greater than 1 hour, and small joint or wrist swelling. The physical examination features that predicted disease persistence included higher number of swollen joints and the presence of metatarsophalangeal compression pain (see **Table 2**).

QUALITATIVE STUDIES

Identifying patients at the earliest stages of inflammatory arthritis and the predictive symptoms for the development of persistent RA is difficult in the setting of cohort studies because the questions are predetermined and often reflect the items in classification criteria. Identifying novel clinical features predictive of persistent disease requires asking questions outside of typical features of established RA such as joint pain, stiffness, and swelling. Stack and colleagues[12] contend that qualitative methods may be informative in this area by exploring patients' experiences in depth and identifying emerging themes. To that end, they performed a systematic review of qualitative studies exploring patients' experiences of the symptoms of RA at the onset of their disease. From their synthesis, they identified several interacting themes emerging from these retrospective studies of patients with RA. Patients reflected that both typical symptoms, such as joint swelling, stiffness, pain, and tenderness, as well as fatigue, weakness, and the emotional impact of those symptoms, preceded the onset of RA. Moreover, joint pain was most commonly described as involving the feet and hands with larger joint involvement being less common. The emotional distress identified in those studies included anger, fearfulness, and depression (**Table 3**). These data suggest that emotional well-being should be explored in patients at risk for RA. Stack and colleagues[12] also described major deficiencies in the current qualitative literature, noting that most studies have retrospectively examined persons with established RA, and that the assessments about symptom onset were secondary to the primary aim of most studies.

In order to improve on existing literature and identify symptoms earlier in the disease process, this group collaborated with the Amsterdam Arthralgia Cohort to perform a qualitative analysis of symptom complexes in 15 seropositive (RF and/or anti–citrullinated protein antigen [ACPA]) patients with arthralgia and 11 newly presenting patients with RA by the 2010 criteria.[13,14] The Amsterdam Arthralgia Cohort is the largest of its kind following adults 18 to 70 years of age with joint pain and ACPA or RF positivity who were initially included even though there was no clinical evidence of synovitis based on a 2-physician examination of 44 joints. This cohort has been followed since June 2004.[15] In their recent publication, they report themes common to patients with arthralgia and early RA. They noted that pain was described not only in reference to the joints but also in muscles and tendons. Symptoms such as tingling sensations; weakness and loss of strength; fatigue and sleeping difficulties; self-reported swelling, redness, and warmth; and joint stiffness were prominent and could be intermittent or palindromic symptoms. The intensity of the symptoms seemed to worsen through the spectrum from arthralgia to early RA. For example, patients with arthralgia only described pain as being bothersome and annoying, whereas the patients with early RA had pain that intensified to excruciating levels before diagnosis, suggesting that pain intensifies as the burden of inflammation increases just before diagnosis. The intermittency of joint symptoms also was a greater theme in patients with arthralgia reporting short episodes of intermittent swelling, pain, and atigue versus more persistent symptoms in patients with RA. Patients with RA described swelling as a significant change, occurring shortly before diagnosis. Both arthralgia-only and early RA groups reported night pain as a troubling theme; however, fatigue and sleep difficulties were dominant symptoms in patients with arthralgia (see **Table 3**). These qualitative studies may help to identify novel symptoms and provide new insights into symptom type, frequency, quality, or intensity that can be used to target patients at more imminent risk of developing classified disease, although further work is needed and should focus on prospective studies of individuals considered to be at risk of RA. Moreover, prospective studies are needed to determine whether these novel symptoms help to discriminate between those who will develop inflammatory arthritis versus those who will remain at risk.

Table 3
Symptoms identified from qualitative studies (X indicates that the symptoms were found)

	Joint Pain	Muscle Pain/Paresthesia	Joint Swelling/Redness	Joint Stiffness	Intermittent Symptoms	Weakness	Fatigue	Sleep Difficulty	Emotional Impact
Systematic review by Stack et al[12]	X	—	X	X	—	X	X	X	X
Amsterdam Arthralgia Cohort[14]	X	X	X	X	X	X	X	X	X

CLINICS AND COHORTS TO STUDY INDIVIDUALS AT RISK

To identify and better understand the period of preclinical autoimmunity, several groups around the world have developed clinics or research cohorts to follow individuals thought to be at increased risk of developing RA. There are 3 different varieties of these clinics: arthralgia clinics, in which individuals have already developed joint discomfort but have no overt signs of inflammatory synovitis, whether that be detected by detailed clinical examination or sensitive imaging techniques (depending on the site); cohorts of FDRs, taking advantage of potential burden of genetic or close familial environmental risk, or asymptomatic autoimmunity (eg, CCP positivity, RF positivity, or both). **Tables 4** and **5** respectively list the different clinics or cohorts that have been developed and the clinical features these clinics are following prospectively. The largest cohort of FDRs of patients with RA in Canada comes from Manitoba where El-Gabalawy and colleagues[16,17] have been prospectively following FDRs of North American Native (NAN) (Cree/Ojibway) patients with RA, which is a population with a high prevalence of RA at 2% to 3% and a remarkably high human leukocyte antigen (HLA)-DRB1 shared epitope (SE) prevalence (86%), suggesting a high genetic and shared environmental susceptibility burden. In this NAN-FDR cohort, individuals are routinely and prospectively asked questions about the presence of pain, swelling, and morning stiffness in hand joints and other joints.[18] The likelihood of developing arthritis in these NAN-FDRs has not yet been published, although increased nonspecific musculoskeletal (MSK) symptoms and biomarkers (eg, anti-CCP antibodies and cytokine levels) in these FDRs have already been reported.[18–20] Although a trend for a higher prevalence of nonspecific MSK symptoms was observed in the seropositive (RF or ACPA) FDRs, the overall seropositivity in this cohort was low (8% ACPA, 33% RF), suggesting that the seronegative FDRs also experience more MSK symptoms than controls; however, the incidence of transition to RA is still unknown in this cohort.

The Studies of the Etiology of Rheumatoid Arthritis (SERA) cohort in Denver, Colorado, and associated sites is the largest cohort of at-risk individuals in the United States. SERA prospectively and routinely queries patients about past and current joint

Table 4
Preclinical arthritis prospective cohorts with published data on symptoms

Number	Location	Type of Cohort	Details
1	Amsterdam, Netherlands	Arthralgia cohort[5,15,32,45–49]	ACPA-positive and/or RF-positive patients with arthralgia
2	Manitoba, Canada	FDR cohort[17–20,50,51]	Unaffected FDR of NAN patients with RA regardless of antibody status of the patients or FDR
3	Colorado (and other sites), United States	Combination (FDR, arthralgia, genetic risk)[21–23,52–58]	1. FDR of patients with RA (regardless of antibody status) 2. Arthralgia (from health fair) 3. HLA-DRB1–positive asymptomatic patients
4	Leeds, United Kingdom	Combination (FDR, arthralgia)[27,59]	1. ACPA-positive FDR of patients with RA 2. Patients with arthralgia
5	Leiden, Netherlands	Arthralgia cohort[24–26]	Clinically suspect arthralgia regardless of seropositivity

Abbreviations: HLA, human leukocyte antigen; NAN, North American Native.

Table 5
Symptoms followed in at-risk clinics (X indicates that the symptoms were found)

| | Joint Involvement | | | | | Duration of | | | | | |
	Joint Pain	Joint Swelling	Joint Stiffness	Intermittency	Symmetry	Symptoms	Pain Intensity	Fatigue	Sleep	Stress	Nodules
NAN-FDR Clinic	X	X	X	—	—	—	—	—	—	—	—
SERA	X	X	X	X	X	X	X	X	X	X	X
Leiden CSA Cohort	X	X	X	—	X	X	X	X	—	X	X
Amsterdam Arthralgia Cohort	X	X	X	X	X	X	X	—	—	—	—
Leeds Cohort	X	X	X	X	X	X	X	—	—	—	—

Abbreviations: CSA, clinically suspect arthralgia; SERA, Studies of the Etiology of RA.

stiffness, swelling, and pain in all joints of the upper and lower extremities as well as asking questions about fatigue, sleep, and stress (Perceived Stress Scale).[21–23] SERA has already reported on the prevalence of RA-related autoantibodies, cytokines, and chemokines in their subjects. The value of this broader range of symptom collection is being investigated in this and other collaborative ongoing cohorts.

The Leiden group follows patients with clinically suspect arthralgia (CSA), defined as individuals with arthralgia of the small joints without clinically evident arthritis, whose symptom character is such that the rheumatologist suspects these individuals will progress to arthritis over time. There were no specific symptoms required for inclusion, and referral to the cohort was based on the decision of the rheumatologist, which more than likely reflected classification criteria (eg, morning stiffness, swollen joints). The Leiden group expressly did not have inclusion symptoms because the symptoms that are predictive of arthritis development are not known. This recruitment strategy may allow greater patient inclusion, but may make reproducing their population difficult for other cohorts. The Leiden CSA cohort follows these individuals regardless of seropositivity, and has reported on magnetic resonance imaging findings in this at-risk stage.[24] The clinical features followed in this CSA cohort include presenting symptoms (location, character, localization), current symptoms (inflammatory character, morning stiffness), fatigue, and stress (perceived stress scale).[25,26]

The Amsterdam Arthralgia Cohort follows seropositive patients with arthralgia (described earlier). This group recently published a prediction rule[5] to identify the features that were predictive of the development of inflammatory arthritis (a single swollen joint) and 2010 classifiable RA. The symptom features that ultimately remained in the multivariate model included duration of symptoms (category <12 months vs $\geq$12 months), intermittent symptoms, location in both upper and lower extremities, pain visual analogue scale (VAS; $\geq$50), morning stiffness ($\geq$1 hour), and patient-reported swollen joints on history. The other nonsymptom variables that remained included having an FDR with RA, never drinking alcohol, and ACPA and RF positivity. This prediction rule classified patients as having high, medium, and low risk of developing swollen joints, with 43% of high-risk individuals developing arthritis by 1 year and 81% by 5 years.

In Leeds, United Kingdom, cohorts of both ACPA-positive FDRs and patients with arthralgia are being followed to determine the proportion of patients with nonspecific musculoskeletal complaints who are ACPA-positive and who develop inflammatory arthritis, and who develop RA. This group has recently published predictors of the development of inflammatory arthritis (defined as any swollen and tender joint) in the Leeds anti-CCP–positive cohort with symptoms without clinical arthritis.[27] In an attempt to validate the Amsterdam Arthralgia clinic prediction rule,[5] they also included the same predictors in their analysis. The potential clinical features examined included symptom duration, intermittency of symptoms, involvement of upper and lower extremities, early morning stiffness, pain (on a VAS), and tenderness of the small joints on physical examination. Their results indicate that the symptoms important for risk stratification include early morning stiffness greater than or equal to 30 minutes, and tenderness of hand or foot joints on examination. The other nonsymptom variables included high titer (>3 times the upper limit of normal) ACPA and/or RF, SE positivity, or power Doppler positivity of the metacarpophalangeal (MCP) or proximal interphalangeal (PIP) joints of the hands on ultrasonography (US-PD+). Further validation of the Amsterdam and Leeds prediction rules and/or the importance of US-PD of the hands in a larger cohort are warranted because there is controversy as to whether arthralgia without detectable swelling may still represent synovitis, particularly if there is a power Doppler signal present in symptomatic joints.

SUMMARY OF SYMPTOMS AND SIGNS THAT REQUIRE ONGOING STUDY

Investigation to date indicates that symptoms often precede the onset of clinical signs of overt physically detectable persistent synovitis. There are no published data that examine the onset of symptoms even those not specific to joints in the period of systemic autoimmunity that precedes the onset of symptoms or classifiable RA. Studies to date examining symptoms heralding persistent arthritis or classifiable RA have been performed in patients earlier and earlier in their trajectory to overt disease, starting from those with undifferentiated clinical synovitis, to newer studies examining nonspecific MSK pain without synovitis. The symptoms captured in these prospective, observational studies still largely reflect the symptoms experienced in patients with classifiable, established RA (see **Table 2**). Newer qualitative studies are striving to identify as yet unexamined, predictive symptoms and may provide clinicians with new methods to more precisely define individual risk. They have identified patient-reported symptoms, such as pain with increasing intensity, periodic or palindromic symptoms, stiffness, difficulty with function, fatigue, disturbance of sleep, and psychological distress as novel candidates for inclusion in prediction models. In addition, one area of study is how best to allow subjects to describe and localize their symptoms. Is having patients identify the specific location of their symptoms on a figure the best approach, or would verbal descriptions of the location of symptoms be adequate? Studies focusing on physical signs have been fewer and thus less informative, which may be because of the issues of reproducibility and specificity across examiners, which has been shown to improve with standardization for some domains (eg, tenderness), but others (eg, swelling) still seem to be difficult to standardize.[28] A thorough joint examination of tender and swollen joints needs to be thoroughly and periodically performed, especially for the small joints including MCPs, because they have been highlighted as being most active in the earliest phases of RA.[29,30] These findings need to be corroborated with imaging studies, especially given early studies in seropositive patients with arthralgia that suggested that subclinical abnormalities can increasingly be detected in individuals who eventually develop inflammatory arthritis, although the predictive ability of these findings needs to be validated.[25–27,31,32] A further difficulty in interpreting studies of physical examination in the preclinical period is that little has been published about the validity of physical examination during this time. More needs to be known about the sensitivity, specificity, reproducibility, and agreement across examiners.

It is clear from retrospective studies examining costs or frequency of accessing care that as the diagnosis of RA approaches, the number of primary care visits and associated health care costs increases well before formal diagnosis.[33] A recent population-based national study from Taiwan confirmed this finding in the 8-year period before diagnosis and examined it further, identifying MSK symptoms as the most significant cause of these increased physician visits. Respiratory and gastrointestinal symptoms were common causes for physician visits in this population.[34] This finding suggests that a host of nonspecific symptoms may predate a diagnosis of RA.

Behaviors and personal circumstances should be included in symptom questionnaires because these may impart genetic and environmental protective or risk factors that contribute significantly to the ability to predict the development of inflammatory arthritis and RA. Based on published data concerning risk factors associated with the onset of RA, these could include the use of tobacco, alcohol, adherence to dental hygiene, travel and migration, family history of RA and autoimmunity, exposure to pollution and particulate matter, and physical and psychological stress.[35] All of these elements need to be incorporated into a model along with escalating intensity and specificity of symptoms to derive a valid model to predict imminent classifiable disease for which an intervention could be considered to prevent RA.

SUMMARY

Signs and symptoms often occur well in advance of a formal diagnosis of RA. However, these do not necessarily represent symptoms that are included in classification criteria. Their intensity, frequency, and persistence over time seem to be important in the spectrum from preclinical autoimmunity to classifiable RA. Prospective study of signs and symptoms in individuals at risk for RA will help to determine their onset and relationship with epitope spreading, cytokine evolution, sensitive imaging, and their usefulness in discriminating between individuals patients who will develop incident inflammatory arthritis versus normal controls.

REFERENCES

1. Eisenbarth GS, Moriyama H, Robles DT, et al. Insulin autoimmunity: prediction/ precipitation/prevention type 1A diabetes. Autoimmun Rev 2002;1(3):139–45.
2. Johnston SD, Watson RG, McMillan SA, et al. Serological markers for coeliac disease: changes with time and relationship to enteropathy. Eur J Gastroenterol Hepatol 1998;10(3):259–64.
3. Arbuckle MR, McClain MT, Rubertone MV, et al. Development of autoantibodies before the clinical onset of systemic lupus erythematosus. N Engl J Med 2003; 349(16):1526–33.
4. Gerlag DM, Raza K, van Baarsen LG, et al. EULAR recommendations for terminology and research in individuals at risk of rheumatoid arthritis: report from the Study Group for Risk Factors for Rheumatoid Arthritis. Ann Rheum Dis 2012; 71(5):638–41.
5. van de Stadt LA, Witte BI, Bos WH, et al. A prediction rule for the development of arthritis in seropositive arthralgia patients. Ann Rheum Dis 2013;72(12):1920–6.
6. Villeneuve E, Nam JL, Bell MJ, et al. A systematic literature review of strategies promoting early referral and reducing delays in the diagnosis and management of inflammatory arthritis. Ann Rheum Dis 2013;72(1):13–22.
7. Karlson EW, Sanchez-Guerrero J, Wright EA, et al. A connective tissue disease screening questionnaire for population studies. Ann Epidemiol 1995;5(4): 297–302.
8. van der Helm-van Mil AH, le Cessie S, van Dongen H, et al. A prediction rule for disease outcome in patients with recent-onset undifferentiated arthritis: how to guide individual treatment decisions. Arthritis Rheum 2007;56(2):433–40.
9. McNally E, Keogh C, Galvin R, et al. Diagnostic accuracy of a clinical prediction rule (CPR) for identifying patients with recent-onset undifferentiated arthritis who are at a high risk of developing rheumatoid arthritis: a systematic review and meta-analysis. Semin Arthritis Rheum 2014;43(4):498–507.
10. Bedran Z, Quiroz C, Rosa J, et al. Validation of a prediction rule for the diagnosis of rheumatoid arthritis in patients with recent onset undifferentiated arthritis. Int J Rheumatol 2013;2013:548502.
11. Kuriya B, Villeneuve E, Bombardier C. Diagnostic and prognostic value of history-taking and physical examination in undifferentiated peripheral inflammatory arthritis: a systematic review. J Rheumatol Suppl 2011;87:10–4.
12. Stack RJ, Sahni M, Mallen CD, et al. Symptom complexes at the earliest phases of rheumatoid arthritis: a synthesis of the qualitative literature. Arthritis Care Res (Hoboken) 2013;65(12):1916–26.

13. van Schaardenburg DJ, Stack RJ, van Tuyl LH, et al. Symptom complexes at the beginning of rheumatoid arthritis: a qualitative exploration in at risk individuals and in new patients prior to diagnosis. Arthritis Rheum 2013;65(Suppl. 10):S960.

14. Stack RJ, van Tuyl LH, Sloots M, et al. Symptom complexes in patients with sero-positive arthralgia and in patients newly diagnosed with rheumatoid arthritis: a qualitative exploration of symptom development. Rheumatology (Oxford) 2014;53(9):1646–53.

15. Bos WH, Wolbink GJ, Boers M, et al. Arthritis development in patients with arthralgia is strongly associated with anti-citrullinated protein antibody status: a prospective cohort study. Ann Rheum Dis 2010;69(3):490–4.

16. Barnabe C, Elias B, Bartlett J, et al. Arthritis in aboriginal Manitobans: evidence for a high burden of disease. J Rheumatol 2008;35(6):1145–50.

17. Oen K, Robinson DB, Nickerson P, et al. Familial seropositive rheumatoid arthritis in North American native families: effects of shared epitope and cyto-kine genotypes. J Rheumatol 2005;32(6):983–91.

18. Smolik I, Robinson DB, Bernstein CN, et al. First-degree relatives of patients with rheumatoid arthritis exhibit high prevalence of joint symptoms. J Rheumatol 2013;40(6):818–24.

19. El-Gabalawy HS, Robinson DB, Hart D, et al. Immunogenetic risks of anti-cyclical citrullinated peptide antibodies in a North American Native population with rheumatoid arthritis and their first-degree relatives. J Rheumatol 2009; 36(6):1130–5.

20. El-Gabalawy HS, Robinson DB, Smolik I, et al. Familial clustering of the serum cytokine profile in the relatives of rheumatoid arthritis patients. Arthritis Rheum 2012;64(6):1720–9.

21. Hughes-Austin JM, Deane KD, Derber LA, et al. Multiple cytokines and chemo-kines are associated with rheumatoid arthritis-related autoimmunity in first-degree relatives without rheumatoid arthritis: Studies of the Aetiology of Rheumatoid Arthritis (SERA). Ann Rheum Dis 2013;72(6):901–7.

22. Demoruelle MK, Weisman MH, Simonian PL, et al. Brief report: airways abnor-malities and rheumatoid arthritis-related autoantibodies in subjects without arthritis: early injury or initiating site of autoimmunity? Arthritis Rheum 2012; 64(6):1756–61.

23. Young KA, Deane KD, Derber LA, et al. Relatives without rheumatoid arthritis show reactivity to anti-citrullinated protein/peptide antibodies that are associ-ated with arthritis-related traits: studies of the etiology of rheumatoid arthritis. Arthritis Rheum 2013;65(8):1995–2004.

24. van Steenbergen HW, Huizinga TW, van der Helm-van Mil AH. The preclinical phase of rheumatoid arthritis: what is acknowledged and what needs to be as-sessed? Arthritis Rheum 2013;65(9):2219–32.

25. van Steenbergen HW, van Nies JA, Huizinga TW, et al. Characterising arthralgia in the preclinical phase of rheumatoid arthritis using MRI. Ann Rheum Dis 2014. [Epub ahead of print].

26. van Steenbergen HW, van Nies JA, Huizinga TW, et al. Subclinical inflamma-tion on MRI of hand and foot of anti-citrullinated peptide antibody-negative arthralgia patients at risk for rheumatoid arthritis. Arthritis Res Ther 2014; 16(2):R92.

27. Rakieh C, Nam JL, Hunt L, et al. Predicting the development of clinical arthritis in anti-CCP positive individuals with non-specific musculoskeletal symptoms: a prospective observational cohort study. Ann Rheum Dis 2014. [Epub ahead of print].

28. Grunke M, Witt MN, Ronneberger M, et al. Use of the 28-joint count yields significantly higher concordance between different examiners than the 66/68-joint count. J Rheumatol 2012;39(7):1334–40.
29. Emery P, Breedveld FC, Dougados M, et al. Early referral recommendation for newly diagnosed rheumatoid arthritis: evidence based development of a clinical guide. Ann Rheum Dis 2002;61(4):290–7.
30. Green M, Marzo-Ortega H, Wakefield RJ, et al. Predictors of outcome in patients with oligoarthritis: results of a protocol of intraarticular corticosteroids to all clinically active joints. Arthritis Rheum 2001;44(5):1177–83.
31. Krabben A, Stomp W, van der Heijde DM, et al. MRI of hand and foot joints of patients with anticitrullinated peptide antibody positive arthralgia without clinical arthritis. Ann Rheum Dis 2013;72(9):1540–4.
32. van de Stadt LA, Bos WH, Meursinge Reynders M, et al. The value of ultrasonography in predicting arthritis in auto-antibody positive arthralgia patients: a prospective cohort study. Arthritis Res Ther 2010;12(3):R98.
33. Morse A. Services for people with rheumatoid arthritis [Report no. 9780102955071]. London: 2009. Available at: http://www.nao.org.uk/report/services-for-people-with-rheumatoid-arthritis/.
34. Lai NS, Tsai TY, Li CY, et al. Increased frequency and costs of ambulatory medical care utilization prior to the diagnosis of rheumatoid arthritis: a national population-based study. Arthritis Care Res (Hoboken) 2014;66(3):371–8.
35. Karlson EW, Deane K. Environmental and gene-environment interactions and risk of rheumatoid arthritis. Rheum Dis Clin North Am 2012;38(2):405–26.
36. Maksymowych W. Development of a web-based Screening Tool for Early Rheumatoid Arthritis-ERASE: the E-triage RA Study in Early Arthritis. 2008.
37. Khraishi M, Uphall E, Mong J. The self-administered Rheumatoid Arthritis (Ra) Screening Questionnaire (RASQ) is a simple and effective tool to detect RA patients. Ann Rheum Dis 2010;69(Suppl. 3):374.
38. Bell MJ, Tavares R, Guillemin F, et al. Development of a self-administered early inflammatory arthritis detection tool. BMC Musculoskelet Disord 2010;11:50.
39. Tavares R, Wells GA, Bykerk VP, et al. Validation of a self-administered inflammatory arthritis detection tool for rheumatology triage. J Rheumatol 2013;40(4):417–24.
40. Callahan LF, Pincus T. A clue from a self-report questionnaire to distinguish rheumatoid arthritis from noninflammatory diffuse musculoskeletal pain. The P-VAS:D-ADL ratio. Arthritis Rheum 1990;33(9):1317–22.
41. Visser H, Le Cessie S, Vos K, et al. How to diagnose rheumatoid arthritis early: a prediction model for persistent (erosive) arthritis. Arthritis Rheum 2002;46(2):357–65.
42. El Miedany Y, Youssef S, Mehanna AN, et al. Development of a scoring system for assessment of outcome of early undifferentiated inflammatory synovitis. Joint Bone Spine 2008;75(2):155–62.
43. Tunn EJ, Bacon PA. Differentiating persistent from self-limiting symmetrical synovitis in an early arthritis clinic. Br J Rheumatol 1993;32(2):97–103.
44. Mjaavatten MD, Uhlig T, Haugen AJ, et al. Positive anti-citrullinated protein antibody status and small joint arthritis are consistent predictors of chronic disease in patients with very early arthritis: results from the NOR-VEAC cohort. Arthritis Res Ther 2009;11(5):R146.
45. Bos WH, Dijkmans BA, Boers M, et al. Effect of dexamethasone on autoantibody levels and arthritis development in patients with arthralgia: a randomised trial. Ann Rheum Dis 2010;69(3):571–4.

46. Bos WH, Ursum J, de Vries N, et al. The role of the shared epitope in arthralgia with anti-cyclic citrullinated peptide antibodies (anti-CCP), and its effect on anti-CCP levels. Ann Rheum Dis 2008;67(9):1347–50.

47. Limper M, van de Stadt L, Bos W, et al. The acute-phase response is not predictive for the development of arthritis in seropositive arthralgia - a prospective cohort study. J Rheumatol 2012;39(10):1914–7.

48. van Baarsen LG, Bos WH, Rustenburg F, et al. Gene expression profiling in autoantibody-positive patients with arthralgia predicts development of arthritis. Arthritis Rheum 2010;62(3):694–704.

49. van de Stadt LA, van der Horst AR, de Koning MH, et al. The extent of the anti-citrullinated protein antibody repertoire is associated with arthritis development in patients with seropositive arthralgia. Ann Rheum Dis 2011;70(1):128–33.

50. El-Gabalawy HS, Robinson DB, Daha NA, et al. Non-HLA genes modulate the risk of rheumatoid arthritis associated with HLA-DRB1 in a susceptible North American Native population. Genes Immun 2011;12(7):568–74.

51. Ferucci ED, Darrah E, Smolik I, et al. Prevalence of anti-peptidylarginine deiminase type 4 antibodies in rheumatoid arthritis and unaffected first-degree relatives in indigenous North American Populations. J Rheumatol 2013;40(9): 1523–8.

52. Demoruelle MK, Parish MC, Derber LA, et al. Performance of anti-cyclic citrullinated Peptide assays differs in subjects at increased risk of rheumatoid arthritis and subjects with established disease. Arthritis Rheum 2013;65(9):2243–52.

53. Feser M, Derber LA, Deane KD, et al. Plasma 25,OH vitamin D concentrations are not associated with rheumatoid arthritis (RA)-related autoantibodies in individuals at elevated risk for RA. J Rheumatol 2009;36(5):943–6.

54. Gan RW, Deane KD, Zerbe GO, et al. Relationship between air pollution and positivity of RA-related autoantibodies in individuals without established RA: a report on SERA. Ann Rheum Dis 2013;72(12):2002–5.

55. Kolfenbach JR, Deane KD, Derber LA, et al. A prospective approach to investigating the natural history of preclinical rheumatoid arthritis (RA) using first-degree relatives of probands with RA. Arthritis Rheum 2009;61(12):1735–42.

56. Mikuls TR, Thiele GM, Deane KD, et al. Porphyromonas gingivalis and disease-related autoantibodies in individuals at increased risk of rheumatoid arthritis. Arthritis Rheum 2012;64(11):3522–30.

57. Willis VC, Demoruelle MK, Derber LA, et al. Sputum autoantibodies in patients with established rheumatoid arthritis and subjects at risk of future clinically apparent disease. Arthritis Rheum 2013;65(10):2545–54.

58. Deane KD, Striebich CC, Goldstein BL, et al. Identification of undiagnosed inflammatory arthritis in a community health fair screen. Arthritis Rheum 2009; 61(12):1642–9.

59. Emery P. The CCP Study: coordinated programme to prevent arthritis - can we identify arthritis at a pre-clinical stage? 2013. March 13, 2014 [cited March 16, 2014]. Available at: http://clinicaltrials.gov/ct2/show/NCT02012764?term=prevent+arthritis&rank=1. Accessed on March 16, 2014.

Recognition of Preclinical and Early Disease in Axial Spondyloarthritis

Dinny Wallis, MBChB[a], Robert D. Inman, MD[b],*

KEYWORDS

- Ankylosing spondylitis • Diagnosis • Magnetic resonance imaging • Genetic testing
- Serology

KEY POINTS

- Early diagnosis of axSpA is important because therapy may retard radiographic progression of disease.
- Targeting specific patient groups, such as those with chronic back pain younger than age of 45 years, or extra-articular manifestations of disease may improve timeliness of diagnosis of axSpA.
- Use of genetic and serologic markers may contribute to identification of patients with preclinical or early axSpA.
- The risks and benefits of detection of early or preclinical disease should be considered.

INTRODUCTION

Axial spondyloarthritis (axSpA) is a chronic, inflammatory disease characterized by back pain, spinal ankylosis, peripheral arthritis, and extra-articular manifestations. AxSpA has generally been considered an autoinflammatory disease in the past, because it was thought to lack the autoantibodies that characterize autoimmune rheumatic diseases, such as rheumatoid arthritis and systemic lupus erythematosus. In those conditions, preclinical detection of diagnostic autoantibodies has made very early detection of incipient disease a possibility, although disease does not develop in all those individuals with autoantibodies. Identification of preclinical and early axSpA is therefore a more complex challenge.

Disclosures: Nil.
[a] Department of Rheumatology, Royal Hampshire County Hospital, Romsey Road, Winchester 50300PP, UK; [b] Division of Rheumatology, Toronto Western Hospital, University of Toronto, 399 Bathurst Street, Toronto M5T 2S8, Ontario, Canada
* Corresponding author.
E-mail address: robert.inman@uhnresearch.ca

WHY SHOULD AXIAL SPONDYLOARTHRITIS BE DIAGNOSED EARLY?

The estimated prevalence of axSpA is between 0.2% and 1.2% in white European populations.[1] The diagnosis is often delayed by up to 8 years, mainly because sacroiliitis, which is considered a hallmark of ankylosing spondylitis (AS), is not visible on plain radiographs in the early stages of the disease.[2] In recent years, the challenge of early diagnosis of axSpA has become a high priority area of research. Although nonsteroidal anti-inflammatory drugs (NSAIDs) and physiotherapy are the cornerstones of management, tumor necrosis factor inhibitors (TNFi) are effective in patients who are resistant to standard therapy and are more effective in younger patients and those with shorter disease duration.[3–6] It has also been shown that TNFi can suppress the inflammation detected on magnetic resonance imaging (MRI).[7,8] Recent studies have demonstrated that TNFi agents can slow radiographic progression of the disease and the effect is most pronounced when treatment is started earlier in the course of disease.[9] This has added to the imperative for early identification of patients with axSpA.

WHAT IS "EARLY ANKYLOSING SPONDYLITIS"? THE CONCEPT OF AXIAL SPONDYLOARTHRITIS

Historically AS has been defined by the modified New York classification criteria,[10] which require the presence of radiographic sacroiliitis. More recently the use of MRI for earlier detection of inflammation in the sacroiliac joints has led to the identification of patients with features of axSpA who do not fulfill the modified New York criteria, and this has introduced the terminology of nonradiographic axSpA (nr-axSpA). Criteria have been developed for the classification of patients with axSpA including those with nr-axSpA.[11,12] It has been proposed that nr-axSpA may represent an early form of AS. This concept is supported by evidence that some patients do progress to AS over time. Data from early axSpA cohorts have demonstrated that over a 2-year period, approximately 10% of patients with undifferentiated SpA or nr-axSpA progress to radiographic AS.[13–16] However, several patients did not progress to AS over the duration of these studies. This finding, along with the identification of genetic and gender differences between AS and nr-axSpA, has led to the concept of nr-axSpA as a distinct disease entity and not just early AS. A lower frequency of HLA-B27 in nr-axSpA than in AS has been observed in the German Spondyloarthritis Inception Cohort (GESPIC)[16] and in two trials of adalimumab in nr-axSpA, one performed in Germany[3,16] and one an international multicenter trial.[17] In GESPIC the rates of HLA-B27 carriage were 72.6% in nr-axSpA and 84.3% in AS. Gender differences between the two groups have been demonstrated in three German studies with the percentage of males ranging from 31% to 43% in nr-axSpA compared with 65% to 77% in AS.[16,18,19] In general, disease activity and burden of symptoms did not differ, although C-reactive protein levels were lower in nr-axSpA.

EARLY RECOGNITION OF ANKYLOSING SPONDYLITIS IN PRIMARY CARE: THE "BACK PAIN POPULATION"

The first presenting feature in AS is usually low back pain, which is typically characterized by such features as early morning stiffness, relief with exercise, lack of improvement with rest, and nocturnal pain. These constellations of clinical features are key elements of inflammatory back pain (IBP). A description of IBP in association with AS was first published in 1977[20] and several criteria for IBP have been proposed since then.[21–23] The sensitivity and specificity of these IBP criteria for axSpA are broadly similar. For example, the Assessment of Spondyloarthritis International Society (ASAS) criteria for IBP have a sensitivity of 79.6% and specificity of 72.4%. However, chronic low back pain is very common in the general population and only approximately 5% of such patients are considered to have SpA.[24,25] Inflammatory low back pain is itself not uncommon: the current prevalence of IBP in the US population as a whole is estimated at 5%.[26] Various strategies and referral algorithms have been proposed to improve the timeliness of referral of patients with suspected SpA from primary care to rheumatologists. Because axSpA is a chronic disease and greater than or equal to 95% of patient are symptomatic by the age of 45 years,[27] the target population for early diagnosis should be those with back pain for more than 3 months and age of onset less than 45 years. Several combinations of parameters have been proposed for recognition of patients with early SpA, which commonly include presence of HLA-B27, IBP, family history of SpA, raised acute-phase reactants, characteristic extra-articular features, suspicion of sacroiliitis on imaging, and response to NSAIDs.[28–31] Although the optimal algorithm has not yet been defined, using the presence of either IBP or HLA-B27 in this population as a trigger for referral to a rheumatologist has proved effective in several studies in identifying patients with axSpA.[32] It should, however, be noted that although approximately 8% of the white population are HLA-B27 positive, only a small proportion (<5%) develop axSpA and the use of HLA-B27 alone as a screening test is not appropriate.

IMAGING FOR EARLIER RECOGNITION OF SPONDYLOARTHRITIS

Although MRI has revolutionized the imaging of axSpA, the specificity of some MRI lesions has not been clearly defined. Sacroiliac MRI lesions considered characteristic of SpA are bone marrow edema, capsulitis, synovitis, and enthesitis. In the spine, corner-based inflammatory lesions, end-plate lesions, diffuse vertebral body lesions, and spinous process bone marrow edema lesions are characteristic.[33,34] However, an evaluation of 174 patients with back pain caused by SpA, degenerative arthritis, or malignancy demonstrated that any of the spinal lesions listed may be present in degenerative arthritis or malignancy.[35] The spinal inflammatory lesions most suggestive of axSpA, as concluded by ASAS/OMERACT,[36] are corner-based inflammatory lesions, anterior/posterior spondylitis in three or more sites, and end-plate lesions. With regard to sacroiliitis, a definition of a positive MRI has been proposed by the same group and is widely used.[37] When applied to a cohort of 29 patients with early IBP and 18 control subjects, the ASAS definition of sacroiliitis gave a sensitivity of 79%, specificity of 89%, and likelihood ratio of 7.1.[38] The MORPHO study found that the ASAS definition of a positive MRI using bone marrow edema only had a sensitivity of 67% and specificity of 88%. In this study, inclusion of erosions in the definition of a positive MRI improved sensitivity.[39] Studies that have included needle biopsy of sacroiliac joints to confirm histologic sacroiliitis have found the specificity of MRI in confirming early sacroiliitis to be high (100%) but sensitivity was low (37.7%).[40] The concept of preclinical (asymptomatic) radiologic disease has not been investigated in detail. However, sacroiliac joint lesions are observed in control subjects with no back pain[35] and in one study of 35 patients with AS and 35 healthy control subjects, inflammatory SpA-like lesions occurred in 26% of control subjects.[41] Asymptomatic radiographic sacroiliitis has been observed in up to 32% of patients with inflammatory bowel disease (IBD).[42–44] Further prospective studies are required to investigate long-term outcomes in young patients presenting with back pain and in asymptomatic individuals with apparent inflammatory lesions on MRI. The definition of an inflammatory lesion may need to be reconsidered in the future.

BIOMARKERS FOR EARLIER RECOGNITION OF SPONDYLOARTHRITIS

An association between AS and IBD has been recognized for many years. Evidence of intestinal inflammation, which may be subclinical, is present in up to 65% of patients with SpA.[45] IBD is associated with a variety of serologic antibodies that suggest loss of tolerance to a subset of commensal microorganisms.[46] These include anti–Saccharomyces cerevesiae antibodies (ASCA), antineutrophil cytoplasmic antibodies, anti-I2 (associated with anti-Pseudomonas activity), anti–Escherichia coli outer membrane porin C, and anti-flagellin (anti-CBir1) antibodies. Circulating antibodies may be useful in distinguishing IBD from healthy control subjects and from other gastrointestinal disorders. For example, sensitivity of ASCA for IBD ranges from 31% to 45% and specificity from 90% to 100%.[47] The role of circulating antibodies in the pathogenesis of IBD is not understood but it is generally accepted that they reflect an aberrant immune response rather than the recognition of specific or pathogenic bacteria. The presence of these antibodies in AS has been investigated in several studies. Patients with AS have been shown to have higher titers than control subjects of anti-I2, ASCA IgG, and total ASCA.[48] Anti-CBir1 (anti-flagellin) antibodies are also elevated in patients with AS compared with patients with mechanical back pain and are associated with elevation of acute phase reactants in patients who have AS without coexisting IBD.[49] It is possible that these patients have subclinical IBD and further studies are required to answer this question. In IBD, the presence of certain antibodies has clinical significance; in Crohn disease, ASCA are associated with younger age of onset and small bowel involvement,[50] whereas antineutrophil cytoplasmic antibodies are associated with ulcerative colitis–like features.[51] Anti-CBir1 antibodies are associated with fibrostenosing disease and complicated small bowel disease.[52] The frequency of subclinical bowel inflammation in axSpA has suggested that a possible triggering event in the immunopathogenesis of axSpA is gut microbial dysbiosis and altered immune response to gut flora. Future work might investigate whether the presence of serum antibodies, such as anti-CBir1, in asymptomatic individuals might predict development of axSpA, or might provide prognostic information in early AS.

Other areas of interest for biomarkers in axSpA are the Wnt/β-catenin and bone morphogenic protein signaling pathways. There is evidence that abnormalities of Wnt/β-catenin signaling may contribute to spinal fusion in axSpA. Sclerostin is an antagonist of Wnt/β-catenin signaling, contributing an inhibitory signal in normal bone homeostasis. The expression of sclerostin is impaired in osteocytes of patients with AS and lower serum levels of sclerostin are seen in patients with axSpA compared with patients with osteoarthritis and healthy control subjects.[53] Enhancement of Wnt/β-catenin signaling has been demonstrated in a mouse model of peripheral and spinal ankylosis.[54] Bone morphogenic protein signaling is a key molecular pathway in bone formation. Noggin is an antagonist of bone morphogenic protein signaling[55] and in a mouse model of ankylosing enthesitis, systemic overexpression of noggin prevented ankylosis.[56]

Recent work has demonstrated that IgG autoantibodies to noggin and sclerostin are present in healthy individuals, but are present at significantly higher levels in patients with AS.[57] Preclinical autoantibody detection has proved valuable for identification of incipient rheumatoid arthritis and systemic lupus erythematosus. It remains to be determined whether immune complexes consisting of autoantibodies to sclerostin and noggin might similarly prove valuable in the identification of preclinical axSpA.

GENETIC TESTING FOR EARLIER RECOGNITION OF SPONDYLOARTHRITIS

AS is a highly heritable disease. A large proportion of the genetic risk is defined by HLA-B27, the major genetic variant of the disease. Approximately 8% of white populations are positive for HLA-B27 and 80% to 90% of patients with AS carry HLA-B27. However, only a small proportion (1%–5%) of individuals positive for HLA-B27 develops AS. Testing healthy individuals for HLA-B27 is therefore not a useful method for identifying patients with preclinical AS. Could other genes contributing to the heritability of AS improve the predictive use of genetic testing? Strong associations have been identified with several genes including *IL23R* and *ERAP1*. The association of *IL23R* with AS has been confirmed in several studies of white populations[58–60] and provides evidence for the role of the T-helper 17 (Th17) lymphocyte pathway in AS. Similar studies have confirmed the association of AS with *ERAP1*,[61,62] although the mechanism by which ERAP1 influences AS susceptibility is not clear. In a mouse model of inflammatory arthritis with enthesitis, it was demonstrated that the entheses and aortic root contain a resident population of interleukin (IL)-23R+ T cells, which allow the tissue to respond to IL-23.[63] A further study of a mouse model in SpA and IBD reported that enthesitis and ileitis were IL-23 dependent and that enthesitis was specifically dependent on IL-17A and IL-22.[64] These findings have contributed to the understanding of the etiopathogenesis of AS. Recent findings from high-density genotyping of immune-related loci have identified more than 20 genetic loci associated with AS.[65] One research challenge at hand is the application of this expanded scope of genetic susceptibility to AS, with a view to addressing whether a distinctive signature of genetic variants would have potential diagnostic use in the detection of preclinical AS.

FUTURE DIRECTIONS: TARGETING HIGH-RISK POPULATIONS
Extra-Articular Manifestations: Inflammatory Bowel Disease, Psoriasis, and Uveitis

In addition to targeting the "back pain population" in primary care for early detection of AS, several recent studies have focused on other patient populations that may be enriched with undiagnosed SpA, specifically patients with IBD, psoriasis, and acute anterior uveitis.

Between 4% and 10% of patients with IBD have AS[66] and up to 22% may have other features of SpA.[67] Patients may present first with either SpA or IBD, or with the two concurrently.[67–69] The Toronto Axial Spondyloarthritis Questionnaire was recently developed as a case-finding tool to be administered to patients with IBD and chronic back pain[70] with the aim of facilitating timely referral of patients with IBD with suspected axSpA from the gastroenterologist to the rheumatologist. The tool includes questions about the response of back pain to biologic drugs used in the management of IBD.

For detection of psoriatic arthritis in patients with psoriasis, several tools have been developed including the Psoriasis Epidemiology Screening Tool (PEST),[71] Psoriatic Arthritis Screening and Evaluation,[72] and the Toronto Psoriatic Arthritis Screen.[73] The sensitivities and specificities of these three tools have been compared in several studies of patients with psoriasis with no known psoriatic arthritis. Coates and colleagues[74] reported in a study based in UK dermatology clinics broadly similar sensitivities and specificities for psoriatic arthritis among the three tools of 74% to 77%

and 29% to 38%, respectively. A US study found higher specificities of 45% to 55%,[75] whereas a study from the Republic of Ireland reported specificities of more than 90% for all three tools but low sensitivities of 24% to 41%.[76] The variation in results between these studies probably reflects the differences in study populations; for example, the prevalence of psoriatic arthritis was significantly higher in the US (64%) than the British (24%) or Irish (29%) study populations.

The association between acute anterior uveitis and SpA is well recognized, with up to 78% of patients with HLA-B27–associated acute anterior uveitis having underlying SpA.[77] The Dublin Uveitis Evaluation Tool is an algorithm recently developed for the detection of undiagnosed SpA in patients presenting with acute anterior uveitis, which was found to have a sensitivity of 96% and specificity 97%.[78] The prevalence of SpA in the study population was approximately 40%.

The clinical potential of these tools for detecting early SpA is starting to be recognized. The use of PEST has been recommended in UK national clinical guidelines for the management of psoriasis, although it should be noted that the tool does not identify axial disease or IBP. Further investigation and validation of these tools for the detection of early SpA in other secondary care patient populations is warranted.

First-Degree Relatives

The strong heritability of axSpA suggests that first-degree relatives should be regarded as at-risk populations for future serologic and genetic testing of preclinical disease. A study using the Icelandic genealogy database and a population-wide survey highlights the potential of this approach.[79] For each AS proband in Iceland, first-degree, second-degree, and third-degree relatives had relative risks of 75.5, 20.2, and 3.5, respectively (all P values <.0001), indicating a significantly increased risk for relatives of the patients with AS to develop AS, suggesting a strong heritable factor, whereas the fourth-degree relatives had a relative risk of 1.04 (P = .476) for having AS.

RISKS AND BENEFITS OF PRECLINICAL AND EARLY IDENTIFICATION

In recent years, the diagnosis of axSpA has increasingly been made at an earlier stage in the disease as a result of increasing use of MRI and awareness of the wide spectrum of disease as described in new classification criteria. As advances are made in the understanding of genetic and serologic markers relating to SpA, these could play an expanding role in the identification of early or even preclinical disease. The prospect of screening certain patient populations for axSpA may become a reality in the near future. Screening is defined as the process of identifying apparently healthy individuals who may be at increased risk of a disease or condition. Ten principles for evaluation of screening programs were proposed by Wilson and Jungner in a report commissioned by the World Health Organization in 1968.[80] Several of these principles pose problems for the early identification of axSpA. An example is the availability of a suitable test or examination: although radiographic AS may be easy to identify, the early diagnosis of nonradiographic axSpA depends on local clinical and radiological expertise. In addition, the natural history of nr-axSpA remains incompletely understood.

These criteria have been reconsidered by the US Preventive Services Task Force with a focus on health outcomes.[81] The US Preventive Services Task Force notes that one of the most important issues in considering screening programs is whether the screening program would result in sufficient net benefit for the population to justify starting the program, given the level of resources required. The task force also lists

> **Box 1**
> **Key research questions for preclinical and very early axSpA**
>
> 1. What is the natural history of early or nonradiographic axSpA?
> 2. What is the best strategy for early identification of axSpA?
> 3. What is the significance of MRI "inflammatory lesions" in healthy individuals and those with early IBP, and how do these lesions evolve over time?
> 4. How may biomarkers and genetic testing be incorporated into clinical practice to aid diagnosis and treatment of axSpA?

several factors to be taken into account when estimating benefits and harms of a screening program. These factors have direct relevance when considering screening for axSpA.

In estimating the magnitude of potential benefits, the probability of an adverse health outcome without screening, and the magnitude of incremental health benefit of earlier versus later treatment, should be considered. In the case of axSpA, it now seems that treatment with a TNFi earlier is more effective than treatment later in the disease course. However, many patients never require a TNFi. There is evidence that sustained NSAID therapy may alter radiographic progression if acute-phase reactants are elevated.[82] Earlier diagnosis could provide relief of symptoms and could avoid unnecessary investigations or ineffective therapies for undiagnosed back pain. But it is not clear whether earlier diagnosis would alter long-term outcomes across the whole spectrum of severity of axSpA. This would require prospective studies of well-characterized axSpA cohorts, with a particular focus on those patients with features predicting progressive disease.

The potential harms of screening relate to overdiagnosis and false-positive tests. Screening should detect patients who would otherwise suffer adverse health

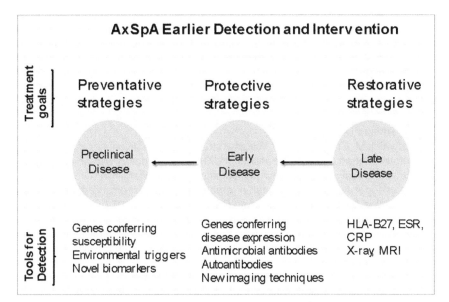

Fig. 1. A model for the future: investigation and treatment of axSpA. CRP, C-reactive protein; ESR, erythrocyte sedimentation rate.

outcomes. Labeling patients who have, for example, sacroiliitis on imaging but no symptoms of axSpA raises ethical and management questions. Would detection of asymptomatic, preclinical disease be beneficial on balance? Would such screening entail any possibility of physical harm (eg, complications from investigations or treatment) or psychological harm (eg, anxiety after a false-positive result)? Are current diagnostic modalities (clinical, serologic, genetic, or imaging) of sufficient sensitivity and specificity that identification of suspected preclinical axSpA would justify initiation of treatment? Is the current understanding of the basic mechanisms underlying the disease sufficient to design preventative interventions before the disease becomes clinically expressed?

SUMMARY

In recent years, several strategies have been used to improve the detection of early AS, including the provision of referral pathways from primary care, increasing availability and understanding of MRI, and case-finding tools in patients with extra-articular manifestations. Questions for future research are listed in **Box 1**. Addressing these questions may lead to alternative methods of early recognition of disease, incorporating genetic and serologic testing for biomarkers that predict the development of axSpA, allowing more precise prognosis and improved management (**Fig. 1**). However, the risks and benefits of preclinical disease identification have to be carefully considered as such screening strategies are formulated and tested.

REFERENCES

1. Sieper J, Rudwaleit M, Khan MA, et al. Concepts and epidemiology of spondyloarthritis. Best Pract Res Clin Rheumatol 2006;20:401.
2. Rudwaleit M, Khan MA, Sieper J. The challenge of diagnosis and classification in early ankylosing spondylitis: do we need new criteria? Arthritis Rheum 2005; 52:1000.
3. Haibel H, Rudwaleit M, Listing J, et al. Efficacy of adalimumab in the treatment of axial spondylarthritis without radiographically defined sacroiliitis: results of a twelve-week randomized, double-blind, placebo-controlled trial followed by an open-label extension up to week fifty-two. Arthritis Rheum 1981;58:2008.
4. Rudwaleit M, Listing J, Brandt J, et al. Prediction of a major clinical response (BASDAI 50) to tumour necrosis factor alpha blockers in ankylosing spondylitis. Ann Rheum Dis 2004;63:665.
5. Rudwaleit M, Claudepierre P, Wordsworth P, et al. Effectiveness, safety, and predictors of good clinical response in 1250 patients treated with adalimumab for active ankylosing spondylitis. J Rheumatol 2009;36:801.
6. Vastesaeger N, van der Heijde D, Inman RD, et al. Predicting the outcome of ankylosing spondylitis therapy. Ann Rheum Dis 2011;70:973.
7. Braun J, Baraliakos X, Golder W, et al. Magnetic resonance imaging examinations of the spine in patients with ankylosing spondylitis, before and after successful therapy with infliximab: evaluation of a new scoring system. Arthritis Rheum 2003;48:1126.
8. Rudwaleit M, Baraliakos X, Listing J, et al. Magnetic resonance imaging of the spine and the sacroiliac joints in ankylosing spondylitis and undifferentiated spondyloarthritis during treatment with etanercept. Ann Rheum Dis 2005;64:1305.

9. Haroon N, Inman RD, Learch TJ, et al. The impact of tumor necrosis factor alpha inhibitors on radiographic progression in ankylosing spondylitis. Arthritis Rheum 2013;65:2645.

10. van der Linden S, Valkenburg HA, Cats A. Evaluation of diagnostic criteria for ankylosing spondylitis. A proposal for modification of the New York criteria. Arthritis Rheum 1984;27:361.

11. Rudwaleit M, Landewe R, van der Heijde D, et al. The development of Assessment of SpondyloArthritis International Society classification criteria for axial spondyloarthritis (part I): classification of paper patients by expert opinion including uncertainty appraisal. Ann Rheum Dis 2009;68:770.

12. Rudwaleit M, van der Heijde D, Landewe R, et al. The development of Assessment of SpondyloArthritis International Society classification criteria for axial spondyloarthritis (part II): validation and final selection. Ann Rheum Dis 2009; 68:777.

13. Mau W, Zeidler H, Mau R, et al. Clinical features and prognosis of patients with possible ankylosing spondylitis. Results of a 10-year followup. J Rheumatol 1988;15:1109.

14. Sampaio-Barros PD, Bertolo MB, Kraemer MH, et al. Undifferentiated spondyloarthropathies: a 2-year follow-up study. Clin Rheumatol 2001;20:201.

15. Sampaio-Barros PD, Bortoluzzo AB, Conde RA, et al. Undifferentiated spondyloarthritis: a longterm followup. J Rheumatol 2010;37:1195.

16. Poddubnyy D, Rudwaleit M, Haibel H, et al. Rates and predictors of radiographic sacroiliitis progression over 2 years in patients with axial spondyloarthritis. Ann Rheum Dis 2011;70:1369.

17. Sieper J, van der Heijde D, Dougados M, et al. Efficacy and safety of adalimumab in patients with non-radiographic axial spondyloarthritis: results of a randomised placebo-controlled trial (ABILITY-1). Ann Rheum Dis 2013;72(6): 815–22.

18. Kiltz U, Baraliakos X, Karakostas P, et al. Do patients with non-radiographic axial spondylarthritis differ from patients with ankylosing spondylitis? Arthritis Care Res (Hoboken) 2012;64:1415.

19. Rudwaleit M, Haibel H, Baraliakos X, et al. The early disease stage in axial spondylarthritis: results from the German Spondyloarthritis Inception Cohort. Arthritis Rheum 2009;60:717.

20. Calin A, Porta J, Fries JF, et al. Clinical history as a screening test for ankylosing spondylitis. JAMA 1977;237:2613.

21. Dougados M, van der Linden S, Juhlin R, et al. The European Spondylarthropathy Study Group preliminary criteria for the classification of spondylarthropathy. Arthritis Rheum 1991;34:1218.

22. Rudwaleit M, Metter A, Listing J, et al. Inflammatory back pain in ankylosing spondylitis: a reassessment of the clinical history for application as classification and diagnostic criteria. Arthritis Rheum 2006;54:569.

23. Sieper J, van der Heijde D, Landewe R, et al. New criteria for inflammatory back pain in patients with chronic back pain: a real patient exercise by experts from the Assessment of SpondyloArthritis International Society (ASAS). Ann Rheum Dis 2009;68:784.

24. Chou R, Qaseem A, Snow V, et al. Diagnosis and treatment of low back pain: a joint clinical practice guideline from the American College of Physicians and the American Pain Society. Ann Intern Med 2007;147:478.

25. Underwood MR, Dawes P. Inflammatory back pain in primary care. Br J Rheumatol 1995;34:1074.

26. Weisman MH, Witter JP, Reveille JD. The prevalence of inflammatory back pain: population-based estimates from the US National Health and Nutrition Examination Survey, 2009-10. Ann Rheum Dis 2013;72:369.

27. Feldtkeller E, Khan MA, van der Heijde D, et al. Age at disease onset and diagnosis delay in HLA-B27 negative vs. positive patients with ankylosing spondylitis. Rheumatol Int 2003;23:61.

28. van den Berg R, de Hooge M, Rudwaleit M, et al. ASAS modification of the Berlin algorithm for diagnosing axial spondyloarthritis: results from the SPondyloArthritis Caught Early (SPACE)-cohort and from the Assessment of SpondyloArthritis International Society (ASAS)-cohort. Ann Rheum Dis 2013;72:1646.

29. Sieper J, Srinivasan S, Zamani O, et al. Comparison of two referral strategies for diagnosis of axial spondyloarthritis: the Recognising and Diagnosing Ankylosing Spondylitis Reliably (RADAR) study. Ann Rheum Dis 2013;72:1621.

30. Poddubnyy D, Vahldiek J, Spiller I, et al. Evaluation of 2 screening strategies for early identification of patients with axial spondyloarthritis in primary care. J Rheumatol 2011;38:2452.

31. Feldtkeller E, Rudwaleit M, Zeidler H. Easy probability estimation of the diagnosis of early axial spondyloarthritis by summing up scores. Rheumatology 2013;52:1648.

32. Rudwaleit M, Sieper J. Referral strategies for early diagnosis of axial spondyloarthritis. Nat Rev Rheumatol 2012;8:262.

33. Maksymowych WP, Lambert RG. Magnetic resonance imaging for spondyloarthritis–avoiding the minefield. J Rheumatol 2007;34:259.

34. Marzo-Ortega H, McGonagle D, O'Connor P, et al. Efficacy of etanercept in the treatment of the entheseal pathology in resistant spondylarthropathy: a clinical and magnetic resonance imaging study. Arthritis Rheum 2001;44:2112.

35. Bennett AN, Rehman A, Hensor EM, et al. Evaluation of the diagnostic utility of spinal magnetic resonance imaging in axial spondylarthritis. Arthritis Rheum 2009;60:1331.

36. Hermann KG, Baraliakos X, van der Heijde DM, et al. Descriptions of spinal MRI lesions and definition of a positive MRI of the spine in axial spondyloarthritis: a consensual approach by the ASAS/OMERACT MRI study group. Ann Rheum Dis 2012;71:1278.

37. Rudwaleit M, Jurik AG, Hermann KG, et al. Defining active sacroiliitis on magnetic resonance imaging (MRI) for classification of axial spondyloarthritis: a consensual approach by the ASAS/OMERACT MRI group. Ann Rheum Dis 2009;68:1520.

38. Aydin SZ, Maksymowych WP, Bennett AN, et al. Validation of the ASAS criteria and definition of a positive MRI of the sacroiliac joint in an inception cohort of axial spondyloarthritis followed up for 8 years. Ann Rheum Dis 2011;71:56.

39. Weber U, Maksymowych WP. Sensitivity and specificity of magnetic resonance imaging for axial spondyloarthritis. Am J Med Sci 2011;341:272.

40. Gong Y, Zheng N, Chen SB, et al. Ten years' experience with needle biopsy in the early diagnosis of sacroiliitis. Arthritis Rheum 2011;64:1399.

41. Weber U, Hodler J, Kubik RA, et al. Sensitivity and specificity of spinal inflammatory lesions assessed by whole-body magnetic resonance imaging in patients with ankylosing spondylitis or recent-onset inflammatory back pain. Arthritis Rheum 2009;61:900.

42. McEniff N, Eustace S, McCarthy C, et al. Asymptomatic sacroiliitis in inflammatory bowel disease. Assessment by computed tomography. Clin Imaging 1995; 19:258.

43. Turkcapar N, Toruner M, Soykan I, et al. The prevalence of extraintestinal manifestations and HLA association in patients with inflammatory bowel disease. Rheumatol Int 2006;26:663.
44. de Vlam K, Mielants H, Cuvelier C, et al. Spondyloarthropathy is underestimated in inflammatory bowel disease: prevalence and HLA association. J Rheumatol 2000;27:2860.
45. Mielants H, Veys EM, Goemaere S, et al. Gut inflammation in the spondyloarthropathies: clinical, radiologic, biologic and genetic features in relation to the type of histology. A prospective study. J Rheumatol 1991;18:1542.
46. Landers CJ, Cohavy O, Misra R, et al. Selected loss of tolerance evidenced by Crohn's disease-associated immune responses to auto- and microbial antigens. Gastroenterology 2002;123:689.
47. Prideaux L, De Cruz P, Ng SC, et al. Serological antibodies in inflammatory bowel disease: a systematic review. Inflamm Bowel Dis 2012;18:1340.
48. Mundwiler ML, Mei L, Landers CJ, et al. Inflammatory bowel disease serologies in ankylosing spondylitis patients: a pilot study. Arthritis Res Ther 2009;11:R177.
49. Wallis D, Asaduzzaman A, Weisman M, et al. Elevated serum anti-flagellin antibodies implicate subclinical bowel inflammation in ankylosing spondylitis: an observational study. Arthritis Res Ther 2013;15:R166.
50. Quinton JF, Sendid B, Reumaux D, et al. Anti-*Saccharomyces cerevisiae* mannan antibodies combined with antineutrophil cytoplasmic autoantibodies in inflammatory bowel disease: prevalence and diagnostic role. Gut 1998; 42:788.
51. Vasiliauskas EA, Plevy SE, Landers CJ, et al. Perinuclear antineutrophil cytoplasmic antibodies in patients with Crohn's disease define a clinical subgroup. Gastroenterology 1996;110:1810.
52. Targan SR, Landers CJ, Yang H, et al. Antibodies to CBir1 flagellin define a unique response that is associated independently with complicated Crohn's disease. Gastroenterology 2005;128:2020.
53. Appel H, Ruiz-Heiland G, Listing J, et al. Altered skeletal expression of sclerostin and its link to radiographic progression in ankylosing spondylitis. Arthritis Rheum 2009;60:3257.
54. Las Heras F, Pritzker KP, So A, et al. Aberrant chondrocyte hypertrophy and activation of beta-catenin signaling precede joint ankylosis in ank/ank mice. J Rheumatol 2012;39:583.
55. Groppe J, Greenwald J, Wiater E, et al. Structural basis of BMP signalling inhibition by the cystine knot protein Noggin. Nature 2002;420:636.
56. Lories RJ, Derese I, Luyten FP. Modulation of bone morphogenetic protein signaling inhibits the onset and progression of ankylosing enthesitis. J Clin Invest 2005;115:1571.
57. Tsui FW, Tsui HW, Las Heras F, et al. Serum levels of novel noggin and sclerostin-immune complexes are elevated in ankylosing spondylitis. Ann Rheum Dis 2013. [Epub ahead of print].
58. Rahman P, Inman RD, Gladman DD, et al. Association of interleukin-23 receptor variants with ankylosing spondylitis. Arthritis Rheum 2008;58:1020.
59. Pimentel-Santos FM, Ligeiro D, Matos M, et al. Association of IL23R and ERAP1 genes with ankylosing spondylitis in a Portuguese population. Clin Exp Rheumatol 2009;27:800.
60. Rueda B, Orozco G, Raya E, et al. The IL23R Arg381Gln non-synonymous polymorphism confers susceptibility to ankylosing spondylitis. Ann Rheum Dis 2008; 67:1451.

61. Maksymowych WP, Inman RD, Gladman DD, et al. Association of a specific ERAP1/ARTS1 haplotype with disease súsceptibility in ankylosing spondylitis. Arthritis Rheum 2009;60:1317.
62. Tsui FW, Haroon N, Reveille JD, et al. Association of an ERAP1 ERAP2 haplotype with familial ankylosing spondylitis. Ann Rheum Dis 2009;69:733.
63. Sherlock JP, Joyce-Shaikh B, Turner SP, et al. IL-23 induces spondyloarthropathy by acting on ROR-gammat+ CD3+CD4-CD8- entheseal resident T cells. Nat Med 2012;18:1069.
64. Benham H, Rehaume LM, Hasnain SZ, et al. IL-23-mediates the intestinal response to microbial beta-glucan and the development of spondyloarthritis pathology in SKG mice. Arthritis Rheumatol 2014. http://dx.doi.org/10.1002/ART.38638.
65. Cortes A, Hadler J, Pointon JP, et al. Identification of multiple risk variants for ankylosing spondylitis through high-density genotyping of immune-related loci. Nat Genet 2013;45:730.
66. Rudwaleit M, Baeten D. Ankylosing spondylitis and bowel disease. Best Pract Res Clin Rheumatol 2006;20:451.
67. Palm O, Moum B, Ongre A, et al. Prevalence of ankylosing spondylitis and other spondyloarthropathies among patients with inflammatory bowel disease: a population study (the IBSEN study). J Rheumatol 2002;29:511.
68. Orchard TR, Wordsworth BP, Jewell DP. Peripheral arthropathies in inflammatory bowel disease: their articular distribution and natural history. Gut 1998;42:387.
69. Meuwissen SG, Dekker-Saeys BJ, Agenant D, et al. Ankylosing spondylitis and inflammatory bowel disease. I. Prevalence of inflammatory bowel disease in patients suffering from ankylosing spondylitis. Ann Rheum Dis 1978;37:30.
70. Alnaqbi KA, Touma Z, Passalent L, et al. Development, sensibility, and reliability of the Toronto Axial Spondyloarthritis Questionnaire in inflammatory bowel disease. J Rheumatol 2013;40:1726.
71. Ibrahim GH, Buch MH, Lawson C, et al. Evaluation of an existing screening tool for psoriatic arthritis in people with psoriasis and the development of a new instrument: the Psoriasis Epidemiology Screening Tool (PEST) questionnaire. Clin Exp Rheumatol 2009;27:469.
72. Husni ME, Meyer KH, Cohen DS, et al. The PASE questionnaire: pilot-testing a psoriatic arthritis screening and evaluation tool. J Am Acad Dermatol 2007; 57:581.
73. Gladman DD, Schentag CT, Tom BD, et al. Development and initial validation of a screening questionnaire for psoriatic arthritis: the Toronto Psoriatic Arthritis Screen (ToPAS). Ann Rheum Dis 2009;68:497.
74. Coates LC, Aslam T, Al Balushi F, et al. Comparison of three screening tools to detect psoriatic arthritis in patients with psoriasis (CONTEST study). Br J Dermatol 2013;168:802.
75. Walsh JA, Callis Duffin K, Krueger GG, et al. Limitations in screening instruments for psoriatic arthritis: a comparison of instruments in patients with psoriasis. J Rheumatol 2013;40:287.
76. Haroon M, Kirby B, FitzGerald O. High prevalence of psoriatic arthritis in patients with severe psoriasis with suboptimal performance of screening questionnaires. Ann Rheum Dis 2013;72:736.
77. Chung YM, Liao HT, Lin KC, et al. Prevalence of spondyloarthritis in 504 Chinese patients with HLA-B27-associated acute anterior uveitis. Scand J Rheumatol 2009;38:84.
78. Haroon M, O'Rourke M, Ramasamy P, et al. A novel evidence-based detection of undiagnosed spondyloarthritis in patients presenting with acute anterior

uveitis: the DUET (Dublin Uveitis Evaluation Tool) algorithm. Arthritis Rheum 2013;65:2779.

79. Geirsson AJ, Kristjansson K, Gudbjornsson B. A strong familiality of ankylosing spondylitis through several generations. Ann Rheum Dis 2010;69:1346.

80. Wilson J, Jungner G. Principles and practice of screening for disease. Geneva (Switzerland): World Health Organization; 1968.

81. Harris R, Sawaya GF, Moyer VA, et al. Reconsidering the criteria for evaluating proposed screening programs: reflections from 4 current and former members of the U.S. Preventive services task force. Epidemiol Rev 2011;33:20.

82. Poddubnyy D, Rudwaleit M, Haibel H, et al. Effect of non-steroidal anti-inflammatory drugs on radiographic spinal progression in patients with axial spondyloarthritis: results from the German Spondyloarthritis Inception Cohort. Ann Rheum Dis 2012;71:1616.

Identifying and Treating Preclinical and Early Osteoarthritis

 CrossMark

David T. Felson, MD, MPH[a,b,c,d],*, Richard Hodgson, BM, PhD[c,d]

KEYWORDS

- Osteoarthritis • Knee pain • Magnetic resonance imaging • Biomarkers

KEY POINTS

- The limited efficacy of current nonsurgical treatments for osteoarthritis (OA) may be due partly to their use at a late point in the evolution of disease when structural deterioration is often advanced; this provides a rationale for identifying persons with early disease or those at high risk.
- Persons at especially high risk of later disease who would be good targets for treatment are those with sports-related major knee injuries, those with anatomic abnormalities of their hips associated with a high rate of later OA, and those from families with an unusually high risk of early disease.
- Chronic knee pain is a harbinger of knee OA.
- Evolving imaging approaches using magnetic resonance imaging hold promise in identifying joints with reversible structural findings that represent early lesions of OA.

INTRODUCTION

Osteoarthritis (OA) is the most common form of arthritis. Although prevalence estimates differ depending on the country and how disease is assessed, OA clearly affects millions of persons in the United States and a similar number in Europe. In developing countries it is also the most common form of arthritis. OA prevalence increases with age and with obesity, and the rapidly increasing demand for knee and hip replacements is due in part to the burgeoning population of those with OA because of the aging of the population and increasing rates of obesity. OA is the most common

Supported by National Institutes of Health AR47785.
Funded by NIHMS-ID: 619172.
[a] Medicine, Boston University School of Medicine, Suite 200, 650 Albany Street, Boston, MA 02118, USA; [b] University of Manchester, Stopford Building, Oxford Road, Manchester M13 9PT, UK; [c] Clinical Epidemiology Unit, Boston University, Boston, MA, USA; [d] NIHR Biomedical Research Unit, University of Manchester, Manchester, UK
* Corresponding author. Medicine, Boston University School of Medicine, Suite 200, 650 Albany Street, Boston, MA 02118.
E-mail address: dfelson@bu.edu

cause of mobility disability in the world, and its overall impact as a cause of years lived with disability and limited quality of life is rising.[1]

One of the central reasons for the increase in demand for knee and hip replacements is that medical and rehabilitative treatments for OA are not very effective. There are no treatments that have been shown consistently to delay the structural progression of disease, and none is approved by regulatory agencies for this purpose. Meta-analyses suggest that nonsurgical treatments such as exercise, anti-inflammatory medications, and others all have modest efficacy at best. New more effective treatments for established disease are badly needed.

One major reason why treatments are not delaying joint replacement surgery may be that treatment begins too late in the course of OA to have an effect. Many of the structural findings uncovered in recent comprehensive cohort studies of persons with knee OA have suggested that most persons with disease have advanced structural findings in the knee by the time they are clinically diagnosed, and have frequent knee pain. Varus or valgus malalignment, meniscal damage such as tears, and prevalent cartilage loss are all common features of middle-aged and older persons with new-onset chronic knee pain.[2] Radiographic evidence of OA is a relatively late phenomenon in the structural evolution of this disease. For example, alterations in the shape of the periarticular bones often precede the development of disease by 5 to 10 years radiographically.[3] Abnormalities seen on magnetic resonance imaging (MRI) are present several years before disease development in most cases. Many of these structural changes are not known to be reversible and, to the extent that they drive disease progression, a patient presenting with knee pain is often on the downslope of such a trajectory.

A recent focus on changes in the peripheral and central nervous system that develop as part of osteoarthritic pain suggests that nervous system–related changes have also occurred in many persons by the time they develop the chronic pain of OA. These changes in the nervous system make treatment more challenging and pain more severe than might have occurred had the disease been identified and treated earlier.[4]

Therefore, the rationale for focusing on early OA is that irreversible structural changes may not yet be established and that chronic nervous system sensitization to pain has not yet evolved. To target early OA, the choice might include those with early disease and those at high risk of disease who do not yet have symptoms or early disease.

The evolution of OA from the earliest evidence of joint injury to end-stage disease is shown in **Fig. 1**. Early osteochondral lesions are usually unaccompanied by symptoms in middle-aged and elderly persons. Even meniscal tears, which are common and occur incidentally, are often not associated with knee pain or other symptoms.[5] The initial defect in cartilage or initial meniscal tear or extrusion is followed by a constellation of features including more damage in the initial location leading to asymmetry of the joint and malalignment, bony remodeling, and damage to adjacent tissues.[6] For example, an incidental meniscal tear puts a knee at high risk of adjacent cartilage damage and of meniscal extrusion. There is tissue loss between the 2 bones and narrowing of the joint on that side, initially to a subtle degree that is not visible on the radiograph. First symptoms occur only after this process is far advanced, and are mild and intermittent. The patient usually does not seek care until symptoms including pain are more troublesome or frequent. By the time symptoms are present, roughly 80% of knees have clinically important frontal plane malalignment (varus or valgus) and even knees without frontal plane malalignment often have patellofemoral malalignment. This malalignment increases stress or focal loading across the affected region of the joint. Cartilage loss and/or meniscal damage is the rule.[7]

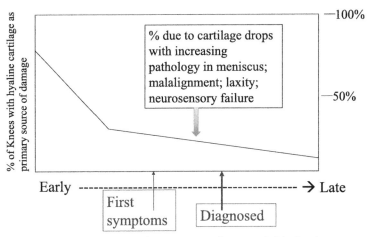

Fig. 1. Source of joint damage according to stage of osteoarthritis development.

Other features of disease that can coexist at the time include ligamentous laxity, proprioceptive deficiencies, muscle weakness, and synovitis. Whereas some of these, such as muscle weakness and synovitis, may be amenable to therapy, for others there is no known therapy. Thus, for early treatment approaches to be successful, at least for knee OA, patients need to be identified at a point before the development of meniscal damage, substantial cartilage loss, or malalignment. Waiting for radiographic evidence of disease for diagnosis is almost certainly too late because many of the irreversible structural findings accompany radiographic changes. Ideally an approach that targets either those at high risk who are willing to consider preventive therapy or those with very early disease constitute the most likely route to success.

RISK FACTORS: IDENTIFYING THOSE AT HIGH RISK OF EARLY OSTEOARTHRITIS
Age

The major risk factor for OA is older age.[8,9] In all joints and among both genders, OA prevalence increases steeply with age, starting at around age 50 to 55 years. A multitude of factors contributes to this increase, including the senescence of cartilage leading to its fragility,[10] the failure of periarticular structures that provide protection against joint damage during weight bearing, increasing muscle weakness with age, neurosensory failure with age, and ligamentous laxity. Because of these changes (many of which are age-related) and the challenge in reversing them, targeting early OA may need to focus on persons of middle age who may be at high risk of developing OA earlier than expected. Because knee and hip replacements are often reserved for older persons, early onset of OA when a person is in their 30s or 40s poses special therapeutic challenges, and the reward for any prevention strategy may be great.

Obesity

Obesity plays a major role in increasing the risk of OA of the knee and, to a lesser extent, the hip. Jiang and colleagues[11] have suggested that eliminating the problem of obesity might prevent up to 50% of knee OA in the United States and a lesser proportion in countries where obesity is not as prevalent. Effects of obesity in causing OA may be complex. Obesity not only increases the risk of knee and hip OA but also increases the risk of hand OA, suggesting that its effects on disease are not completely mediated by effects on mechanical load. Indeed, adipokines have been linked with OA occurrence, although there are no clear-cut data as yet to suggest that the effects of leptin or other adipokines are independent of the loading effect of weight. Convincing evidence demonstrating the role of adipokines might point to an opportunity for slowing the rate of progression of disease in those who are obese.

Gender

Women are at substantially higher risk than men of contracting OA in all joints except the hips. Women are more likely than men to develop structural disease in their joints, and, for a given level of structural disease, women are also more likely to have joint pain.[12] Although women have higher rates of OA than men, this gender difference does not develop until the sixth decade, when women have just gone through or are going through the menopause. This fact has obviously raised questions about whether estrogen or hormonal loss triggers OA, a matter as yet unresolved despite many studies.

Traumatic Joint Injury

Among the most potent risk factors for OA is major injury, such as from sports, leading to an anterior cruciate ligament (ACL) or meniscal tear. In the knee, such major injuries account for approximately 10% of all OA, but in joints that are rarely affected by OA such as the ankles, injuries account for more than 70% of OA cases.[13] Meniscal damage, including tears and extrusion, has been consistently shown to be among the most potent risk factors for later development of OA. Even incidental tears with no recollected injury pose a very high risk of later disease, and a partial meniscectomy does not necessarily reduce this risk. Similarly, ACL tears even without concomitant meniscal tears increase the risk of OA later, and surgical treatment does not seem to lessen this risk.

Injuries such as ACL and meniscal tears may represent a special opportunity to prevent OA. These injuries occur in young persons whose joints are otherwise normal, without the coexisting pathomechanics and bone-shape alterations that typify clinical OA. Animal studies[14] have identified a superhealer strain of mouse which, faced with traumatic joint injury, heals without arthritis. Characteristics of these mice include a blunted inflammatory response, suggesting that prolific inflammation may be a major cause of permanent joint damage after an injury, and that ablating this inflammatory response may lessen the ultimate joint damage. There are ongoing trials testing whether disease can be prevented by administering potent anti-inflammatory treatments at an early stage after either ACL or meniscal tears.

In the knee, frontal plane malalignment (**Fig. 2**), in either the varus or valgus direction, is a major cause of disease progression. Usually malalignment develops as a consequence of disease when cartilage loss or meniscal extrusion narrows one side of the joint. However, even among normal prediseased knees there is a modest variation in alignment status, and some normal people have varus or valgus knees without any preexisting knee damage. Recent studies[15,16] have shown definitively that prediseased knees with malalignment are at modestly increased risk of developing OA, probably because such knees experience increased focal loads at the site of malalignment and these loads ultimately lead to tissue breakdown, especially as a person becomes older and their intra-articular soft tissue becomes more fragile.

The Hip and Congenital Abnormalities

The hip is a special case whereby joints at high risk of OA may be readily identified. A large percentage of hip OA cases occur against the background of preexisting

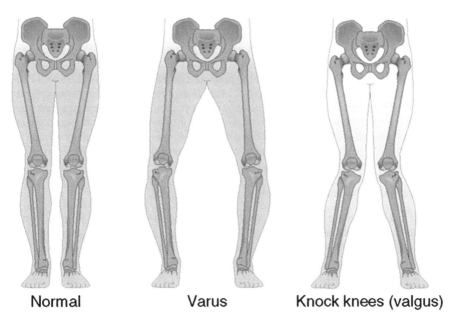

| Normal | Varus | Knock knees (valgus) |

Fig. 2. Different frontal plane alignments. Varus and valgus alignments increase stress across medial and lateral knee compartments, respectively.

anatomic abnormalities. Such abnormalities include hip dysplasia, which when severe, is detected and corrected at birth, but when present on a mild basis, often persists into adulthood. Other developmental abnormalities include slipped capital femoral epiphysis and Legg-Perthes disease, which occur more commonly in boys than in girls. Lastly, recent years have seen the identification and characterization of the major hip anatomic abnormality, femoroacetabular impingement (FAI),[17] which clearly predilects to later hip OA. FAI has 2 often coexisting subtypes, cam deformity and pincer deformity, the latter being more common in girls. Cam deformities may arise before the closure of the epiphysis and be brought on by athletic or other activities. FAI symptoms may occur in teenage years or early adulthood and may be correctable with osteotomy surgery, although the efficacy of this surgery is yet to be proved. Such surgery, if effective, might prevent OA from developing later.

Genetic Risk

After combining data from multiple large-scale studies of OA in which genetic material was obtained from subjects, Zeggini and colleagues[18] uncovered a set of genetic abnormalities associated with an increased risk of OA, most prominently among them an abnormality in the gene GDF5. Neither GDF5 nor other genes currently identified as predisposing to OA is associated with a high risk of disease. One compelling hypothesis is that these genes increases the risk of disease by altering joint shape[19] and, if so, they may inform us of joint shapes that predispose to later OA and help to identify persons at high risk of OA. The genes so far identified are more commonly associated with joint-specific OA than with generalized OA.

THE ROLE OF INFLAMMATION IN OSTEOARTHRITIS

Inflammation is a clearly a component of OA, whether defined as the presence of inflammatory cytokines in joint tissues such as cartilage matrix and synovial fluid, or as histologic evidence of synovitis, which is present variably in OA knees and hands.[20,21] Though present in most joints with OA to some extent, the impact of inflammation on OA joints is not clear, as any effects in clinical OA may be overwhelmed by disease mechanopathology. Synovitis clearly increases the risk of joint pain and its severity,[21] and it is likely that inflammation within the joint contributes to pain sensitization, which occurs in many persons with chronic OA.[4] However, there is no consistent evidence that synovitis leads to cartilage loss independent of other structural findings that drive this loss (eg, meniscal tears). Moreover, studies consistently show that persons with radiographically identified OA do not have elevated systemic levels of acute-phase reactants.[22-24] Trials testing different anti-inflammatory approaches for OA, many used in rheumatoid arthritis, are ongoing.

THE FEASIBILITY OF IDENTIFYING EARLY OSTEOARTHRITIS

Several strategies have been tested to determine whether persons with early OA can be successfully identified. The best test is to examine persons with a few months of knee pain at a point when their radiographs are either normal or show only very mild disease and follow them to determine if they are likely to develop OA, and whether there are any predictors that might identify those who do develop disease. Of 2 such studies, 1 with only a 3-year follow-up found that 42% had incident radiographic OA at follow-up and reported that there were no factors that identified persons at highest risk.[25] On the other hand, Thorstensson and colleagues[26] followed 143 subjects with limited history of chronic knee pain and found that 86% developed radiographic OA over 12 years. In work from the Framingham Study,[27] those with unilateral knee OA had a greater than 90% likelihood of developing OA in the contralateral knee over a 10-year follow-up, and most of those contralateral knees that developed OA were also frequently painful. These data collectively suggest that chronic knee pain accurately identifies middle-aged persons at high risk of later OA, although the disease may not develop immediately, and that those with unilateral disease are at extremely high risk of developing bilateral disease. In these studies, developing OA is defined as a radiograph positive for OA and, as noted earlier, radiographic positivity is a relatively late feature of disease.

MRI findings suggestive of OA are present in most middle-aged persons with chronic knee pain, including even most of those whose radiographs do not show OA.[28] In a study of 255 persons drawn from the community with knee pain, 124 (49%) had negative radiographs but clear-cut evidence of OA on MRI. Thirty-eight percent had radiographic OA and only 13% (33 subjects) had no OA by either imaging modality. Thus, either chronic knee pain alone or knee pain coupled with MRI findings suggesting OA (eg, cartilage loss) might accurately identify early disease. The salient concern is whether even these preradiographic MRI-based findings are revealed early enough that treatment can prevent further damage.

SPECIAL HIGH-RISK GROUPS

There are unique groups at especially high risk of OA who might be excellent targets for disease prevention. Among these are young people who have sustained major knee injuries, including those with meniscal or ACL tears. Such persons are at extremely high risk of developing OA within 10 to 20 years, and their disease evolves often by the fourth decade or even earlier. Because inflammatory response to the injury may drive some of the later destructive joint changes, exciting opportunities to prevent disease may include suppressing the inflammatory response to the injury as suggested by animal models of disease (see earlier discussion).

As noted earlier, hip OA is often preceded by a variety of prearthritic anatomic abnormalities. Surgery to correct these developmental abnormalities, including FAI, may possibly prevent later hip OA, although there is currently no evidence that correction of the abnormalities actually does. Identification of factors that prevent the development of these abnormalities could ultimately also prevent the later development of disease. Therefore hip anatomic abnormalities offer a special case whereby early changes that predispose to OA might be prevented.

Other persons at risk include those who come from families in which there is a high risk of OA. Commonly these are families with an inheritance of joint-specific disease such as hip OA or thumb-base OA. Unusually, there are families with generalized disease in which young persons not yet affected are at high risk of developing disease, especially if they carry the gene that predisposes to disease. Most genetic factors identified so far do not increase the risk of disease sufficiently to characterize persons with these genes as at high risk.[18,29] However, as in rheumatoid arthritis, persons carrying a combination of genes, each conferring a modest increased risk of disease, are at high risk of disease.

Another opportunity for disease prevention is available in persons who present with one joint affected with OA. Their risk of developing disease in other joints, especially the contralateral as yet unaffected joint, is high. To the extent that prevention strategies can be developed, these persons are certainly at risk and would benefit from such opportunities.

IMAGING APPROACHES TO IDENTIFY PERSONS WITH EARLY DISEASE

Imaging techniques have become available to detect the earliest changes in cartilage that might represent compositional alterations of early disease. The use of these techniques assumes that disease begins in cartilage. It is now recognized[10] that the process of disease even early on clearly involves interplay between cartilage and other structures within the joint, and that all of these are acted on by loading, with levels of excessive focal loading often driving the process. Even so, to the extent that cartilage plays a role in its own destruction or that abnormalities within cartilage provide evidence that abnormal loading is causing damage, imaging that detects subtle cartilage abnormalities may provide strong evidence that early OA exists regardless of cause. Imaging of intra-articular structures such as cartilage, synovium, and bone can show early evidence of disease before the irreversible pathomechanics of disease are established.

An appreciation for the information provided by imaging necessitates a brief exposition of cartilage biology. The 2 major molecular components of cartilage are type II collagen, which provides the skeleton of cartilage, and aggrecan, a macromolecular aggregate consisting of a core hyaluronic acid molecule surrounded by glycosaminoglycan (GAG) side chains that are highly negatively charged. The GAG molecules are covalently bound through link proteins to the hyaluronic acid; when cartilage is compressed, the electrostatic repulsion that ensues derives from these negative charges being forced into close proximity. When this pressure is released, the electric charges can dissipate. The negative charges from GAGs in aggrecan provide cartilage with its compressive stiffness.

The process of aggrecan degradation is mediated by 2 enzymes, ADAMTS4 and ADAMTS5, with the latter probably the more important. By contrast, collagen degradation is mediated by a series of matrix metalloproteinases, especially 1, 8, and 13, with the last of these being critical. In terms of early disruption of cartilage matrix, the loss of aggrecan is almost certainly reversible, whereas the loss of collagen matrix is not.[30] With the loss of aggrecan comes a loss of compressive stiffness, a physical softening of cartilage, and a tendency for that local area to swell as it imbibes proton ions from water. Imaging or other physical diagnostic tests that depend on measuring softness or local swelling might successfully identify early compositional changes in cartilage that are reversible, as might attempts to detect a depletion of negative charges that especially occur in cartilage after aggrecan depletion.

Although conventional MRI is clearly superior to radiographs in revealing evidence of damage to intra-articular structures such as cartilage and menisci, it does not generally reveal compositional changes in these tissues. It only shows evidence of damage to the tissues when cartilage has been worn away or menisci torn. Using an MRI approach, techniques have been developed that identify regional abnormalities within cartilage based on either the disruption to their collagen network or loss of aggrecan.

When aggrecan is depleted, the high concentration and negative charges become less homogeneous and diminish in some regions. MRI techniques that take advantage of this heterogeneity, and the depletion of GAGs and their negative charges within regions of cartilage, can successfully identify regions of compositional damage.[31]

The best validated of these techniques is delayed gadolinium-enhanced MRI of cartilage (dGEMRIC). dGEMRIC involves measuring the T1 relaxation time of cartilage some time (typically 90 minutes) after the intravenous injection of a contrast agent consisting of gadolinium with diethylenetriamine penta-acetic acid (Gd-DTPA). Because both the Gd-DTPA and the proteoglycans are negatively charged, the concentration of gadolinium in cartilage depends on proteoglycan content. As gadolinium reduces the T1 relaxation time, a T1 map acquired after administration of Gd-DTPA should be related to the proteoglycan content.

In vivo dGEMRIC of autologous chondrocyte implantation cartilage has been validated against GAG concentration of biopsies. In OA, in vivo dGEMRIC has been shown to correlate well with GAG content measured after joint replacement. dGEMRIC of ex vivo cartilage specimens from patients with OA correlates with GAG content to a greater extent than morphologic measures, although the applicability of ex vivo results is limited. Results comparing dGEMRIC with arthroscopic findings have been mixed. The reproducibility of dGEMRIC measurements has been high in healthy volunteers, patients with early OA, and patients with a history of ACL injury.

dGEMRIC differentiates between normal and osteoarthritic cartilage and correlates with severity of disease. It may also predict the development of OA changes. Changes have been demonstrated in association with meniscal abnormality, acetabular dysplasia, FAI, ACL injury, and patellar dislocation. Improvement in dGEMRIC values has been seen in patients after weight loss, collagen hydrolysate, and exercise.

In sum, dGEMRIC is a reproducible technique that can be implemented on standard clinical MRI scanners. It depends on the proteoglycan concentration and is therefore potentially useful in early OA. Unfortunately, it is practically challenging; it typically requires a double dose of gadolinium-based contrast agent, which is already implicated as a cause of serious (though rare) adverse events. Furthermore, one cannot image a joint immediately after gadolinium injection; rather, for knees at least, the patient needs to walk around for 90 minutes to allow the gadolinium to diffuse into cartilage. The type and duration of activity may affect the results of the scan because dGEMRIC is probably influenced by other factors in addition to proteoglycan concentration, such as transport mechanisms and cartilage thickness, although in early OA these may act synergistically to increase its sensitivity.

Given the inconvenience and possible risk of gadolinium as a contrast agent, other approaches have been developed that offer promise in the evaluation of early cartilage injury, although these have not been as well validated or studied as dGEMRIC.

T2 measurements of articular cartilage have been widely used in clinical studies of OA, including the large Osteoarthritis Initiative Study. Measurements are straightforward and relatively swift to acquire using multiple spin-echo sequences.

T2 has been linked to collagen, proteoglycan, and water content. Its reproducibility has been high in OA patients and normal controls. T2 is increased in OA, including early OA, and is related to OA severity. It has been shown to predict radiographic OA. However, the relationships between T2 increases and subsequent cartilage loss, although statistically significant in at least one study, are inconsistent and weak. T2 is increased in a variety of conditions including FAI and ACL injury, and after partial meniscectomy.

Although straightforward to measure and used in many clinical studies, the disadvantages of T2 are its complex and incompletely understood dependence on underlying structure and composition, and the change in measurements with orientation resulting from the magic-angle effect. Furthermore, if T2 mapping predominantly reflects disruption or destruction of collagen, T2 mapping may not be ideal for assessing reversible cartilage disease because once collagen is destroyed the matrix is thought to be irreversibly damaged.

T1-rho has been advocated as a measurement that is more sensitive than T2 to GAG concentration (and hence better for assessing early OA), but which does not require intravenous contrast. T1-rho is the relaxation time under the influence of a spin-lock pulse, and is calculated from multiple images acquired with different spin-lock pulse durations.

Several studies have demonstrated a correlation between T1-rho measured in vivo and GAG measurements after joint replacement in OA, although the strength of the correlation has differed. Correlations have also been shown with macroscopic grade of cartilage damage. Reproducibility of T1-rho measurements has been variable.

T1-rho has been shown to be increased in OA, including early OA, and to increase with disease severity. It also predicts the progression of morphologic changes. T1-rho is increased in the presence of FAI, patellar maltracking, ACL injury, and meniscal injury. Progression has been demonstrated after ACL reconstruction and partial meniscectomy.

Several studies have looked at both T1-rho and T2 measurements. Although outcomes from both have often been broadly similar, T1-rho may be more sensitive with larger changes; however, this may be partly offset by poorer reproducibility.

T1-rho therefore has the advantage that it may be more sensitive than T2 for assessing early cartilage change and, unlike dGEMRIC, it does not require intravenous contrast agent. Its disadvantages include sensitivity to field inhomogeneities, which make it technically challenging and time-consuming.

Sodium MRI is an attractive means of assessing early cartilage change in OA because the positively charged sodium ions map to negatively charged GAGs. Because the sodium nuclei resonate at a lower frequency than the hydrogen nuclei at a particular magnetic field strength, different hardware, including a different radio-frequency coil, is required. Signal from sodium is inherently very low, so images are of low resolution and are time-consuming to acquire.

In vitro sodium imaging of cartilage has shown good correlation with GAG measurements. Reproducibility has been demonstrated in healthy volunteers and OA patients. Sodium MRI of cartilage has shown differences from controls in OA, including early OA. It has been used to study cartilage repair tissue, and correlates strongly with T1-rho and dGEMRIC.

Sodium MRI has the advantage of being a more direct measure of GAG content. However, it is technically challenging, requires high field strengths and specialist hardware, and has the major limitation of low signal-to-noise ratio and, hence, resolution.

GAG chemical exchange saturation transfer (gagCEST) imaging makes use of the hydrogen nuclei of amide and hydroxyl groups in GAGs, which resonate at a slightly different frequency to those of water. Although these cannot be imaged directly, they can be saturated by a radiofrequency pulse at the appropriate frequency; this saturation is then transferred to nearby water protons, reducing the signal from the bulk water that forms the image. Static and radiofrequency field inhomogeneities make this technique technically challenging, particularly at lower field strengths, and gagCEST is often performed at 7 T. gagCEST has been shown to correlate well with sodium imaging in patients who have undergone cartilage repair surgery. Although not yet widely used, gagCEST may be useful in early OA, as it offers the potential to map GAG content at higher resolution than sodium MRI. However, it is technically demanding and will probably require high magnetic field strengths.

SUMMARY AND FUTURE CONSIDERATIONS

Identifying those at high risk of or with early OA may offer an opportunity to successfully intervene to lessen the burden of disease on patients and society. Those with chronic joint pain but with no radiographic features of OA and those drawn from high-risk groups with imaging studies suggesting early structural changes of disease may be good candidates for treatment. Future studies need to test strategies to treat these persons and to identify who among them would benefit most from any treatment.

REFERENCES

1. Murray CJ, Vos T, Lozano R, et al. Disability-adjusted life years (DALYs) for 291 diseases and injuries in 21 regions, 1990-2010: a systematic analysis for the Global Burden of Disease Study 2010. Lancet 2012;380(9859):2197–223.
2. Sharma L, Chmiel JS, Almagor O, et al. The role of varus and valgus alignment in the initial development of knee cartilage damage by MRI: the MOST study. Ann Rheum Dis 2013;72(2):235–40.
3. Neogi T, Bowes M, Niu J, et al. MRI-based three-dimensional bone shape of the knee predicts onset of knee osteoarthritis: data from the Osteoarthritis Initiative. Arthritis Rheum 2013;65:2048–58.
4. Neogi T, Frey-Law L, Scholz J, et al. Sensitivity and sensitisation in relation to pain severity in knee osteoarthritis: trait or state? Ann Rheum Dis 2013. [Epub ahead of print].
5. Englund M, Guermazi A, Gale D, et al. Incidental meniscal findings on knee MRI in middle aged and elderly persons in the United States. N Engl J Med 2008; 359(11):1108–15.
6. Roemer FW, Felson DT, Yang T, et al. The association between meniscal damage of the posterior horns and localized posterior synovitis detected on T1-weighted contrast-enhanced MRI–the MOST study. Semin Arthritis Rheum 2013;42(6):573–81.
7. Sharma L, Chmiel JS, Almagor O, et al. Significance of pre-radiographic MRI lesions in persons at higher risk for knee osteoarthritis. Arthritis Rheum 2014; 66:1811–9.
8. Lawrence RC, Felson DT, Helmick CG, et al. Estimates of the prevalence of arthritis and other rheumatic conditions in the United States. Part II. Arthritis Rheum 2008;58(1):26–35.
9. Zhang Y, Xu L, Nevitt MC, et al. Comparison of the prevalence of knee osteoarthritis between the elderly Chinese population in Beijing and whites in the United States: The Beijing Osteoarthritis Study. Arthritis Rheum 2001;44(9):2065–71.

10. Loeser RF. Aging and osteoarthritis: the role of chondrocyte senescence and aging changes in the cartilage matrix. Osteoarthr Cartil 2009;17(8):971–9.

11. Jiang L, Tian W, Wang Y, et al. Body mass index and susceptibility to knee osteoarthritis: a systematic review and meta-analysis. Joint Bone Spine 2012;79(3): 291–7.

12. Segal NA, Glass NA, Torner J, et al. Quadriceps weakness predicts risk for knee joint space narrowing in women in the MOST cohort. Osteoarthr Cartil 2010;18(6): 769–75.

13. Valderrabano V, Horisberger M, Russell I, et al. Etiology of ankle osteoarthritis. Clin Orthop Relat Res 2009;467(7):1800–6.

14. Ward BD, Furman BD, Huebner JL, et al. Absence of posttraumatic arthritis following intraarticular fracture in the MRL/MpJ mouse. Arthritis Rheum 2008; 58(3):744–53.

15. Sharma L, Eckstein F, Song J, et al. Relationship of meniscal damage, meniscal extrusion, malalignment, and joint laxity to subsequent cartilage loss in osteoarthritic knees. Arthritis Rheum 2008;58(6):1716–26.

16. Felson DT, Niu J, Gross KD, et al. Valgus malalignment is a risk factor for lateral knee osteoarthritis incidence and progression: findings from the Multicenter Osteoarthritis Study and the Osteoarthritis Initiative. Arthritis Rheum 2013;65(2):355–62.

17. Nicholls AS, Kiran A, Pollard TC, et al. The association between hip morphology parameters and nineteen-year risk of end-stage osteoarthritis of the hip: a nested case-control study. Arthritis Rheum 2011;63(11):3392–400.

18. Zeggini E, Panoutsopoulou K, Southam L, et al. Identification of new susceptibility loci for osteoarthritis (arcOGEN): a genome-wide association study. Lancet 2012; 380(9844):815–23.

19. Sandell LJ. Etiology of osteoarthritis: genetics and synovial joint development. Nat Rev Rheumatol 2012;8(2):77–89.

20. Haugen IK, Boyesen P, Slatkowsky-Christensen B, et al. Associations between MRI-defined synovitis, bone marrow lesions and structural features and measures of pain and physical function in hand osteoarthritis. Ann Rheum Dis 2012;71(6):899–904.

21. Baker K, Grainger A, Niu J, et al. Relation of synovitis to knee pain using contrast-enhanced MRIs. Ann Rheum Dis 2010;69(10):1779–83.

22. Vlad SC, Neogi T, Aliabadi P, et al. No association between markers of inflammation and osteoarthritis of the hands and knees. J Rheumatol 2011;38(8):1665–70.

23. Kerkhof HJ, Bierma-Zeinstra SM, Castano-Betancourt MC, et al. Serum C reactive protein levels and genetic variation in the CRP gene are not associated with the prevalence, incidence or progression of osteoarthritis independent of body mass index. Ann Rheum Dis 2010;69(11):1976–82.

24. Jin X, Beguerie JR, Zhang W, et al. Circulating C reactive protein in osteoarthritis: a systematic review and meta-analysis. Ann Rheum Dis 2013. [Epub ahead of print].

25. Peat G, Thomas E, Duncan R, et al. Is a "false-positive" clinical diagnosis of knee osteoarthritis just the early diagnosis of pre-radiographic disease? Arthritis Care Res (Hoboken) 2010;62(10):1502–6.

26. Thorstensson CA, Andersson ML, Jonsson H, et al. Natural course of knee osteoarthritis in middle-aged subjects with knee pain: 12-year follow-up using clinical and radiographic criteria. Ann Rheum Dis 2009;68(12):1890–3.

27. Jones RK, Chapman GJ, Findlow AH, et al. A new approach to prevention of knee osteoarthritis: reducing medial load in the contralateral knee. J Rheumatol 2013; 40(3):309–15.

28. Cibere J, Zhang H, Thorne A, et al. Association of clinical findings with pre-radiographic and radiographic knee osteoarthritis in a population-based study. Arthritis Care Res (Hoboken) 2010;62(12):1691–8.

29. van Meurs JB, Uitterlinden AG. Osteoarthritis year 2012 in review: genetics and genomics. Osteoarthr Cartil 2012;20(12):1470–6.

30. Loeser RF, Goldring SR, Scanzello CR, et al. Osteoarthritis: a disease of the joint as an organ. Arthritis Rheum 2012;64(6):1697–707.

31. Oei EH, van TJ, Robinson WH, et al. Quantitative radiological imaging techniques for articular cartilage composition: towards early diagnosis and development of disease-modifying therapeutics for osteoarthritis. Arthritis Care Res (Hoboken) 2014;66(8):1129–41.

Mucosal Immune Responses to Microbiota in the Development of Autoimmune Disease

CrossMark

Kristine A. Kuhn, MD, PhD[a], Isabel Pedraza, MD[b],
M. Kristen Demoruelle, MD[a],*

KEYWORDS

- Microbiota • Pathogenesis • Mucosal immunity • Autoimmune disease

KEY POINTS

- Mucosal microbiota can generate autoimmunity through a variety of mechanisms, including molecular mimicry, alteration of host antigens, exposure of self-antigens, bystander activation, modulation of immune reactivity, and breach of the mucosal firewall.
- Autoimmune disease may be triggered by a single microorganism or alterations of the host microbial community.
- Microbiota changes associated with autoimmune disease may represent causality or a change to the mucosal environment associated with systemic inflammation.
- Prospective studies that evaluate microbial changes at each mucosal site during the pre-clinical period of autoimmunity are needed to better understand the influence of microorganisms in the pathogenesis of autoimmune disease.
- If specific microbiota are found causal or protective in the development of autoimmune disease, novel strategies can be developed that may ultimately prevent disease.

INTRODUCTION

Humans live in symbiosis with greater than or equal to 10^{14} microorganisms that reside on epithelial surfaces of the body, including the skin and mucosal surfaces of the respiratory, gastrointestinal (GI), and genitourinary (GU) tracts.[1] These microbiota can be pathogenic or nonpathogenic, and they include a diverse community of

Disclosure: The authors declare no conflicts of interest.
[a] Division of Rheumatology, University of Colorado School of Medicine, 13001 E. 17th Place, Aurora, CO 80045, USA; [b] Division of Pulmonary/Critical Care Medicine, Cedars-Sinai Medical Center, 8700 Beverly Boulevard, Los Angeles, CA 90048, USA
* Corresponding author. Division of Rheumatology, University of Colorado School of Medicine, 1775 Aurora Court, Mail Stop B-115, Aurora, CO 80045.
E-mail address: Kristen.Demoruelle@UCDenver.edu

Rheum Dis Clin N Am 40 (2014) 711–725
http://dx.doi.org/10.1016/j.rdc.2014.07.013
0889-857X/14/$ – see front matter © 2014 Elsevier Inc. All rights reserved.
rheumatic.theclinics.com

bacteria, viruses, and fungi. The symbiotic nature of the host-microbial relationship implies a mutual benefit. Microbes gain access to habitats and nutrients important for their survival. Humans need microbes for certain metabolic functions as well as proper immune system development and maintenance.

Healthy individuals maintain a well-balanced microbial composition. Although the exact composition of a normal healthy microbiota is currently undefined, it is the focus of the National Institutes of Health–sponsored Human Microbiome Project.[2] Of particular interest for this review, alterations of what may be considered normal healthy microbiota may result in inflammation and autoimmunity, termed *dysbiosis*.[3] Such an imbalance may include an overgrowth or elimination of a single microbial species or changes in the relative abundance (increase or decrease) of multiple microorganisms within the community as a whole. Over the past decade, rapid advances in DNA sequencing technologies have allowed expanding knowledge of this intricate relationship and its potential association with disease. This article reviews data supporting the role of mucosal microbiota in the development of autoimmune disease.

OVERVIEW OF MUCOSAL IMMUNITY

The mucosal immune system (**Fig. 1**) evolved to prevent invasion of resident and pathogenic microbes. The first line of defense is the physical barrier established by a mucus layer overlying epithelial cells. The epithelial layer is typically composed of several cell types, depending on anatomic location. Within the epithelial layer, there are secretory cells that synthesize and secrete proteoglycans to generate mucus as well as other cells that aid in microbial defense. Almost all epithelial cells produce antimicrobial proteins that are retained in the mucus layer.[4] The GI tract, skin, and lung epithelial layers also contain intraepithelial lymphocytes (IELs) that participate in microbial defense (reviewed in Refs.[5,6]). IELs are a heterogeneous group of antigen-experienced T cells that function to protect from microbial invasion and maintain epithelial homeostasis,[7] and similar cells may also be present at other mucosal sites. Not only do the cells of the epithelial layer participate in direct microbial defense but also they aid in communication with other members of the mucosal immune system through cytokine and chemokine production.

Just beneath the epithelial layer is a network of innate immune cells primed for antigen exposure.[8] If microorganisms do breach the epithelial barrier, they are quickly phagocytosed by macrophages; macrophage activation leads to neutrophil, B-cell, and T-cell recruitment. Furthermore, tissue-resident macrophages and dendritic cells continually sample mucosal antigens in the lung and GI lamina propria and migrate to the mediastinal and mesenteric lymph nodes, respectively. Many of these innate cells do not circulate systemically and, therefore, compartmentalize immune responses to the mucosal system. These mucosal draining lymph nodes thus act as a firewall, which allows the host to continuously sample and respond to mucosal microbiota without generating a systemic inflammatory response.[9]

In mucosal lymph nodes, antigen-loaded dendritic cells induce specific IgA+ B cells to differentiate into plasma cells.[8] The plasma cells then migrate back to the mucosal lamina propria and produce IgA that is transcytosed across the epithelial barrier. IgD antibodies can also be generated and secreted in response to bacteria, specifically the nasal and respiratory mucosa.[10] These mucosal IgD antibodies are often polyreactive in response to bacteria and, of interest, can frequently be autoreactive. Also, within the draining lymph nodes of mucosal sites, T cells are activated and differentiate into one of several subtypes, in particular T-regulatory (Treg) and Th17 T-cell

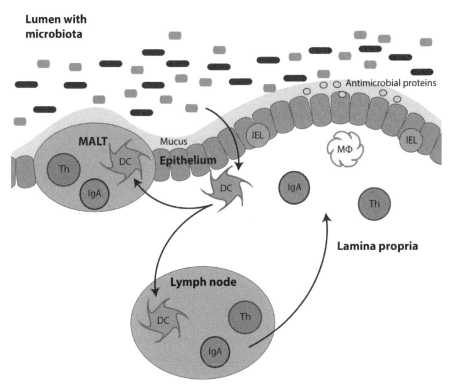

Fig. 1. Overview of the mucosal immune system. The mucosal barrier prevents invasion from commensal bacteria through generation of a mucus layer with antimicrobial proteins. Epithelial cells provide a second physical barrier and can signal to the immune system through secretion of chemokines and cytokines. Innate cells, such as DCs and Mφ, continually sample antigens that are able to cross the barrier and migrate to MALT or the local draining lymph nodes. There the innate cells present antigen to Th and IgA and activate adaptive immune responses. Activated T and B cells return to the lamia propria to direct further immune responses. Few cells migrate out of the mucosal system into systemic circulation. The general microanatomy shown in the cartoon is similar across all mucosal sites, but there are minor differences in each mucosal site (gut, lung, skin, etc.) with regard to specialized cell types, antimicrobial proteins, and relative numbers of immune cell populations (see text). DC, dendritic cell; IgA, B cell; Mφ, macrophage; Th, T cell.

subsets.[11] These activated T cells can also migrate back to the mucosa into the tissue lamina propria, where they partake in mucosal defense.

Mucosal sites also harbor lymphoid aggregates that are well organized into secondary and tertiary lymph structures, known as mucosal-associated lymphoid tissues (MALTs).[8] For some mucosal sites, such as the GI and nasopharyngeal tract, MALT is constitutive; these include GI-associated lymphoid tissue, to which Peyer patches belong, and nasal-associated lymph tissue, which includes Waldeyer's ring. In contrast, other areas of MALT are not preprogrammed and develop in response to inflammation or infection. Such areas include the lung mucosa that contains inducible bronchus-associated lymphoid tissue.[12] In these lymphoid follicles, B and T cells mature after antigen exposure, differentiate, and expand.

Importantly, even in MALT that is constitutive, colonization with microorganisms is required for normal immune development. Studies using germ-free mice have demonstrated significant immunologic alterations. Secondary lymph organs are hypoplastic in germ-free mice, and the absolute numbers of innate and adaptive cells are dramatically reduced.[13] Commensal microbes are required to prime innate cells (neutrophils, dendritic cells, and natural killer cells) for reactivity against invasive pathogens.[14,15] Mature B cells and class switching from IgM to IgG or IgA requires the presence of microbiota.[16,17] Finally, T-cell differentiation into Treg and Th17 cells has been shown critically dependent on specific microbial populations.[18–22]

MICROORGANISMS MAY INITIATE SYSTEMIC AUTOIMMUNITY

The etiology for most systemic autoimmune diseases is currently unknown, although both genetic and environmental factors likely play a role. For systemic autoimmune diseases, such as rheumatoid arthritis (RA) and systemic lupus erythematosus (SLE), data demonstrate a period of preclinical autoimmunity, during which systemic inflammatory markers and autoantibodies specific for disease are abnormally elevated in the blood years prior to the onset of clinically classifiable disease manifestations.[23–27] The mechanisms as well as anatomic site(s) for the generation of preclinical autoreactivity are, however, unknown.

Advances in technologies, including DNA sequencing, have led to culture-independent nonbiased approaches that evaluate the total composition of microbiota present at a mucosal site, even in absence of overt pathologic infection.[28,29] These advances have led to an increased focus on evaluating the mucosal microbial community as a whole, including consideration of the presence/increase of potentially bad bacteria as well as the elimination/decrease of potentially good bacteria. Therefore, the microbial influence on autoimmune disease can now be evaluated as potentially triggered by a single microbe or alterations of the larger microbial community.

Potential Mechanisms By Which Microbiota Could Induce Autoimmunity

Because of the significant effects microbiota exert on immune development, it is easy to speculate that dysbiosis at a mucosal site can alter immune function and result in autoimmune disease. There are several potential mechanisms by which microorganisms could shape the immune system to generate autoimmunity (**Table 1**). These include molecular mimicry, generation of neoantigens, bystander activation, modulation of immune reactivity, and a breach of the mucosal firewall. Understanding the details of how each pathway could contribute to systemic autoimmunity at different mucosal sites may lead to novel mechanism-specific or microbial-specific targets for disease prevention.

Molecular mimicry

Molecular mimicry is the development of an antibody that cross-reacts with a microbial protein as well as normal host tissue. A classic example of molecular mimicry triggering autoimmunity is acute rheumatic fever. In acute rheumatic fever, T cells respond to a specific peptide epitope of *Streptococcus pyogenes*.[30] During pharyngitis with *S pyogenes*, these specific T cells stimulate B-cell generation of a cross-reactive antibody to human cardiac myosin, resulting in acute rheumatic fever–associated carditis. Because not all infections with *S pyogenes* result in rheumatic fever, genetics and the specific site of infection seem to play a critical role in generating an autoimmune response.[31] Although acute rheumatic fever is a well-established example of molecular mimicry, such a process may occur in the pathogenesis of other autoimmune diseases.

Table 1
Potential mechanisms of mucosal microbiota generation of autoimmunity

Mucosal Immune Response	Definition	Example
Molecular mimicry	Generation of a cross-reactive antibody that recognizes shared epitopes of microbial and host tissue proteins	S pyogenes in acute rheumatic fever
Microbial alteration of host antigens	Microbial-induced modification of host proteins creating neoantigens	P gingivalis and citrullinated proteins in RA
Microbial-induced exposure of self-antigens	Externalization of previously intracellular self-proteins that generate autoimmune responses	Bacterial-induced NET formation and citrullinated proteins in RA
Bystander activation	Mucosal responses to microbiota producing inflammatory cytokines that spill over and activate nearby autoreactive cells	S aureus and ANCA-associated vasculitis
Modulation of immune reactivity	Specific microorganisms shaping the development of the host immune system	Clostridia species influence mucosal Treg cell development
Breach of the mucosal firewall	Mucosal-limited immune responses to microbiota that aberrantly move beyond the mucosa	Antigliadin antibodies in celiac disease

Microbial alteration of host antigens

Some microbes are able to modify host proteins, thereby creating neoantigens that are recognized as foreign to the adaptive immune system and could generate autoimmunity. For example, *Porphyromonas gingivalis* is uniquely found to express a peptidylarginine deiminase (PAD) enzyme capable of citrullinating host proteins (eg, fibrinogen and α-enolase).[32,33] By generating citrullinated fibrinogen and α-enolase, neoantigens are generated that can bind with high affinity to major histocompatibility complex class II HLA-DR4 shared epitopes.[34] Therefore, these protein alterations by *P gingivalis* could potentially lead to autoimmunity in RA in the form of antibodies to citrullinated protein antigens (ACPAs).

Microbial-induced exposure of self-antigens

In RA and SLE, autoantibodies can be generated to intracellular self-proteins, although these proteins must first be externalized to generate an immune response. Such a phenomenon can occur at the mucosal surface with the induction of neutrophil extracellular traps (NETs). NETs are a mechanism by which neutrophils decondense and expel their chromatin in response to inflammation or bacteria. For example, during NET formation, antibacterial and citrullinated proteins that were previously intracellular are now externalized, and these citrullinated proteins may trigger mucosal ACPA responses. In addition, specific bacterial species can have differential effects on inducing NETs (eg, *Lactobacillus rhamnosus* inhibits NET formation[35]). Therefore, certain microbial changes can affect the rate of NET formation and as such may be associated with increases or decreases in generation of autoimmunity.

Bystander activation

Microbial infection at a mucosal site results in activation of innate and then adaptive immune responses. Both microbe-specific and nonspecific B and T cells are recruited to an inflamed mucosal site.[11] Bystander activation occurs when the cytokines of the inflammatory milieu activate the nonspecific adaptive cells in addition to the microbe-specific B and/or T cells. Alternatively, some bacteria express superantigens that can activate T cells in a T-cell receptor–independent manner. In such a fashion, autoreactive B or T cells can be activated, partake in tissue damage, and perpetuate autoimmune disease.[8] One hypothesized example of bystander activation is the association between Staphlococcus aureus and antineutrophil cytoplasmic antibody (ANCA)-associated vasculitis. Methylation motifs within S aureus DNA can activate ANCA-producing B cells via Toll-like receptors (TLRs) in patients with ANCA-associated vasculitis.[36] Similarly, bacterial and viral DNA can signal through TLRs, generating exacerbated type I interferon (IFN) responses and polyclonal B-cell activation in patients with SLE.[37]

Modulation of immune reactivity

As discussed previously, commensal microbiota have a significant impact on immune maturation, and specific bacteria can modulate immune responses. For example, selected Clostridia species increase mucosal Treg cell development[18,19] whereas segmented filamentous bacteria (SFB), also members of the Clostridia family, allow generation of Th17 cells.[20] SFB or similar species, however, have not been identified in humans by sequencing studies.[20] Furthermore, one microbial species may affect development of T cells in different compartments. Intestinal polysaccharide antigen A from Bacteroides fragilis promotes splenic Th1 responses whereas in the intestinal lamina propria it promotes Treg cells.[21,22] Therefore, changes in commensal microbiota can have significant impacts on immune reactivity both locally and systemically; these effects may diverge based on immunologic site. It can be projected that these and other microbiota changes, either single organism or community alterations, may be sufficient in the setting of genetic predisposition to shape the immune system, resulting in autoimmunity.

Breach of the mucosal firewall

As discussed previously, inflammatory reactions are generally limited to the mucosa during the body's natural response to environmental antigens and microbes. This represents a mucosal firewall within which mucosal responses are contained and do not move beyond the regional lymph nodes.[9] If this mucosal firewall is compromised, however, immune responses that once were limited to the mucosa could become systemic. For example, in celiac disease, antibodies to gliadin that are generated in response to the presence of gliadin (a wheat protein) in the gut can become systemic rather than remaining contained within the gut mucosa.

Furthermore, in localized mucosal immune responses to microbiota, autoantibodies are generated locally as part of the body's natural immune response and can serve as broad protection against microorganisms.[38] Such a phenomenon has been demonstrated in the lung mucosa because autoantibodies, including rheumatoid factor and antinuclear antibodies, have been found in airway sections in response to bacteria.[39] Furthermore, in a study by Willis colleagues[40] that evaluated ACPA responses in the lung, arthritis-free subjects at risk for future RA had sputum RA-related autoantibody positivity found generated in the lung. Some individuals, these natural mucosal-generated autoantibodies may become systemic, perhaps related to genetic or other environmental factors.

Although there are several different mechanisms by which microorganisms could generate autoimmunity, further study is needed to determine the role of each in the development of specific autoimmune diseases. As such, prospective natural history studies are critical to define the specific microorganisms, mechanisms, and additional factors involved in disease pathogenesis.

The Role of Mucosal Microbiota in Specific Systemic Autoimmune Diseases

Rheumatoid arthritis and mucosal microbiota

Mucosal dysbiosis has long been suggested as playing a role in the development of RA,[41,42] and numerous microorganisms resident to a variety of host mucosal sites have been linked to RA pathogenesis. Therefore, unlike rheumatic fever in which a single bacterium has been found to trigger disease, the connection of mucosal microbiota and the development of RA is likely more complex. Some studies have identified associations of RA and viruses, such as Epstein-Barr virus (EBV). A majority of associations of microorganisms and RA have focused on bacteria, including older studies that demonstrated associations between RA and *Mycoplasma, Proteus*, and *Escherichia*[43–52] as well as a study by Eerola and colleagues[53] that identified the total composition of gut microbiota differed in newly diagnosed RA compared with controls.

In more recent studies, Scher and colleagues demonstrated that patients with recent-onset RA had an increased abundance of *Prevotella* and a decreased abundance of *Bacteroides* compared with subjects with chronic treated RA, those with psoriatic arthritis, and healthy controls.[54] This study further identified *Prevotella copri* as the most abundant *Prevotella* species present in a majority of patients with recent-onset RA. Murine gut colonization with *P copri* led, however, to increased severity of colitis and not increased susceptibility for inflammatory arthritis. In accordance with Koch postulates, if a microbe is causal for disease it should be able to cause disease when introduced into a healthy organism. Although this may suggest *P copri* is not causal for RA, it may also represent the difficulty of applying Koch postulates if disease due to dysbiosis is a community effect and not a single species. Other human RA studies have identified different patterns of gut dysbiosis associated with RA. For example, Liu and colleagues[55] found an increased abundance of fecal *Lactobacillus* in RA, and Vaahtovuo and colleagues[56] demonstrated decreased *Bacteroides* in RA compared with controls.

Investigations of RA and microbiota have also placed significant focus on the oral mucosa because RA patients have a significantly higher prevalence and severity of periodontal disease.[57] Specific focus has centered on *P gingivalis* because, as discussed previously, it is capable of generating neoantigens, such as citrullinated α-enolase, due to its unique expression of PAD.[32,33] Studies have found ACPAs to human citrullinated α-enolase that are specific for RA and are also reactive to citrullinated bacterial α-enolase, suggesting the possibility of molecular mimicry.[58] Furthermore, elevations of antibodies to *P gingivalis* were associated with RA-related autoantibody elevations in subjects in the preclinical period of RA, suggesting a possible role in initiation of autoimmunity.[59] De Smit and colleagues,[60] however, recently demonstrated elevations of anti–*P gingivalis* antibodies in preclinical RA subjects with arthralgias did not predict future onset of inflammatory arthritis.

Furthermore, recent studies suggest that variation in the oral microbiome and *P gingivalis* are associated with severity of periodontal disease and not specific for RA.[57,61] For example, Mikuls and colleagues[57] found that serum anti–*P gingivalis* antibody levels were similar in patients with RA and controls, but they were significantly elevated in those with periodontal disease. Similarly, Scher and colleagues[61] evaluated subjects with new-onset RA and found that subgingival microbial communities were different between RA and controls, but this difference was explained by the presence of periodontal disease and was not specific to RA. This study reported alternative bacterial associations with RA, including increased abundance of *Prevotella* and *Leptotrichia*, as well as *Anaeroglobus geminatus* that was specifically associated with RA-related autoantibody positivity.[61] Therefore, it may be that the association of periodontal disease and *P gingivalis* in RA does not trigger autoimmunity, but periodontal disease–associated inflammation and/or *P gingivalis*–related PAD activity may generate local citrullinated peptides in the gingival tissue, which are targeted by autoantibodies generated elsewhere. Further studies are needed to determine how each of these factors contributes to the pathogenesis of RA.

In addition, the lung mucosa has been suggested as playing a role in the development of RA.[62–64] Lung microbiota have a more limited repertoire than other mucosal sites, but lung dysbiosis has been associated with chronic diseases, such as asthma and emphysema.[65,66] Previous studies have identified associations between RA and *Mycoplasma pneumonia*.[43,67] Also, heat shock proteins (HSPs) have been suggested as a potential cross-reactive antigen associated with bacterial infection and synovitis in RA,[51,68] and recent studies identified an association of serum anti-HSP antibodies and RA-related lung disease.[69] Therefore, lung microbiota may also play a role in development of RA-related autoimmunity, but additional studies are needed.

Spondylarthritis and microbial associations of disease

A causal relationship may exist between microbes and disease in the spondyloarthridities (SpA), in particularly reactive arthritis (ReA), during which infection clearly precedes the onset of arthritis. ReA can develop after infection with various GI and GU infections, including *Salmonella*, *Shigella*, *Yersinia*, *Campylobacter*, and *Chlamydia*.[70] Bacterial products, such as strain-specific lipopolysaccharides, have been found within the synovium of patients with ReA due to *Yersinia*, *Salmonella*, and *Chlamydia*,[71–73] suggesting the disease is due to persistent inflammation of the target tissue driven by the bacterial products.[74] In these cases, the bacterium may generate an arthritogenic peptide via mechanisms (discussed previously), such as molecular mimicry or neoantigen formation that can be presented by HLA-B27 to CD8[+] T cells, and this hypothesis is supported by bacteria-specific CD8[+] T cells that are found to be expanded in the synovial fluid of patients with ReA.[75,76]

In the same fashion, it has been suggested that *Klebsiella pneumonia* is the causative agent for ankylosing spondyloarthritis (AS),[77] a view that is controversial. Another line of studies, using denaturing gel gradient electrophoresis, failed to show a difference in the microbiota in a cohort of 15 AS patients with a median duration of 14 years compared with controls.[78] More rigorous studies using 16S ribosomal RNA sequencing demonstrate microbial associations in AS may be similar to inflammatory bowel disease, a disease in which alterations within the intestinal microbial community have been identified.[79,80] An abstract presented by Stoll and colleagues[79] demonstrated that among 28 children ages 7 to 14 with SpA, there was a decreased abundance in *Faecalibacterium prausnitzii*, which is hypothesized to have a regulatory effect on the mucosal immune system.[81] These studies are greatly limited, however, by population size and/or microbial analysis methodology. Again, rigorous preclinical natural history studies are essential in understanding the link between the microbiota and disease.

Lupus, Sjögren syndrome, and viral microorganisms

Microorganisms have also been hypothesized to trigger SLE and primary Sjögren syndrome, although a majority of these studies have focused on viral rather than bacterial microorganisms. Viral microorganisms, similar to bacteria, have the potential to induce autoimmune responses through the mechanisms (described previously), such as molecular mimicry, bystander activation, and so forth.

Multiple viruses have been linked to SLE, including EBV, cytomegalovirus (CMV), and parvovirus B19.[82–85] In these studies, SLE patients have higher prevalence of viral antibodies and higher viral PCR levels compared with controls. SLE-associated antibodies can be elevated, however, in the serum years prior to disease onset, and the association of these microorganisms with the generation of autoimmunity in the preclinical period of SLE is unclear. In addition, for EBV, molecular mimicry and bystander activation have been suggested as viral-induced mechanisms of SLE pathogenesis. Specifically, similar amino acid sequences have been identified between an EBV peptide and SLE autoantigen,[84] and EBV can generate polyclonal activation as well as transactivate superantigen.[86]

In Sjögren syndrome, disease pathogenesis induced by molecular mimicry and bystander activation has also been suggested with EBV, CMV, and human T-lymphotropic virus type 1.[87–90] Furthermore, increased serum type I IFN levels have been identified in individuals with SLE and Sjögren syndrome and may be related to viral induced immune responses.[91–93] Also, the antigenic protein La/SSB, often targeted in patients with SLE and Sjögren syndrome, is increased in virally infected cells and involved in viral RNA processing, suggesting molecular mimicry may play a role in disease development.[92]

Unfortunately, understanding of the human virome is limited. As more research evolves in this area, it will be interesting to see how exposures to specific commensal viruses can influence immunity similar to what is observed with commensal bacteria.

BARRIERS TO UNCOVERING THE LINK BETWEEN MICROBIOTA AND AUTOIMMUNE DISEASE

Although the established and emerging data presented herein are intriguing, several methodologic and biologic issues make investigations in this area challenging. Advances in culture-independent methods for identification and quantification of microbiota have revolutionized the field. Yet, these advances also lead to challenges in comparing studies. Currently, differences in techniques of data acquisition as well as analytical approaches applied to the large metadata generated have made comparison between studies difficult. Furthermore, new technologies can evaluate metabolomics and enzymatic activity of microorganisms; the function and activity of specific microbial genes may provide further detail to determine the potential role of microbiota in the development of autoimmune disease. Future efforts need to focus on incorporating these multiple facets by which microbiota may generate autoimmunity.

Sampling mucosal sites is also a challenge. In the gut, fecal samples do not allow determination from which specific part of the GI tract a particular microorganism came. In addition, biospecimens from the lung can include upper airway microbes depending on collection techniques. Furthermore, although these mucosal fluid biospecimens are feasible to collect, they may not adequately represent the microorganisms adjacent to and actively interacting with the mucosal immune system.

Furthermore, much of the understanding of the microbial effects on mucosal and systemic immunity is based on animal studies. Yet, these studies are not always relevant to human physiology. For example, SFB, which are required for Th17 development in mice, have not been identified in humans.[20]

Finally, many studies of microbial association with autoimmune disease evaluate subjects after diagnosis (ie, after the onset of clinically classifiable disease). Systemic preclinical autoantibodies are often elevated, however, several years prior. Therefore, if mucosal microbiota are the cause of autoimmunity, their influence on the immune system would likely occur years prior to diagnosis. As such, a central issue related to understanding the role of microbiota in disease is that microbial changes at clinical disease diagnosis may be causal, but they may also represent a change to the mucosal environment associated with systemic inflammation, such that different microorganisms are more likely to inhabit and propagate in this new inflammatory environment. Therefore, to determine causality, it is crucial for future studies to include subjects in the preclinical period of disease who are prospectively followed in natural history studies.

IMPLICATIONS FOR PREVENTION OR TREATMENT OF AUTOIMMUNE DISEASE

It has long been suggested that microorganisms may play a role in the development of systemic autoimmune disease. If specific microbes are found causal of disease, targeted treatments can be designed to more effectively treat and even prevent systemic disease onset. Such an approach is demonstrated in rheumatic fever, in which it is now understood that a specific bacteria, S pyogenes, triggers disease pathogenesis. As such, appropriate antibiotic treatment has reduced the incidence of acute rheumatic fever and, even further, has set the stage for the development of more accurate biomarkers for diagnosis and potential vaccines that may prevent disease in high-risk individuals.[94] In addition, it may be altered microbial communities that trigger autoimmunity for some diseases, and, if so, an approach that replaces and restores normal healthy mucosal microbiota may be needed. Such approaches could include replacement of normal healthy microbiota, as is the case in fecal transplant, or introduction of antiinflammatory microbiota to the community through probiotics or alterations in the diet. More thorough studies addressing the therapeutic potential of microbial modulation are required.

FUTURE DIRECTIONS

Understanding of the synergism between commensal microorganisms and health is rapidly expanding. As the field moves forward, additional variables, including genetics, diet, and other environmental factors, need to be addressed. For example, much attention is currently paid to the way in which microbiota shape immune function. The role of the immune system, however, in shaping microbiota is now only being unearthed. Furthermore, in an era of genome-wide association studies, it is important to consider the role of genetic polymorphisms on immune and mucosal barrier functions as well as how these may influence microbiota. Finally, dietary and other environmental factors may influence commensal microbial populations and/or physiologic responses to microbiota. These factors, and perhaps others yet to be identified, may play an essential role in determining how microbiota may influence the development of autoimmune disease in some but not all individuals.

REFERENCES

1. Backhed F, Ley RE, Sonnenburg JL, et al. Host-bacterial mutualism in the human intestine. Science 2005;307:1915–20.

2. Shafquat A, Joice R, Simmons SL, et al. Functional and phylogenetic assembly of microbial communities in the human microbiome. Trends Microbiol 2014;22:261–6.
3. Ivanov II, Honda K. Intestinal commensal microbes as immune modulators. Cell Host Microbe 2012;12:496–508.
4. Gallo RL, Hooper LV. Epithelial antimicrobial defence of the skin and intestine. Nat Rev Immunol 2012;12:503–16.
5. Cheroutre H. IELs: enforcing law and order in the court of the intestinal epithelium. Immunol Rev 2005;206:114–31.
6. Erle DJ, Pabst R. Intraepithelial lymphocytes in the lung: a neglected lymphocyte population. Am J Respir Cell Mol Biol 2000;22:398–400.
7. Cheroutre H, Lambolez F, Mucida D. The light and dark sides of intestinal intraepithelial lymphocytes. Nat Rev Immunol 2011;11:445–56.
8. Murphy K, Travers P, Walport M, et al. Janeway's immunobiology. 8th edition. New York: Garland Science; 2012.
9. Macpherson AJ, Slack E, Geuking MB, et al. The mucosal firewalls against commensal intestinal microbes. Semin Immunopathol 2009;31:145–9.
10. Zheng NY, Wilson K, Wang X, et al. Human immunoglobulin selection associated with class switch and possible tolerogenic origins for C delta class-switched B cells. J Clin Invest 2004;113:1188–201.
11. Hooper LV, Littman DR, Macpherson AJ. Interactions between the microbiota and the immune system. Science 2012;336:1268–73.
12. Foo SY, Phipps S. Regulation of inducible BALT formation and contribution to immunity and pathology. Mucosal Immunol 2010;3:537–44.
13. Bauer H, Horowitz RE, Levenson SM, et al. The response of the lymphatic tissue to the microbial flora. Studies on germfree mice. Am J Pathol 1963;42:471–83.
14. Clarke TB, Davis KM, Lysenko ES, et al. Recognition of peptidoglycan from the microbiota by Nod1 enhances systemic innate immunity. Nat Med 2010;16:228–31.
15. Ganal SC, Sanos SL, Kallfass C, et al. Priming of natural killer cells by non-mucosal mononuclear phagocytes requires instructive signals from commensal microbiota. Immunity 2012;37:171–86.
16. Pereira P, Forni L, Larsson EL, et al. Autonomous activation of B and T cells in antigen-free mice. Eur J Immunol 1986;16:685–8.
17. Hooijkaas H, Benner R, Pleasants JR, et al. Isotypes and specificities of immunoglobulins produced by germ-free mice fed chemically defined ultrafiltered "antigen-free" diet. Eur J Immunol 1984;14:1127–30.
18. Atarashi K, Tanoue T, Oshima K, et al. Treg induction by a rationally selected mixture of Clostridia strains from the human microbiota. Nature 2013;500:232–6.
19. Atarashi K, Tanoue T, Shima T, et al. Induction of colonic regulatory T cells by indigenous Clostridium species. Science 2011;331:337–41.
20. Ivanov II, Atarashi K, Manel N, et al. Induction of intestinal Th17 cells by segmented filamentous bacteria. Cell 2009;139:485–98.
21. Mazmanian SK, Liu CH, Tzianabos AO, et al. An immunomodulatory molecule of symbiotic bacteria directs maturation of the host immune system. Cell 2005;122:107–18.
22. Mazmanian SK, Round JL, Kasper DL. A microbial symbiosis factor prevents intestinal inflammatory disease. Nature 2008;453:620–5.
23. Rantapaa-Dahlqvist S, de Jong BA, Berglin E, et al. Antibodies against cyclic citrullinated peptide and IgA rheumatoid factor predict the development of rheumatoid arthritis. Arthritis Rheum 2003;48:2741–9.

24. Arbuckle MR, McClain MT, Rubertone MV, et al. Development of autoantibodies before the clinical onset of systemic lupus erythematosus. N Engl J Med 2003; 349:1526–33.
25. Demoruelle MK, Parish MC, Derber LA, et al. Performance of anti-cyclic citrullinated peptide assays differs in subjects at increased risk of rheumatoid arthritis and subjects with established disease. Arthritis Rheum 2013;65:2243–52.
26. Deane KD, El-Gabalawy H. Pathogenesis and prevention of rheumatic disease: focus on preclinical RA and SLE. Nat Rev Rheumatol 2014;10:212–28.
27. Olsen NJ, Karp DR. Autoantibodies and SLE–the threshold for disease. Nat Rev Rheumatol 2014;10:181–6.
28. Weisburg WG, Barns SM, Pelletier DA, et al. 16S ribosomal DNA amplification for phylogenetic study. J Bacteriol 1991;173:697–703.
29. Preheim SP, Perrotta AR, Friedman J, et al. Computational methods for high-throughput comparative analyses of natural microbial communities. Meth Enzymol 2013;531:353–70.
30. Goldstein I, Rebeyrotte P, Parlebas J, et al. Isolation from heart valves of glycopeptides which share immunological properties with Streptococcus haemolyticus group A polysaccharides. Nature 1968;219:866–8.
31. Bryant PA, Smyth GK, Gooding T, et al. Susceptibility to acute rheumatic fever based on differential expression of genes involved in cytotoxicity, chemotaxis, and apoptosis. Infect Immun 2014;82:753–61.
32. McGraw WT, Potempa J, Farley D, et al. Purification, characterization, and sequence analysis of a potential virulence factor from Porphyromonas gingivalis, peptidylarginine deiminase. Infect Immun 1999;67:3248–56.
33. Wegner N, Wait R, Sroka A, et al. Peptidylarginine deiminase from Porphyromonas gingivalis citrullinates human fibrinogen and alpha-enolase: implications for autoimmunity in rheumatoid arthritis. Arthritis and Rheum 2010;62:2662–72.
34. Hill JA, Southwood S, Sette A, et al. Cutting edge: the conversion of arginine to citrulline allows for a high-affinity peptide interaction with the rheumatoid arthritis-associated HLA-DRB1*0401 MHC class II molecule. J Immunol 2003; 171:538–41.
35. Vong L, Lorentz RJ, Assa A, et al. Probiotic Lactobacillus rhamnosus inhibits the formation of neutrophil extracellular traps. J Immunol 2014;192:1870–7.
36. Tadema H, Abdulahad WH, Lepse N, et al. Bacterial DNA motifs trigger ANCA production in ANCA-associated vasculitis in remission. Rheumatology 2011;50: 689–96.
37. Giordani L, Sanchez M, Libri I, et al. IFN-alpha amplifies human naive B cell TLR-9-mediated activation and Ig production. J Leukoc Biol 2009;86:261–71.
38. Kato A, Hulse KE, Tan BK, et al. B-lymphocyte lineage cells and the respiratory system. J Allergy Clin Immunol 2013;131:933–57 [quiz: 58].
39. Schiotz PO, Egeskjold EM, Hoiby N, et al. Autoantibodies in serum and sputum from patients with cystic fibrosis. Acta pathologica et microbiologica Scandinavica Section C. Immunology 1979;87:319–24.
40. Willis VC, Demoruelle MK, Derber LA, et al. Sputum autoantibodies in patients with established rheumatoid arthritis and subjects at risk of future clinically apparent disease. Arthritis and Rheum 2013;65:2545–54.
41. Svartz N. The primary cause of rheumatoid arthritis is an infection–the infectious agent exists in milk. Acta Med Scand 1972;192:231–9.
42. Murray GR. Discussion on focal sepsis as a factor in disease. Proc R Soc Med 1926;19:26.

43. Ramirez AS, Rosas A, Hernandez-Beriain JA, et al. Relationship between rheumatoid arthritis and Mycoplasma pneumoniae: a case-control study. Rheumatology (Oxford) 2005;44:912–4.
44. Newkirk MM, Goldbach-Mansky R, Senior BW, et al. Elevated levels of IgM and IgA antibodies to Proteus mirabilis and IgM antibodies to Escherichia coli are associated with early rheumatoid factor (RF)-positive rheumatoid arthritis. Rheumatology (Oxford) 2005;44:1433–41.
45. Rashid T, Ebringer A. Rheumatoid arthritis is linked to Proteus–the evidence. Clin Rheumatol 2007;26:1036–43.
46. Silman AJ, Pearson JE. Epidemiology and genetics of rheumatoid arthritis. Arthritis Res 2002;4(Suppl 3):S265–72.
47. Aoki S, Yoshikawa K, Yokoyama T, et al. Role of enteric bacteria in the pathogenesis of rheumatoid arthritis: evidence for antibodies to enterobacterial common antigens in rheumatoid sera and synovial fluids. Ann Rheum Dis 1996;55:363–9.
48. Ebringer A, Wilson C, Tiwana H. Is rheumatoid arthritis a form of reactive arthritis? J Rheumatol 2000;27:559–63.
49. Rashid T, Darlington G, Kjeldsen-Kragh J, et al. Proteus IgG antibodies and C-reactive protein in English, Norwegian and Spanish patients with rheumatoid arthritis. Clin Rheumatol 1999;18:190–5.
50. Roudier J, Petersen J, Rhodes GH, et al. Susceptibility to rheumatoid arthritis maps to a T-cell epitope shared by the HLA-Dw4 DR beta-1 chain and the Epstein-Barr virus glycoprotein gp110. Proc Natl Acad Sci U S A 1989;86: 5104–8.
51. Albani S, Keystone EC, Nelson JL, et al. Positive selection in autoimmunity: abnormal immune responses to a bacterial dnaJ antigenic determinant in patients with early rheumatoid arthritis. Nat Med 1995;1:448–52.
52. Alspaugh MA, Henle G, Lennette ET, et al. Elevated levels of antibodies to Epstein-Barr virus antigens in sera and synovial fluids of patients with rheumatoid arthritis. J Clin Invest 1981;67:1134–40.
53. Eerola E, Mottonen T, Hannonen P, et al. Intestinal flora in early rheumatoid arthritis. Br J Rheumatol 1994;33:1030–8.
54. Scher JU, Sczesnak A, Longman RS, et al. Expansion of intestinal Prevotella copri correlates with enhanced susceptibility to arthritis. Elife (Cambridge) 2013;2:e01202.
55. Liu X, Zou Q, Zeng B, et al. Analysis of fecal lactobacillus community structure in patients with early rheumatoid arthritis. Curr Microbiol 2013;67:170–6.
56. Vaahtovuo J, Munukka E, Korkeamaki M, et al. Fecal microbiota in early rheumatoid arthritis. J Rheumatol 2008;35:1500–5.
57. Mikuls TR, Payne JB, Yu F, et al. Periodontitis and Porphyromonas gingivalis in patients with rheumatoid arthritis. Arthritis Rheumatol 2014;66:1090–100.
58. Lundberg K, Kinloch A, Fisher BA, et al. Antibodies to citrullinated alpha-enolase peptide 1 are specific for rheumatoid arthritis and cross-react with bacterial enolase. Arthritis Rheum 2008;58:3009–19.
59. Mikuls TR, Thiele GM, Deane KD, et al. Porphyromonas gingivalis and disease-related autoantibodies in individuals at increased risk of rheumatoid arthritis. Arthritis and Rheum 2012;64:3522–30.
60. de Smit M, van de Stadt LA, Janssen KM, et al. Antibodies against Porphyromonas gingivalis in seropositive arthralgia patients do not predict development of rheumatoid arthritis. Ann Rheum Dis 2014;73:1277–9.

61. Scher JU, Ubeda C, Equinda M, et al. Periodontal disease and the oral microbiota in new-onset rheumatoid arthritis. Arthritis and Rheum 2012;64:3083–94.
62. Demoruelle MK, Weisman MH, Simonian PL, et al. Brief report: airways abnormalities and rheumatoid arthritis-related autoantibodies in subjects without arthritis: early injury or initiating site of autoimmunity? Arthritis Rheum 2012;64: 1756–61.
63. Fischer A, Solomon JJ, du Bois RM, et al. Lung disease with anti-CCP antibodies but not rheumatoid arthritis or connective tissue disease. Respir Med 2012;106: 1040–7.
64. Klareskog L, Stolt P, Lundberg K, et al. A new model for an etiology of rheumatoid arthritis: smoking may trigger HLA-DR (shared epitope)-restricted immune reactions to autoantigens modified by citrullination. Arthritis Rheum 2006;54: 38–46.
65. Abrahamsson TR, Jakobsson HE, Andersson AF, et al. Low gut microbiota diversity in early infancy precedes asthma at school age. Clin Exp Allergy 2014; 44(6):842–50.
66. Zakharkina T, Heinzel E, Koczulla RA, et al. Analysis of the airway microbiota of healthy individuals and patients with chronic obstructive pulmonary disease by T-RFLP and clone sequencing. PLoS One 2013;8:e68302.
67. Haier J, Nasralla M, Franco AR, et al. Detection of mycoplasmal infections in blood of patients with rheumatoid arthritis. Rheumatology (Oxford) 1999;38: 504–9.
68. van Eden W. Heat-shock proteins as immunogenic bacterial antigens with the potential to induce and regulate autoimmune arthritis. Immunol Rev 1991;121: 5–28.
69. Harlow L, Rosas IO, Gochuico BR, et al. Identification of citrullinated hsp90 isoforms as novel autoantigens in rheumatoid arthritis-associated interstitial lung disease. Arthritis and Rheum 2013;65:869–79.
70. Keat A. Reiter's syndrome and reactive arthritis in perspective. N Engl J Med 1983;309:1606–15.
71. Granfors K, Jalkanen S, von Essen R, et al. Yersinia antigens in synovial-fluid cells from patients with reactive arthritis. N Engl J Med 1989;320:216–21.
72. Granfors K, Jalkanen S, Lindberg AA, et al. Salmonella lipopolysaccharide in synovial cells from patients with reactive arthritis. Lancet 1990;335:685–8.
73. Nanagara R, Li F, Beutler A, et al. Alteration of Chlamydia trachomatis biologic behavior in synovial membranes. Suppression of surface antigen production in reactive arthritis and Reiter's syndrome. Arthritis Rheum 1995;38:1410–7.
74. Gerard HC, Branigan PJ, Schumacher HR Jr, et al. Synovial Chlamydia trachomatis in patients with reactive arthritis/Reiter's syndrome are viable but show aberrant gene expression. J Rheumatol 1998;25:734–42.
75. Kuon W, Holzhutter HG, Appel H, et al. Identification of HLA-B27-restricted peptides from the Chlamydia trachomatis proteome with possible relevance to HLA-B27-associated diseases. J Immunol 2001;167:4738–46.
76. Ugrinovic S, Mertz A, Wu P, et al. A single nonamer from the Yersinia 60-kDa heat shock protein is the target of HLA-B27-restricted CTL response in Yersinia-induced reactive arthritis. J Immunol 1997;159:5715–23.
77. Rashid T, Ebringer A. Ankylosing spondylitis is linked to Klebsiella–the evidence. Clin Rheumatol 2007;26:858–64.
78. Stebbings S, Munro K, Simon MA, et al. Comparison of the faecal microflora of patients with ankylosing spondylitis and controls using molecular methods of analysis. Rheumatology 2002;41:1395–401.

79. Stoll ML, Kumar R, Morrow C, et al. A175: dysbiosis of the enteric microbiota in pediatric spondyloarthritis. Arthritis Rheumatol 2014;66(Suppl 11):S228–9.
80. Morgan XC, Tickle TL, Sokol H, et al. Dysfunction of the intestinal microbiome in inflammatory bowel disease and treatment. Genome Biol 2012;13:R79.
81. Miquel S, Martin R, Rossi O, et al. Faecalibacterium prausnitzii and human intestinal health. Curr Opin Microbiol 2013;16:255–61.
82. James JA, Kaufman KM, Farris AD, et al. An increased prevalence of Epstein-Barr virus infection in young patients suggests a possible etiology for systemic lupus erythematosus. J Clin Invest 1997;100:3019–26.
83. Pavlovic M, Kats A, Cavallo M, et al. Clinical and molecular evidence for association of SLE with parvovirus B19. Lupus 2010;19:783–92.
84. Moon UY, Park SJ, Oh ST, et al. Patients with systemic lupus erythematosus have abnormally elevated Epstein-Barr virus load in blood. Arthritis Res Ther 2004;6:R295–302.
85. Nawata M, Seta N, Yamada M, et al. Possible triggering effect of cytomegalovirus infection on systemic lupus erythematosus. Scand J Rheumatol 2001;30:360–2.
86. Sutkowski N, Conrad B, Thorley-Lawson DA, et al. Epstein-Barr virus transactivates the human endogenous retrovirus HERV-K18 that encodes a superantigen. Immunity 2001;15:579–89.
87. Ohyama Y, Carroll VA, Deshmukh U, et al. Severe focal sialadenitis and dacryoadenitis in NZM2328 mice induced by MCMV: a novel model for human Sjogren's syndrome. J Immunol 2006;177:7391–7.
88. Shattles WG, Brookes SM, Venables PJ, et al. Expression of antigen reactive with a monoclonal antibody to HTLV-1 P19 in salivary glands in Sjogren's syndrome. Clin Exp Immunol 1992;89:46–51.
89. Eguchi K, Matsuoka N, Ida H, et al. Primary Sjogren's syndrome with antibodies to HTLV-I: clinical and laboratory features. Ann Rheum Dis 1992;51:769–76.
90. Horiuchi M, Yamano S, Inoue H, et al. Possible involvement of IL-12 expression by Epstein-Barr virus in Sjogren syndrome. J Clin Pathol 1999;52:833–7.
91. Zheng L, Yu C, Zhang Z, et al. Expression of interferon regulatory factor 1, 3, and 7 in primary Sjogren syndrome. Oral Surg Oral Med Oral Pathol Oral Radiol Endod 2009;107:661–8.
92. Mavragani CP, Crow MK. Activation of the type I interferon pathway in primary Sjogren's syndrome. J Autoimmun 2010;35:225–31.
93. Pascual V, Chaussabel D, Banchereau J. A genomic approach to human autoimmune diseases. Annu Rev Immunol 2010;28:535–71.
94. Guilherme L, Ferreira FM, Kohler KF, et al. A vaccine against Streptococcus pyogenes: the potential to prevent rheumatic fever and rheumatic heart disease. Am J Cardiovasc Drugs 2013;13:1–4.

Challenges in Imaging in Preclinical Rheumatoid Arthritis

Daniel P. Marcusa, BA, Lisa A. Mandl, MD, MPH*

KEYWORDS

- Imaging • Preclinical • Inflammatory arthritis

KEY POINTS

- Imaging can identify evidence of synovitis in patients with autoimmunity without clinical arthritis.
- Imaging could be used to risk-stratify patients most at risk of progressing to rheumatoid arthritis.
- More work needs to be done in evaluating and comparing different imaging modalities.

INTRODUCTION

Rheumatoid arthritis (RA) is an autoimmune disease affecting up to 1% of the developed world's population.[1] Because early treatment can limit joint erosion and impede disease progression, it has been important to detect clinical RA at its earliest presentation and to treat with disease-modifying therapy (DMARDs) or biological therapy early, as it has been convincingly shown that delaying therapy in RA patients leads to worse outcomes.[2]

This aspect has led investigators to hypothesize that there may be an even earlier point in RA pathogenesis, when there is evidence of autoimmunity but not yet any evidence of clinical arthritis, and when treatment may be able to abort overt manifestations of the disease altogether (**Fig. 1**).[3] Imaging, therefore, would play a crucial role in identifying preclinical RA patients from those with noninflammatory arthralgias and myalgias.

Does the Preclinical Phase of Rheumatoid Arthritis Exist?

There is clear evidence that preclinical RA exists. Kraan and colleagues[4] have studied the synovial tissue from patients with RA and have found that synovial tissue from

The authors declare no financial or other conflict of interests pertaining to the article, and the funding agencies had no influence into the study design, results, or content of the article.
Department of Medicine, Hospital for Special Surgery, 535 E70th Street, New York City, NY 10021, USA
* Corresponding author.
E-mail address: MandlL@hss.edu

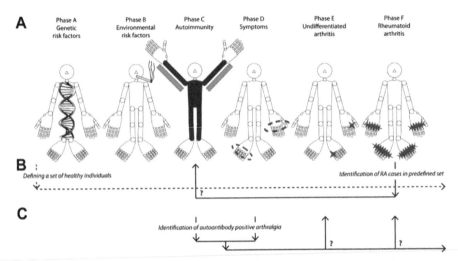

Fig. 1. Pathogenesis of rheumatoid arthritis (RA). (*From* van Steenbergen HW, Huizinga TW, van der Helm-van Mil AH. The preclinical phase of rheumatoid arthritis, what is acknowledged and what needs to be assessed? Arthritis Rheum 2013;65:2219–32; with permission.)

clinically uninvolved knee joints shows infiltration with macrophages and expresses macrophage-derived cytokines. In addition, the uninvolved knee had significantly higher CD68[+] macrophages when compared with tissue biopsies from control patients without RA ($P<.005$). Animal studies have similarly demonstrated that pathologic inflammation can exist in joints before the onset of clinical arthritis. Rhesus monkeys were immunized with type II collagen from bovine hyaline cartilage to model the development of arthritis. Serial synovial arthroscopic biopsies were then performed on their knee joints at 3 time points: before immunization with collagen, 2 weeks after immunization but before the onset of clinical disease, and after the development of clinical arthritis. An influx of macrophages was observed in all knees during the second time course, before the occurrence of arthritis.[4] These findings confirm that there is objective synovial abnormality present in joints before the development of clinically evident arthritis.

Is Imaging an Effective Noninvasive Method of Identifying Preclinical Inflammatory Arthritis?

The question then becomes: is it possible to accurately identify patients with preclinical inflammatory arthritis (IA)? The gold standard would be a synovial biopsy, performed at the first sign of arthralgia. Although this may be feasible under research protocols, it is neither practical nor ethical to routinely perform such biopsies on patients as part of routine clinical care. Imaging, however, is noninvasive and could avoid the risks associated with biopsies, such as infection, bleeding, nerve and tissue damage, or prolonged pain. Because it would be unreasonable to perform gold-standard synovial biopsies on every arthralgia patient, it will be important to evaluate and validate different imaging techniques to discern which, if any, can accurately identify patients with autoimmunity that have imaging evidence of synovitis but no overt clinical synovitis. It will also be important to compare modalities and determine which are most sensitive. Once validated, investigators will be able to ascertain the additive benefit of imaging above and beyond a history and clinical examination in predicting which preclinical patients progress to IA. Determining whether imaging can effectively risk-stratify patients with preclinical inflammatory arthritis would have important implications for both clinical trials and routine clinical care.

ULTRASONOGRAPHY AND POWER DOPPLER

Van de Stadt and colleagues[5] assessed the utility of ultrasonography (US) and power Doppler (PD) in the setting of preclinical RA. In a cohort of 192 arthralgia patients without clinical arthritis but with a positive anti-citrullinated peptide antibody (ACPA) and/or immunoglobulin M rheumatoid factor (IgM-RF), joints that were tender on examination or painful by history were scanned in 2 planes with both US and PD. Two blinded radiologists scored synovitis, joint effusions, and tenosynovitis on a semi-quantitative scale. These patients were then followed for a median of 11 months. Joint effusions, synovitis, and positive PD findings were seen in up to 13% of patients, and 23% of the cohort developed arthritis in 1 or more joints, most commonly in the wrist, metacarpophalangeal (MCP), proximal interphalangeal (PIP), or metatarsophalangeal (MTP) joints. The presence of pain in a joint at the baseline physical examination was associated with arthritis development in that joint, with an odds ratio (OR) of 3.2 (95% confidence interval [CI] 1.8–5.9; $P<.001$). The positive predictive value (PPV) of pain predicting arthritis was 11%, and the negative predictive value (NPV) was 96%. However, when positive findings of synovitis on US and PD were both present, the PPV increased to 35%. This study suggests that in fact when US/PD are used together they are better than clinical examination findings alone at predicting the progression to arthritis in a joint. Although this is a promising result, these findings were only found to have statistical significance at the joint level, not at the patient level. There was also only moderate interobserver reliability ($\kappa = 0.46$, 0.56, 0.23 for synovitis, PD, and joint effusions, respectively).

The same group went on to evaluate 374 IgM-RF–positive and/or ACPA-positive arthralgia patients.[6] After a median follow-up of 12 months, 131 had developed clinical arthritis. Using a multivariate Cox regression, the group developed a prediction rule using the following 9 baseline variables to stratify patients into low-, intermediate-, and high-risk tiers. Increased risk of developing RA was associated with having a first-degree relative with RA, abstaining from alcohol, symptom duration of less than 12 months, intermittent symptoms, symptoms in both upper and lower extremities, a visual analog scale pain score greater than or equal to 50, morning stiffness duration of at least 1 hour, reported joint swelling, and a positive IgM-RF or ACPA (**Fig. 2**). The area under the curve of this model was 0.82 (95% CI 0.75–0.89). Using this risk-calculation rule, 41% had a low risk, 27% had an intermediate risk, and 31% had a high risk of developing arthritis. Compared with the low-risk group, the medium-risk and high-risk groups were both more likely to develop IA, with hazard ratios (HR) of 4.52 (95% CI 2.42–8.77) and 14.86 (95% CI 8.40–28.32), respectively. After 5 years, 12% of the low-risk group developed arthritis, compared with 43% of the intermediate-risk group and 81% of the high-risk group.

This prediction rule was good at identifying low-risk and high-risk patients, suggesting that information routinely available as part of clinical care can effectively risk-stratify patients at the extremes of risk. However, for the 27% in the intermediate-risk group there was still a high level of uncertainty, as 43% developed arthritis within 5 years. These data suggest that perhaps it is in these intermediate-risk patients that incorporating imaging as part of a prediction rule might be particularly informative, and that additional precision is needed to accurately predict progression to clinical RA. Other groups that might also benefit from the addition of imaging to aid with risk stratification

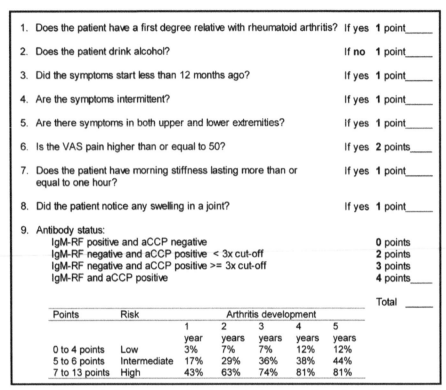

1. Does the patient have a first degree relative with rheumatoid arthritis? If yes **1 point**_____

2. Does the patient drink alcohol? If **no** **1 point**_____

3. Did the symptoms start less than 12 months ago? If yes **1 point**_____

4. Are the symptoms intermittent? If yes **1 point**_____

5. Are there symptoms in both upper and lower extremities? If yes **1 point**_____

6. Is the VAS pain higher than or equal to 50? If yes **2 points**____

7. Does the patient have morning stiffness lasting more than or equal to one hour? If yes **1 point**_____

8. Did the patient notice any swelling in a joint? If yes **1 point**_____

9. Antibody status:
   IgM-RF positive and aCCP negative — **0 points**
   IgM-RF negative and aCCP positive < 3x cut-off — **2 points**
   IgM-RF negative and aCCP positive >= 3x cut-off — **3 points**
   IgM-RF and aCCP positive — **4 points**____

Total _____

Points	Risk	Arthritis development				
		1 year	2 years	3 years	4 years	5 years
0 to 4 points	Low	3%	7%	7%	12%	12%
5 to 6 points	Intermediate	17%	29%	36%	38%	44%
7 to 13 points	High	43%	63%	74%	81%	81%

Fig. 2. Prediction rule for RA using 9 baseline variables to stratify patients into low-, intermediate-, and high-risk tiers. aCCP, anticyclic citrullinated peptide; IgM-RF, immunoglobulin M rheumatoid factor; VAS, visual analog scale. (*From* van de Stadt LA, Witte BI, Bos WH, et al. A prediction rule for the development of arthritis in seropositive arthralgia patients. Ann Rheum Dis 2013;72:1925; with permission.)

include seronegative patients or first-degree relatives of RA patients. Because much of the work in early IA has been done in Europe in ethnically homogeneous cohorts, it will also be important to evaluate the benefit of imaging in patients from a variety of ethnic or racial backgrounds.[7]

Ultrasonography Pros and Cons

US is attractive because it is inexpensive and easy to learn, and individual joints can be scanned quickly. PD adds information on real-time blood flow, and the technique can be easily incorporated into routine care (**Table 1**). However, results are user-dependent and equipment-dependent, and visualizing multiple joints can be very time-consuming.

MAGNETIC RESONANCE IMAGING

It is known that magnetic resonance imaging (MRI) is more sensitive than a clinical examination in patients with established RA. For example, in a cohort of 107 RA patients in clinical remission, 52% of joints with no clinical synovitis had synovitis on MRI.[8] However, its use in preclinical RA remains to be elucidated.

One small study had 13 IgM-RF–positive patients (with or without +/− ACPA) undergo a knee MRI 1 week before arthroscopy.[9] A standard 1.5-T scanner using a

Table 1
Pros and cons of currently available imaging modalities for preclinical rheumatoid arthritis

Modality	Pros	Cons
Ultrasonography	Inexpensive Easy technique to learn Office-based Individual joints are quickly scanned PD aids visualization of synovitis Easily incorporated into routine care	Results are user- and equipment-dependent Time-consuming to visualize multiple involved joint
MRI	More sensitive than ultrasonography Excellent visualization of bone and soft tissue	Expensive Scans can be time-consuming Not office-based, so difficult to incorporate into routine care
PET	Good association with macrophage activity and development of IA Low radiation dose Short C-11 half-life High spatial resolution scanner can detect very low levels of synovitis	Significant nonspecific binding in soft tissue May mask low-level activity in adjacent joints High-resolution scanning can only be done in certain anatomic locations, so may have false negatives Not office-based, so difficult to incorporate into routine care

Abbreviations: IA, inflammatory arthritis; MRI, magnetic resonance imaging; PD, power Doppler; PET, positron emission tomography.

3-dimensional T1-weighted gradient-echo dynamic sequence with contrast-enhanced Gd-DTPA (gadolinium–diethylenetriamine penta-acetic acid complex) was used. These patients then received yearly follow-up after surgery. If a patient developed arthritis, a second arthroscopy was then performed. Synovial tissue was extracted and stained for multiple immune markers. None of the patients had clinical swelling, and although "most patients had arthralgia in more than one joint," only 6 had knee arthralgia (ie, pain in the joint corresponding to the pathologic specimen); all were DMARD and steroid naïve. The MR images from these patients were compared with those from 6 healthy patients without joint symptoms and a normal clinical knee examination. In addition, synovial biopsies were compared with those from 10 non-IA patients having arthroscopy for knee pain, and who had no signs or symptoms of IA at their 5-year follow-up. Four autoantibody-positive arthralgia patients developed arthritis. However, there was no difference in any immunohistochemical findings between autoantibody-positive patients who developed arthritis, autoantibody-positive patients who did not develop arthritis, and the normal arthroscopy controls. Similarly, no difference was found in any MRI parameters between autoantibody-positive patients who neither did nor did not develop arthritis and normal arthroscopy controls. Therefore, although these data suggest that MRI reflects immunohistochemistry, and that autoimmunity precedes inflammation, this study did not indicate a useful role for MRI in the risk stratification of patients with preclinical RA. However, this was a small 13-patient study in which only 5 patients were both ACPA and anti-RF positive. It was also unclear if the index knee was the site of arthralgias in the patients who developed knee arthritis, and knees are not typically the first joints involved in RA. It was helpful, however, in underscoring that imaging studies in preclinical RA should focus on imaging painful joints, and that cohorts being studied should be enriched with patients at high risk of progressing to RA.[9]

Another MRI study evaluated 21 ACPA-positive preclinical RA patients who had arthralgias of the hand or foot joints but no clinical arthritis.[10] The investigators imaged the most painful joints among the PIP 2-5, MCP 2-5, wrist, or MTP 1-5, and compared the results with those of 22 ACPA-positive early RA patients and 19 healthy subjects without joint complaints. There was clear evidence of synovitis in the pre-RA patients. Next, bone marrow edema, synovitis, and erosion were compared in the 3 patient groups. In general, the preclinical RA patients had scores in between those of the healthy controls and the RA cases. These data show clearly that local subclinical inflammation does occur in ACPA-positive arthralgia patients, and that MRI can accurately stratify patients based on synovitis, bone marrow edema, and erosions.

MRI Pros and Cons

Overall MRI is more sensitive than US, and additionally has excellent visualization of bone and soft tissue. However, it is expensive and time-consuming, and patients can become claustrophobic in closed coils. It is also not office-based, making it challenging to incorporate into routine care. (**Table 1**) Because of these concerns, more studies need to be done to identify clinical scenarios whereby MRI might effectively affect patient outcomes. Until such data become available, MRIs should only be ordered sparingly, in situations where results would directly affect disease management.[11]

POSITRON EMISSION TOMOGRAPHY

Positron emission tomography (PET) scanning is a novel imaging technique for the investigation of subclinical arthritis in preclinical RA. One such promising PET method uses the compound ^{11}C-(R)-PK11195 to target the 18-kDa translocator protein, a mitochondrial membrane protein that is upregulated in activated macrophages. Because macrophages infiltrate synovial tissue during the early development of RA, an imaging modality that identifies this cellular subset could prove valuable in the detection of subclinical synovitis.

Gent and colleagues[12] evaluated 29 ACPA positive arthralgia patients, 38% of whom were RF positive, with ^{11}C-(R)-PK11195 PET scans. Median duration of arthralgia was 15 months. These patients were compared with both patients with established RA and healthy controls. Of the 29 arthralgia patients, 4 had positive PET scans, each of whom had between 1 and 5 joints with tracer uptake, and 3 of whom had joints with high tracer uptake. By comparison, all RA patients had positive uptake in all clinically inflamed joints, and none of the 6 healthy controls had uptake in any joint. Of those 4 arthralgia patients with positive PET scans, all developed IA within 14 months: 3 RA and 1 oligoarthritis. However, 5 of the remaining patients with negative PET also developed IA: 3 developed IA in joints that were not scanned by PET while 2 developed IA in joints that had been scanned. Of those 2 false-negative patients, the first developed clinical oligoarthritis and the second developed IA in 1 PIP joint, which spontaneously resolved within 1 year.

This study showed that PET scanning is able to identify synovitis in preclinical RA. However, at the individual joint level, there was no association between development of IA and positive uptake: of the 683 joints scanned there were 14 positive joints, of which 4 developed IA. Of the 671 negative scans, 2 developed IA. However, importantly it remains unclear whether PET scanning confers any additional information over and above existing data. Specifically, it is unclear whether there is an added benefit above ACPA. Of the PET-positive joints, the mean ACPA level was 1180 AU (interquartile range [IQR] 131–2473), compared with 120 AU (IQR 76–474) for the negative joints. Further studies need to be done to explore the best uses of this technology.

For example, it may be that serial PET scans are more informative, in that they could capture the evolution of early synovitis beyond the static information provided by a single scan.

PET Pros and Cons

There is a strong relationship between macrophage activity, identifiable with PET scanning, and development of IA. There are also relatively low risks associated with PET scanning, because of the short half-life of carbon-11 and its low radiation dose. PET scanning also offers high spatial resolution, and can identify very low levels of synovitis.

However, there is significant nonspecific binding of ^{11}C-(R)-PK11195 in soft tissues, which may mask low-level activity in adjacent joints. The high-resolution scanning unique to PET techniques may also only be performed in specific anatomic areas, and can result in possible false-negative scans because of missed activity in non-scanned joints. Conversely, whole-body scanning does not allow for precise evaluation of uptake in small joints. In addition, PET scanning is not an office-based imaging modality, and it is therefore challenging to incorporate it into routine care in nonhospital settings (**Table 1**).

FUTURE DIRECTIONS

There are several potential modalities which, while not currently available outside experimental protocols, may one day provide important insights into patients presenting with autoimmunity but no overt synovitis. These modalities include a variety of radionucleotide imaging techniques, targeted imaging agents that take advantage of antibody-ligand interactions, micro–computed tomography (CT), single-photon emission computed tomography (SPECT), image coregistration techniques combining anatomic and molecular data, such as PET/CT, SPECT/CT, bioluminescence or fluorescence imaging, and optical imaging.[13,14] This exciting area has great potential for the evaluation of preclinical RA.

CHALLENGES IN IMAGING IN PRECLINICAL RHEUMATOID ARTHRITIS

Several challenges remain in the use of imaging in the evaluation of preclinical RA. Many of the studies to date have been small, making it difficult to discern true associations from statistical noise. Large cohorts of patients at high risk for developing RA are needed, to allow investigators to effectively study this patient population. These cohorts have been enrolled, most successfully in Europe, but more work needs to be done, especially in the establishment of cohorts with greater ethnic and racial diversity. In addition, there have been many positive findings in normal control subjects, suggesting issues with discriminative validity when using these high-sensitivity imaging techniques in the preclinical setting. More clear guidelines to establish which findings warrant concern will be needed before these modalities can be integrated into widespread clinical care.

In addition, many of these imaging techniques and their interpretation can be very user-dependent. There is often, at best, only moderate agreement between expert radiologists. The dissemination of standardized techniques and an emphasis on reporting results using standardized methods (eg, RAMRIS) would greatly improve the usefulness of these techniques and of studies evaluating their effectiveness.

There exists an assumption that preclinical imaging demonstrating evidence of subclinical inflammation is proof of the "window of opportunity" during which proper treatment could prevent the development of IA. Studies evaluating the long-term outcomes of patients treated in this early window, compared with those who are not, will be needed to test this assumption and prove its clinical usefulness. In addition, there is some debate on the ethics of treating preclinical RA patients with nonbenign pharmacologic agents. There remains a great need for large prospective trials to convincingly identify subgroups of preclinical RA patients with a high enough risk for further disease progression to justify exposure to a potentially toxic therapy.

Modern imaging techniques can identify synovial inflammation after the development of autoimmunity, but before overt clinical synovitis. How imaging can provide meaningful risk stratification remains a work in progress. Head-to-head studies comparing these imaging modalities are needed to determine which are the most sensitive and specific for local joint inflammation.

REFERENCES

1. Scott DL, Wolfe F, Huizing TW. Rheumatoid arthritis. Lancet 2010;376:1094–108.
2. Lard LR, Visser H, Speyer I, et al. Early versus delayed treatment in patients with recent-onset rheumatoid arthritis: comparison of two cohorts who received different treatment strategies. Am J Med 2001;111(6):446–51.
3. van Steenbergen HW, Huizinga TW, van der Helm-van Mil AH. The preclinical phase of rheumatoid arthritis, what is acknowledged and what needs to be assessed? Arthritis Rheum 2013;65:2219–32.
4. Kraan MC, Versendaal H, Jonker M, et al. Asymptomatic synovitis precedes clinically manifest arthritis. Arthritis Rheum 1998;41(8):1481–8.
5. van de Stadt LA, Bos WH, Reynders MM, et al. The value of ultrasonography in predicting arthritis in auto-antibody positive arthralgia patients: a prospective cohort study. Arthritis Res Ther 2010;12(3):R98.
6. van de Stadt LA, Witte BI, Bos WH, et al. A prediction rule for the development of arthritis in seropositive arthralgia patients. Ann Rheum Dis 2013;72:1920–6.
7. Kochi Y, Suzuki A, Yamada R, et al. Genetics of rheumatoid arthritis: underlying evidence of ethnic differences. J Autoimmun 2009;32(3–4):158–62.
8. Brown AK, Quinn MA, Karim Z, et al. Presence of significant synovitis in rheumatoid arthritis patients with disease-modifying antirheumatic drug-induced clinical remission: evidence from an imaging study may explain structural progression. Arthritis Rheum 2006;54(12):3761–73.
9. van de Sande MG, de Hair MJ, van der Leig C, et al. Different stages of rheumatoid arthritis: features of the synovium in the preclinical phase. Ann Rheum Dis 2011;70(5):772–7.
10. Krabben A, Stomp W, van der Heijde DM, et al. MRI of hand and foot joints of patients with anticitrullinated peptide antibody positive arthralgia without clinical arthritis. Ann Rheum Dis 2013;72(9):1540–4.
11. Yazdany J, Schmajuk G, Robbins M, et al. Choosing wisely: The American College of Rheumatology's top 5 list of things physicians and patients should question. Arthritis Care Res 2013;65(3):329–39.
12. Gent YY, Voskuyl AE, Kloet RW, et al. Macrophage positron emission tomography imaging as a biomarker for preclinical rheumatoid arthritis: findings of a prospective pilot study. Arthritis Rheum 2012;64(1):62–6.
13. Gompels LL, Paleolog EM. A window on disease pathogenesis and potential therapeutic strategies: molecular imaging for arthritis. Arthritis Res Ther 2011;13(1):201.
14. Tremoleda JL, Khalil M, Gompels LL, et al. Imaging technologies for preclinical models of bone and joint disorders. EJNMMI Res 2011;1(1):11.

Identification of Self-antigen–specific T Cells Reflecting Loss of Tolerance in Autoimmune Disease Underpins Preventative Immunotherapeutic Strategies in Rheumatoid Arthritis

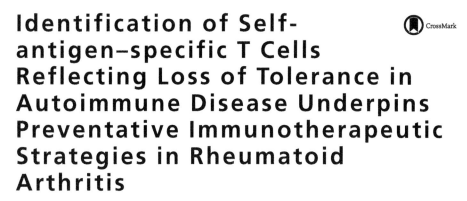 CrossMark

Soi-Cheng Law, BSc (Hons)[a],
Helen Benham, B.App.Sci, MBBS (Hons), FRACP, PhD[a,b],
Hugh H. Reid, BSc (Hons), PhD[c], Jamie Rossjohn, BSc (Hons), PhD[c,d],
Ranjeny Thomas, MBBS, MD[a,*]

KEYWORDS

- Immune tolerance • Regulatory T cells • pMHC tetramers • Rheumatoid arthritis
- Type 1 diabetes • HLA susceptibility

KEY POINTS

- pMHC tetramers specific for citrullinated autoantigens identify antigen-specific T cells in *HLA-DRB1*0401*+ rheumatoid arthritis (RA) patients and healthy controls. In type 1 diabetes, antigen-specific T cells are emerging as diagnostic biomarkers.
- In patients with RA, the frequency of self-antigen–specific CD4+ T cells is correlated with disease activity, similar to findings in collagen-induced arthritis and type 1 diabetes models.

Continued

Declaration: Ranjeny Thomas is supported by Arthritis Queensland. She has filed provisional patents surrounding technology for targeting dendritic cells for antigen-specific tolerance and is a director of a spin-off company, which is commercializing vaccines that target dendritic cells to suppress autoimmune diseases.
[a] The University of Queensland Diamantina Institute, 37 Kent Street, Woolloongabba, Queensland 4102, Australia; [b] The University of Queensland School of Medicine, Translational Research Institute, 37 Kent Street, Woolloongabba, Queensland 4102, Australia; [c] Department of Biochemistry and Molecular Biology, School of Biomedical Sciences, Monash University, Clayton, Victoria 3800, Australia; [d] Institute of Infection and Immunity, School of Medicine, Cardiff University, Heath Park, Cardiff CF14 4XN, UK
* Corresponding author. Translational Research Institute, Princess Alexandra Hospital, The University of Queensland Diamantina Institute, 37 Kent Street, Woolloongabba, Queensland 4102, Australia.
E-mail address: Ranjeny.thomas@uq.edu.au

Rheum Dis Clin N Am 40 (2014) 735–752
http://dx.doi.org/10.1016/j.rdc.2014.07.015
0889-857X/14/$ – see front matter © 2014 Elsevier Inc. All rights reserved.
rheumatic.theclinics.com

Continued

- In RA patients, the proportion of self-antigen–specific CD4$^+$ regulatory T cells is reduced relative to healthy controls, suggesting the hypothesis that *HLA-DRB1* susceptibility alleles fail to promote citrullinated peptide–specific T cell regulation to prevent the development of RA in the face of genetic, environmental, or inflammatory pressures on regulatory T cells.

INTRODUCTION

Rheumatoid arthritis (RA) is a common and incurable systemic inflammatory autoimmune disease affecting 1% to 2% of the population.[1,2] RA is characterized by inflammation of joint synovial tissues and extra-articular sites, with complications of erosive joint damage, lung fibrosis, atherosclerosis, and infection.[3] Current treatments such as disease-modifying antirheumatic drugs and biologic inhibitors of tumor necrosis factor (TNF), interleukin 6 (IL-6), T cells, and B cells are nonspecific and are associated with side effects. Although current drugs block inflammation, they induce long-term remission in less than 50% of patients on treatment. Thus, despite treatment advances, RA is still associated with significant disability, decreased work capacity, and reduced life expectancy, leading to enormous social and economic burden.[4,5]

Effective immunotherapies to restore immune tolerance are considered the "Holy Grail" in autoimmune diseases. Such strategies promise greater specificity, lower toxicity, and a longer-term solution to controlling and preventing RA. However, antigen-specific tolerizing immunotherapy has been more difficult to achieve than blocking inflammation.[6] Design of effective therapies requires a fundamental understanding of the critical immunopathogenetic pathways in RA. The preclinical phase of RA represents a valuable period of time to understand the relationships between genetics, environment, and immune dysregulation in the development of RA and to evaluate preclinical interventions and novel immunomodulation including antigen-specific therapy. The capacity to visualize and characterize antigen-specific autoreactive T cells longitudinally during this period is central to understand dysregulation of adaptive immunity in autoimmune diseases such as RA.

In this article, the authors review advances in understanding self-antigen–specific autoreactive T cells in RA. These developments bring exciting insights to the mechanisms underpinning loss of tolerance and how tolerance could be restored to bring us closer to the goal of RA prevention in the preclinical or recent-onset period.

PRECLINICAL RHEUMATOID ARTHRITIS

The preclinical phase of RA encompasses an initial phase of risk secondary to genetic and environmental factors, characterized by asymptomatic autoimmunity. Multiple genetic and environmental factors influence RA pathogenesis and progression. First-degree relatives (FDR) of patients with RA are a known, high-risk population with a 5- to 7-fold increased risk for incident RA.[7,8] FDR as well as cohorts of unrelated individuals with high genetic and environmental risk factors for RA represent valuable, enriched populations in which to further investigate asymptomatic autoimmunity and preclinical RA and to examine the factors influencing the development and progression of autoimmunity, using appropriate biomarkers. Further, immunotherapeutic interventions aimed at disease prevention can be explored in such populations before the onset of disease.

THE MOLECULAR MECHANISM OF SHARED EPITOPE AND ANTICITRULLINATED PROTEIN ANTIBODIES+ RHEUMATOID ARTHRITIS

Historically, alleles associated with seropositive RA such as *HLA-DRB1*0401, *0404, *0101* molecules in Caucasians, *HLA-DRB1*0405* in Asians, and *HLA-DRB1*1402* in North American Natives (NAN)[9–12] were proposed to share a conserved epitope around amino acids 70 to 74. This epitope is commonly known as the "shared susceptibility epitope" (SE) and includes a positively charged residue at position 71 (see entries in bold in **Table 1**).[9] The positively charged residue at position 71 has been proposed to dictate the nature of amino acid that can be accommodated in the P4 pocket.[13] In line with this observation, 70% of RA patients have the disease-specific anticitrullinated protein antibodies (ACPA). Several citrullinated (cit) autoantigens, including fibrinogen, aggrecan, vimentin, collagen type II, and α-enolase have been described in RA.[14–17] Citrulline is a post-translational modification of arginine, which occurs during inflammation, endoplasmic reticulum stress, and autophagy.[18,19] Presence of ACPA in RA serum implies the presentation of cit-antigens to T cells by dendritic cells (DC) and B cells to support ACPA production by B cells.

Table 1
Classical HLA-DRB1 alleles associated with ACPA+ RA and critical peptide contact residues

HLA-DRB1 Amino Acid at Position					Odds Ratio
11	13	71	74	Classical HLA-DRB1 Alleles	ACPA+ RA
Val	His	**Lys**	Ala	*0401	3.3
Val	His/Phe	**Arg**	Ala	*0408, *0405, *0404, *1001	2.8–10.3
Leu	Phe	**Arg**	Ala	*0102, *0101	1.5
Pro	Arg	**Arg**	Ala	*1601	1.2
Val	His	Arg	Glu	*0403, *0407	0.5–0.7
Asp	Phe	Arg	Glu	*0901	2.1
Ser	Ser	**Arg**	Ala	*1402	>1
Val	His	Glu	Ala	*0402	1.2
Ser	Ser	Lys	Ala	*1303	0.6
Pro	Arg	Ala	Ala	*1501, *1502	0.9
Gly	Tyr	Arg	Gln	*0701	0.7
Ser	Ser/Gly	Arg	Ala	*1101, *1104, *1201	0.5–0.7
Ser	Ser	Arg	Glu	*1401	0.6
Leu	Phe	Glu	Ala	*0103	<1
Ser	Gly	Arg	Leu	*0801, *0804	0.4
Ser	Ser	Lys	Arg	*0301	0.5
Ser	Ser	Glu	Ala	*1102, *1103, *1301, *1302	0.5–0.6

The SE are in bold.
Adapted from Raychaudhuri S, Sandor C, Stahl EA, et al. Five amino acids in three HLA proteins explain most of the association between MHC and seropositive rheumatoid arthritis. Nat Genet 2012;44(3):291–6; and Balandraud N, Picard C, Reviron D, et al. HLA-DRB1 genotypes and the risk of developing anti citrullinated protein antibody (ACPA) positive rheumatoid arthritis. PLoS One 2013;8(5):e64108.

In 2012, a large haplotype association study reported by Raychaudhuri and colleagues[20] attributed most of the DR-associated risk of RA to positions 11, 13, 71, and 74 of DRβ, effectively extending the SE to additional amino acids in the floor of the antigen-binding groove surrounding pocket 4. Unexpectedly, positions 11 and 13 had the highest statistical association with RA risk; the reasons for this are not yet clear.

The prediction that RA risk allomorphs permit binding and presentation of citrullinated peptides was confirmed by solution of the crystal structure of several cit-self-peptides bound to SE⁺ HLA-DRB1*0401 and 0404.[21] Citrulline occupies the P4 pocket and interacts with Lys71β through a hydrogen-bonding network. In contrast, arginine could not be accommodated at P4. His13β forms van der Waals contacts with the P4 citrulline aliphatic moiety. Moreover, a His13βSer polymorphism, present in RA-resistant allomorphs such as HLA-DRB1*1301, is predicted to affect the packing of citrulline in this location. Curiously, the NAN RA risk allele HLA-DRB1*1402 contains the SE, as well as Ser11β and Ser13β. Individuals carrying the non-SE allele HLA-DRB1*0402 have been previously proposed to be protected from RA development. In contrast to HLA-DRB1*0401 or *0404, which did not accommodate Arg, HLA-DRB1*0402 was able to accommodate both citrullinated and native vimentin due to the presence of negatively charged aspartic acid and glutamic acid at positions 70 and 71, respectively.[21] The knowledge from understanding the molecular association of SE and RA warrants further investigation on how the differential presentation of peptides influence the T-cell response.

IMMUNE TOLERANCE AND THE DEVELOPMENT OF AUTOIMMUNITY

Thymic deletion of immature self-reactive T cells with high-affinity T cell receptors (TCRs) constitutes a major mechanism of self-tolerance during neonatal life. Such overtly autoreactive T cells can also be silenced or anergised, either as immature thymocytes or as mature T cells in the periphery.[22,23] These "recessive" tolerance mechanisms reduce the likelihood of autoimmunity resulting from high-affinity autoreactive T cells. However, low-affinity autoreactive T cells escape the deletion threshold and persist, requiring "dominant" tolerance mechanisms involving regulatory T cells (Treg) for their control.[24] Foxp3⁺ Treg may be selected intrathymically or in the periphery in response to antigen presentation by specialized subsets of DC.[6] Autoimmune diseases, including RA and type 1 diabetes (T1D), are associated with genetic variants such as IL2, ILI2RA, and CTLA4, which perturb Treg generation, proliferation, or function.[25] Moreover, RA is associated with genetic variants such as TNFAIP3 that enhance the proinflammatory environment and may promote Treg dysfunction.[26] However, despite the evidence that HLA is the strongest genetic association with RA and that the susceptibility allomorphs preferentially bind cit-autoantigens, it is not yet clear how the recognition of self-antigens presented by susceptibility or protective HLA molecules influences Treg development or function. The dominant protection associated with the inheritance of protective HLA alleles in RA suggests that these alleles promote cit-peptide–specific T-cell regulation to prevent the development of RA more effectively than alleles associated with RA susceptibility.

MEASURING ANTIGEN-SPECIFIC T-CELL RESPONSES

Antigen-specific CD4⁺ and CD8⁺ T cells are key players in autoimmune diseases such as RA and T1D; however, the frequencies and roles of antigen-specific T cells in disease pathogenesis have been difficult to elucidate. T cell responses have typically been measured in bulk T cell populations using indirect methods such as enzyme-linked immunospot assay (ELISpot), flow cytometry–based intracellular cytokine, and activation markers (eg, CD69, CD154, and CD25). However, these methods require in vitro stimulation, which may alter their phenotype and functionality.[27] Furthermore, these methods can only detect antigen-experienced T cells that are capable of producing cytokines on restimulation, ignoring T cells that produce little cytokine on stimulation and overestimating cells stimulated nonspecifically in vitro.[28] Therefore, relying on these techniques to enumerate and characterize the T cell response may be inadequate. The development of multimeric peptide-bound major histocompatibility complex (pMHC) complexes (tetramers) has revolutionized the detection of antigen-specific T cells in mice and humans. Altman and colleagues[29] first described tetramers in 1996, which allowed ex vivo detection of virus-specific T cells by flow cytometry. Since then both class I and class II pMHC tetramers in combination with other staining techniques have been used to study CD8[+] and CD4[+] T cells respectively in viral infections, tumor responses, and autoimmune diseases.[21,30–34]

TETRAMERS: TOOLS OF THE TRADE

$\alpha\beta$ TCR recognize peptides derived from pathogens, tumors, and self that are presented in the context of MHC molecules on antigen-presenting cells. This recognition is very specific for the MHC molecule and peptide.[35] It is therefore possible to detect antigen-specific T cells using soluble pMHC labeled with fluorochromes directly by flow cytometry. The interaction between TCR and pMHC complex is characterized by low affinity and fast off-rate, which are necessary for each TCR to make serial contacts with multiple pMHC complexes.[36] However, these features represent a

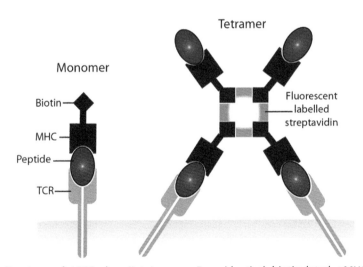

Fig. 1. Structure of MHC class II tetramers. Four identical biotinylated pMHC class II molecules are linked to a central streptavidin molecule to form a tetrameric complex. MHC-TCR interaction is characterized by low affinity and fast dissociation of peptide-MHC complex from the TCR. By binding 2 or more TCRs simultaneously, the affinity of tetramer for TCR is increased compared with monomeric MHC-TCR interaction. The central streptavidin can be labeled with fluorochromes of interest, thus allowing flow cytometric or immunocytochemical use of the tetramer reagents.

challenge for staining antigen-specific T cells with monomeric pMHC complexes. Higher-order multimer construction resulted in increased pMHC-binding affinity, decreased off-rate, and successful staining of T cells. One of the most commonly used pMHC multimers is a tetramer, consisting of 4 identical biotinylated MHC molecules, each loaded with a single peptide linked to a central streptavidin molecule and coupled to a fluorochrome (**Fig. 1**).

Tetramers have become an essential tool in flow cytometric studies, but use in histologic sections has been limited in human studies due to technical challenges.[37,38] The advantages are that they have high specificity and sensitivity, discriminating extremely rare antigen-specific T cells when used sequentially with cell enrichment (10 antigen-specific T cells in 2.5×10^8 mixed populations of cells).[39] Therefore, tetramer assays can be used to enumerate and characterize antigen-specific T cells ex vivo without in vitro stimulation. For example, a recent study found that greater than 50% viral antigen–specific CD4$^+$ T cells displayed a memory phenotype in adults naïve to those viral infections.[34] This phenomenon was attributed to the strong propensity of $\alpha\beta$ TCRs to cross-react with different pMHC complexes due to their flexible binding sites.[40–42] In support of this, the study found an extensive cross-recognition of viral antigen-specific T cells with other microbial peptides.[34]

The major limitation of tetramer assays in human studies is that prior knowledge of specific epitopes for each HLA allele is required to construct the tetramers. This limitation is not so critical when an immunodominant epitope is known, for example, hemagglutinin protein of influenza (HA$_{306-318}$) restricted by the SE allomorph DRB1*0401. CD4$^+$ T cells specific for HA$_{306-318}$ acquired through natural exposure or annual flu vaccination can be readily detected in peripheral blood (PB) of *HLA-DRB1*0401$^+$* individuals.[43] However, when there is a set of complex epitopes recognized by T cells, or when the epitope is unknown, alternative strategies are needed to identify binding epitopes. Identification of MHC-binding epitopes has traditionally involved screening large libraries of peptides with functional assays such as interferon gamma ELISpot, which is laborious and prone to overestimation in diseases such as RA, where background cytokine production is high.[14,44] An unbiased approach known as the tetramer-guided epitope mapping (TGEM) has been designed to identify T cell epitopes. Briefly, a panel of overlapping peptides is divided into pools and each peptide pool is then loaded onto soluble MHC molecules to generate pooled peptide tetramers. The pooled peptide tetramers are then used to stain PB mononuclear cells (PBMC) that have been stimulated with the corresponding whole antigen; this allows the identification of peptide tetramers with positive staining within the pool. Each peptide in the pool is then loaded individually onto MHC molecules and the PBMC staining is repeated to identify the antigenic epitopes (**Fig. 2**).[45] However, TGEM lacks the ability to identify post-translational modified epitopes. A recent strategy that combined TCR selection of highly diverse yeast-displayed peptide-MHC libraries with deep sequencing identified activating microbial and self-ligands for human autoimmune diseases.[46]

TETRAMER APPLICATION: PEPTIDE-BOUND MAJOR HISTOCOMPATIBILITY COMPLEX CLASS I TETRAMERS

An effective CD8$^+$ T cell response after infection or vaccination depends on the size and speed of the response. The dynamics of CD8$^+$ T cell responses may be important to disease progression. With the advent of pMHC class I tetramers, antigen-specific CD8$^+$ T cell responses have been well studied in viral infections and tumor immunology in both animal models and human.[47,48] pMHC class I tetramers have also been used to study antigen-specific CD8[+] autoreactive T cells in T1D in human and the nonobese diabetic (NOD) mouse model for T1D. The frequency of autoantigen-specific CD8[+] T cells in NOD mice was correlated with the degree of insulitis, which predicted of the onset of overt diabetes before the detection of hyperglycemia.[49] In human studies, pMHC class I tetramer[+] CD8[+] T cells were found in recent-onset diabetic but not in healthy donors. In a longitudinal study investigating the reactivity of peripheral CD4[+] and CD8[+] T cells in T1D and T2D patients, CD8[+] T-cell autoreactivity was specific to T1D.[50] Furthermore, autoreactive CD8[+] T cells in recent-onset diabetic patients were correlated with insulin dependence after islet transplantation.[51] In addition to their potential as diagnostic biomarkers, pMHC class I tetramers have also been used to monitor therapeutic responses in T1D patients.[52]

Visualization of antigen-specific T cells in target organs can provide information on their spatial relationship with other subsets of immune cells that flow cytometry cannot. In situ tetramer staining using both pMHC class I and II tetramers has been achieved in pancreatic sections from NOD mice and humans with T1D. Autoreactive CD4[+] and CD8[+] T cells were detected in lymphoid organs and/or islets in diabetic mice and islets in diabetic patients.[37,53,54] In NOD mice, specific autoantigen reactivity can become immunodominant over time.[55,56] This phenomenon is known as "avidity maturation", in which higher-avidity T cells expand within islets over time. In humans, however, no single immunodominant T cell autoreactivity is observed, potentially due to "epitope spreading".[57] It has been observed that a single CD8 autoreactivity was present soon after diagnosis and that specificities expanded as disease progressed. Furthermore, only single CD8 autoreactivity was observed within an islet at particular focal plane.[37] The heterogeneity of autoreactive T cells in target organs represents a challenge to the design of antigen-specific therapy. These data collectively suggest that pMHC class I tetramers make an invaluable tool to probe the diagnosis and prognosis of disease and to understand the underlying pathogenesis of CD8[+] T cell–mediated diseases.

PEPTIDE-BOUND MAJOR HISTOCOMPATIBILITY COMPLEX CLASS II TETRAMERS

In contrast, the use of pMHC class II to characterize CD4[+] T cells in infectious and autoimmune diseases is still rudimentary. The obstacles preventing the wider application of pMHC class II tetramers in autoimmune diseases are (1) difficulties in pMHC class II tetramer production, (2) low frequencies of CD4[+] T cells of any given specificity in PB, (3) the low affinity interaction between TCR and pMHC in autoreactive T cells that have escaped thymic negative selection, and (4) the internalization of TCR-pMHC tetramer complexes after cross-linking, resulting in nonproductive tetramer engagement. These are particularly challenging when dealing with autoantigen-specific CD4[+] T cells. With improvements in tetramer production and strategies to overcome these obstacles in pMHC class II tetramer staining, data are now accumulating in autoimmune diseases.[39,58–60] Briefly, the frequency of antigen-specific CD4[+] T cells is often below 0.2%, which significantly overlaps with the 0.1% background staining obtained using tetramers loaded with an irrelevant peptide. Although an immunomagnetic enrichment protocol allowed the detection of low-frequency pMHC class II tetramer[+] CD4[+] T cells,[39] the authors observed that immunomagnetic enrichment selectively enriched for pMHC class II tetramer[+] CD4[+] T cells with high affinity, which they found to skew the phenotype of the antigen-specific CD4[+] T cells detected after immunomagnetic enrichment.[21] Although the low-binding affinity of TCR was improved by multimerizing the pMHC complexes, there are CD4[+] T cells with MHC-TCR affinity too weak to support tetramer staining. In these cases,

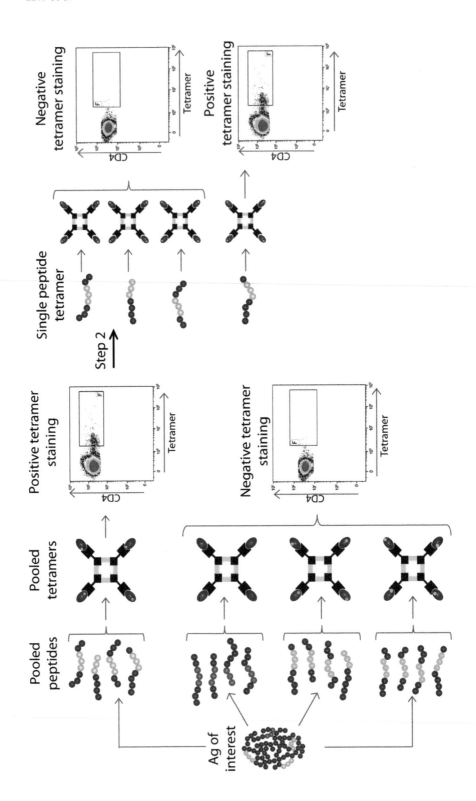

in vitro expansion was necessary to detect the antigen-specific T cells. Such data must be carefully interpreted due to changes in phenotype and preferential expansion of cells with either higher- or lower-affinity TCRs in culture.[61] Another method to detect low-affinity T cells without the need for in vitro stimulation is to incorporate the protein-tyrosine kinase inhibitor, dasatinib (**Fig. 3**). Dasatinib enhances the staining intensity of low-affinity T cells by blocking the internalization of cross-linked TCR-pMHC tetramer complexes from the cell surface, resulting in productive tetramer engagement (**Fig. 4**). A productive engagement requires a second pMHC molecule in the tetramer to bind to a second TCR before the first one dissociates. Nonproductive engagement is often observed when low-affinity ligands dissociate rapidly from cell surface TCR. Both of these engagements downregulate TCR expression. Dasatinib thereby maintains the TCR on the cell surface to increase the likelihood of a productive tetramer engagement (see **Fig. 4**). Furthermore, dasatinib reduces tetramer-induced cell death and the tetramer-negative background, thus increasing detection of rare antigen-specific T cells.[59] Collectively, these improvements have made it possible to use pMHC class II tetramers to study the role of antigen-specific CD4+ T cells in autoimmune responses. Data to date in T1D and RA are discussed later in this article.

TYPE 1 DIABETES

The development of T1D is usually predated by the presence of autoantibodies specific for insulin, glutamate decarboxylase 65 (GAD65), and protein-tyrosine phosphatase 2 (IA-2), which are used as predictive markers for T1D progression.[62,63] GAD65- and proinsulin-specific CD4+ T cells were detected in the PB of T1D and at-risk subjects but not in healthy controls.[54,64,65] Interestingly, tetramer staining in at-risk subjects revealed appearance and disappearance of antigen-specific CD4+ T cells in PB over time, potentially reflecting clonal expansion and target organ homing during the inflammatory process.[49] These studies also demonstrated that some of the GAD65-specific CD4+ T cells were of high avidity.[65,66] T cell avidities are determined by intrinsic TCR affinity for the pMHC complex and the expression levels of TCR, CD4, costimulatory and adhesion molecules.[67] T cells with high avidity toward self-antigen are usually deleted in the thymus; however, the thymic selection process is incomplete and thus T cells with a range of avidities persist, and this was demonstrated for GAD65-specific CD4+ T cells in PB of T1D patients. The high-avidity cells were more susceptible to activation-induced cell death and reflected a biased expression of TCR genes, suggesting clonal expansion of GAD65-specific CD4+ T cells in response to autoantigen exposure during T1D progression.[65] It is known that avidity of T cells can change over time following multiple antigen encounters, a process known as avidity maturation.[66] One mechanism is through selective expansion of T cells expressing optimal

---

Fig. 2. Tetramer-guided epitope mapping as a way to identify immunogenic T cell epitopes from a complex whole antigen. A panel of overlapping peptides is divided into different pools (strings of *purple* and *green; purple* and *pink, purple,* and *orange; purple* and *blue spheres*), and each peptide pool is loaded onto soluble MHC molecules to generate pooled peptide tetramers. The pooled peptide tetramers are then used to stain PBMC that were stimulated with the corresponding whole antigen. Peptides from the pool that gave positive staining are then loaded individually onto MHC molecules to stain the stimulated PBMC, thus allowing the identification of immunogenic epitopes.

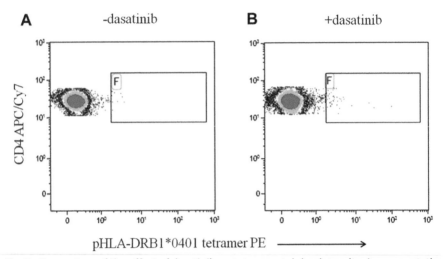

Fig. 3. Comparison of the effect of dasatinib on tetramer staining intensity. A representative sample of PBMC from an RA patient was either pretreated without (*A*) or with (*B*) 50 nM of dasatinib before tetramer staining at room temperature. Tetramer+ cells were gated based on fluorescence minus one. In PBMC pretreated with dasatinib, the tetramer staining intensity was stronger than without dasatinib pretreatment.

affinity for antigens.[68,69] In a cohort of autoantibody-positive subjects at high risk of progression to T1D, avidity and TCR Vβ bias increased over time.[66] Avidity maturation was not observed in autoantibody-negative first-degree relatives or T1D patients. These data collectively suggest that the presence of autoantigen-specific CD4+ T cells may not be sufficient for disease development; however, self-reactive CD4+ T cells with optimal autoantigen affinity might undergo clonal expansion and become pathogenic as autoimmunity progresses. Thus the avidity of autoantigen-specific CD4+ T cells, measured using pMHC class II tetramers, may serve as a predictive marker for progression in T1D.

RHEUMATOID ARTHRITIS

The authors recently demonstrated the molecular mechanism of cit-self-peptide binding to antigen-presenting HLA-DR molecules through solution of high-resolution crystal structures of SE HLA-DRB1 molecules complexed to cit-vimentin and cit-aggrecan peptides in individuals with genetic susceptibility to RA.[21] In the same study, they found reduced protease susceptibility of cit-vimentin relative to vimentin, leading to cit-self-epitope generation, and using pMHC class II tetramers, cit-vimentin and cit-aggrecan-specific CD4+ T cells in PB of *HLA-DRB1*0401+* RA patients and healthy controls. The authors found that the frequency of autoreactive cells specific for cit–self-epitopes correlated with disease activity in RA patients. Interestingly, RA patients were deficient in tetramer+ cit-antigen-specific Tregs but had higher proportions of naive and effector/memory self-antigen–specific T cells relative to healthy individuals. CD4+tetramer+ T cells expressing CD45RO and CXCR3 (characteristic of a Th1 memory phenotype) specific for a range of cit–self-peptides were similarly shown to be increased in enriched PBMC of *HLA-DRB1*0401+* RA patients relative to healthy controls (**Fig. 5**).[17]

An established view in the field of RA is that the inflammatory disease cascade is triggered by the presentation of a post-translationally modified cit-peptide to

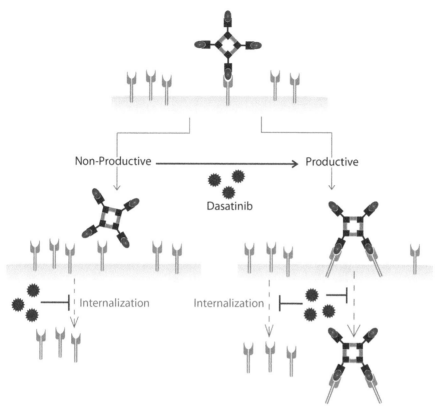

Fig. 4. Productive or nonproductive tetramer engagement with the TCR. A productive tetramer engagement requires 2 or more TCR to be interacting with the tetramer. Nonproductive engagement occurs when only one of the pMHC molecules is in contact with a TCR, leading to a rapid off-rate. Both types of engagements result in TCR downregulation and thus internalization of the tetramer complexes. Dasatinib maintains the TCR on the cell surface, increasing the likelihood of a productive tetramer engagement in T cells with low affinity for the pMHC tetrameric complex.

circulating T cells by HLA-DRβ1 molecules containing the conserved residues of the SE, that is, neo-self cit-epitopes break tolerance. However, this model is inconsistent with the observation that HLA-DRB1*0402 also binds cit-peptides, yet this allele is protective. The reduction in antigen-specific Tregs observed in RA patients rather suggests that they fail to regulate inflammation driven by autoimmunity toward cit-peptides. Reduced protease susceptibility of cit-protein and increased expression of cit-antigens at the joint inflammatory site, particularly in the face of reduced regulation, would increase the opportunity for expansion of autoreactive T cells, as observed in RA patients with active disease. Hence, the authors postulate that *HLA-DRB1* alleles associated with RA susceptibility fail to promote cit-peptide-specific T cell regulation to prevent the development of RA in the face of genetic, environmental, or inflammatory pressures on Treg number or function. Citrullination is catalyzed by the family of calcium-dependent peptidylarginine deiminase (PAD) enzymes.[70] Citrullination of antigens by PAD is constitutive in autophagosomes of macrophages and DC and is upregulated under conditions of endoplasmic reticulum

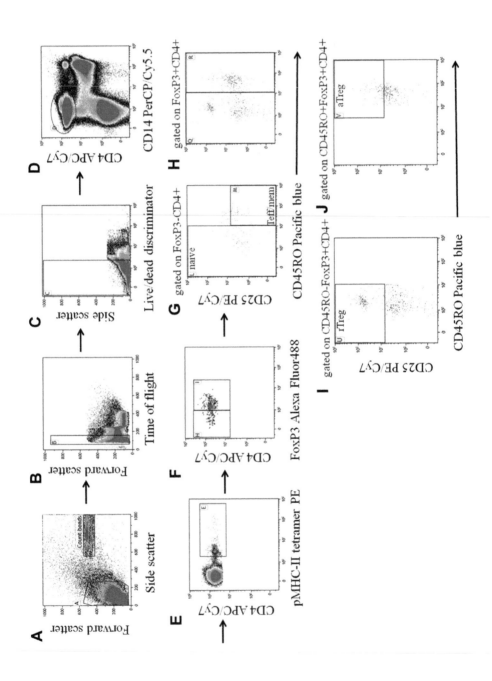

(ER) stress in B cells.[18] A recent article demonstrated that ER stress was constitutive in CD8[+] DC, which induces Foxp3[+] Treg in lymph nodes draining mucosal tissues and cross-present exogenous antigen to CD8[+] T cells. Prevention of ER stress impaired the capacity of CD8[+] DC to present antigen.[71] Taken together, these data suggest that Foxp3[+] Treg specific for cit-autoantigens should be induced in lymph nodes draining mucosal sites such as lung and gut in individuals carrying the HLA-SE. It will be important to determine the lung and gut microbial influences on cit-antigen-specific Treg in the RA preclinical period.

The consequence of selective presentation of cit-antigens by HLA-SE on T cell would be reflected in the TCR usage. Although tremendous effort has been devoted to define the TCR diversity in RA patients, so far there is no consensus on the biased TCR usage between studies. It is possible that only a small fraction of autoreactive T cells are present in the periphery and skewing the TCR repertoire. These studies used different sets of primer sets in bulk T cells or fractionated T cells in patients with various disease durations. There is evidence in human subjects demonstrating that there is a limited heterogeneity of TCR Vα and/or Vβ transcript in early RA,[72] whereas a polyclonal T cell population has been observed in chronic RA.[73,74] This evidence is further supported collagen-induced arthritis (CIA) model that autoreactive T cells can only be seen in lymph nodes after first clinical signs of arthritis,[75] thus stressing the importance to focus on early RA in future studies. These results could undermine the importance of antigen-specific T cells in disease pathogenesis, which can be addressed by sequencing TCR at the single-cell level to reveal the true diversity of the TCR repertoire.

Demonstration of the presence of antigen-specific CD4[+] T cells in synovial target organ would represent an important proof of the role of autoreactive T cells in RA disease pathogenesis. In situ tetramer staining for antigen-specific CD4 T cells in synovial tissue of RA patients thus far has very limited success, even in murine studies.[76,77] Nonetheless, murine studies of arthritic joints have highlighted some important findings. A model of CIA in HLA-DR1 transgenic humanized mice interrogated the CD4[+] T cell population isolated from arthritic joints using tetramers and demonstrated that collagen-specific CD4[+] T cells in peripheral lymphoid organs have biased TCR gene usage. HLA-DR1 molecules did not select for collagen-specific CD4[+] T cells with biased TCR gene usage in the thymus. Rather, the autoreactive T cells expanded during the autoimmune response.[78,79] The data indicate

---

Fig. 5. Representative gating strategy for the characterization of citrullinated antigen-specific CD4[+] T cells in RA patients detailed in Scally et al., 2013, JEM. From 6 × 105 CD4[+] T cells, live CD4[+] T cells were gated, excluding doublets (*B*) and cells of other lineages (*C,D*). CD4[+] HLA-DRB1*0401-vimentin-64Cit59-71 tetramer[+] cells were gated based on fluorescence minus one controls (*E*). To investigate the expression of FoxP3, total tetramer[+] cells were divided into FoxP3[−] and FoxP3[+] populations (*F*). The expression of CD25 and CD45RO were analysed in the FoxP3-CD4[+]tetramer[+] (*G*) and FoxP3[+]CD4[+]tetramer[+] (*H*). From the FoxP3[−]CD4[+]tetramer[+] population (*G*), 2 populations were gated based on the expression of CD45RO, which were naïve T cells (CD45RO-CD25-FoxP3-) and effector/memory (CD45RO[+]CD25-FoxP3-, Teff/mem). From the FoxP3[+]CD4[+]tetramer[+] population (*H*), 2 populations were gated based on the expression of CD45RO: rTreg (CD45RO-CD25[+]FoxP3[+]) (*I*) and aTreg (CD45RO[+]CD25[+]FoxP3[+]) (*J*).The number of tetramer[+] cells was calculated by the addition of flow count beads (*A*). (*Adapted from* Miyara M, Yoshioka Y, Kitoh A, et al. Functional delineation and differentiation dynamics of human CD4 1 T cells expressing the FoxP3 transcription factor. Immunity 2009;30(6):899–911.)

that autoantigen-specific CD4$^+$ T cells can be detected in arthritic joints and have biased TCR usage, which indicates antigen selection and expansion.

SUMMARY

In summary, the role of autoantigen-specific CD4$^+$ T cells in RA disease pathogenesis is becoming clearer with the advent of several technologies, including TCR sequencing, humanized mice, improvements in pMHC class II tetramer production, epitope determination, and staining techniques, as well as single-cell flow cytometric and TCR analysis. pMHC class II tetramers have great potential to probe the phenotype and function of autoreactive T cells in patients with RA and individuals at risk. Through the analysis of cit-antigen-specific autoreactive T cells in RA patients thus far, the authors propose a novel concept for the role of the SE in the pathogenesis of RA: *HLA-DRB1* susceptibility alleles fail to promote cit-peptide-specific T cell-regulation to prevent the development of RA in the face of genetic, environmental, or inflammatory pressures on Treg number or function. Furthermore, the dominant protection associated with inheritance of RA-protective *HLA* alleles suggests that these alleles promote cit-peptide-specific T cell regulation to prevent the development of RA more effectively than alleles associated with RA susceptibility. With expansion in availability of tetramers and application of new technologies to T cell analysis, these fundamental questions will be tractable. In addition, tetramers and novel T-cell technologies will be a great boon to assess the outcome of various antigen-specific immunotherapeutic strategies aiming to restore regulation in the recent-onset or pre-RA period. The study of antigen-specific T cell responses in predisease holds particular promise to understand the mechanisms by which autoimmunity develops and the timing for intervention. The authors anticipate that the distant ideal of tolerance restoration will become progressively more achievable with the innovative application of good investigative tools.

ACKNOWLEDGMENTS

The authors thank Amelie Casgrain for execution of **Figs. 1**, **2**, and **4**.

REFERENCES

1. Helmick CG, Felson DT, Lawrence RC, et al. Estimates of the prevalence of arthritis and other rheumatic conditions in the United States. Part I. Arthritis Rheum 2008;58(1):15–25.
2. Rasch EK, Hirsch R, Paulose-Ram R, et al. Prevalence of rheumatoid arthritis in persons 60 years of age and older in the United States: effect of different methods of case classification. Arthritis Rheum 2003;48(4):917–26.
3. Thomas R, Cope AP. Pathogenesis of rheumatoid arthritis. In: Isaacs JD, editor. Oxford textbook of rheumatology. 4th edition. Oxford (United Kingdom): Oxford University Press; 2013. p. 839–48.
4. Pincus T, Callahan LF, Sale WG, et al. Severe functional declines, work disability, and increased mortality in seventy-five rheumatoid arthritis patients studied over nine years. Arthritis Rheum 1984;27(8):864–72.
5. Michaud K, Messer J, Choi HK, et al. Direct medical costs and their predictors in patients with rheumatoid arthritis: a three-year study of 7,527 patients. Arthritis Rheum 2003;48(10):2750–62.
6. Thomas R. Dendritic cells and the promise of antigen-specific therapy in rheumatoid arthritis. Arthritis Res Ther 2013;15(1):204.

7. Frisell T, Holmqvist M, Kallberg H, et al. Familial risks and heritability of rheumatoid arthritis: role of rheumatoid factor/anti-citrullinated protein antibody status, number and type of affected relatives, sex, and age. Arthritis Rheum 2013; 65(11):2773–82.

8. Hemminki K, Li X, Sundquist J, et al. Familial associations of rheumatoid arthritis with autoimmune diseases and related conditions. Arthritis Rheum 2009;60(3): 661–8.

9. Gregersen PK, Silver J, Winchester RJ. The shared epitope hypothesis: an approach to understanding the molecular genetics of suseptibility to rheumatoid arthritis. Arthritis Rheum 1987;30:1205–13.

10. El-Gabalawy HS, Robinson DB, Daha NA, et al. Non-HLA genes modulate the risk of rheumatoid arthritis associated with HLA-DRB1 in a susceptible North American Native population. Genes Immun 2011;12(7):568–74.

11. Williams RC, Jacobsson LT, Knowler WC, et al. Meta-analysis reveals association between most common class II haplotype in full-heritage Native Americans and rheumatoid arthritis. Hum Immunol 1995;42(1):90–4.

12. Fisher BA, Bang SY, Chowdhury M, et al. Smoking, the HLA-DRB1 shared epitope and ACPA fine-specificity in Koreans with rheumatoid arthritis: evidence for more than one pathogenic pathway linking smoking to disease. Ann Rheum Dis 2014;73:741–7.

13. Hammer J, Gallazzi F, Bono E, et al. Peptide binding specificity of HLA-DR4 molecules: correlation with rheumatoid arthritis association. J Exp Med 1995;181(5): 1847–55.

14. Law SC, Street S, Yu CH, et al. T-cell autoreactivity to citrullinated autoantigenic peptides in rheumatoid arthritis patients carrying HLA-DRB1 shared epitope alleles. Arthritis Res Ther 2012;14(3):R118.

15. Snir O, Rieck M, Gebe JA, et al. Identification and functional characterization of T cells reactive to citrullinated vimentin in HLA-DRB1*0401-positive humanized mice and rheumatoid arthritis patients. Arthritis Rheum 2011;63(10):2873–83.

16. von Delwig A, Locke J, Robinson JH, et al. Response of Th17 cells to a citrullinated arthritogenic aggrecan peptide in patients with rheumatoid arthritis. Arthritis Rheum 2010;62(1):143–9.

17. James E, Rieck M, Pieper J, et al. Citrulline specific Th1 cells are increased in rheumatoid arthritis and their frequency is influenced by disease duration and therapy. Arthritis Rheum 2014;66:1712–22.

18. Ireland JM, Unanue ER. Autophagy in antigen-presenting cells results in presentation of citrullinated peptides to CD4 T cells. J Exp Med 2011;208(13):2625–32.

19. Ireland JM, Unanue ER. Processing of proteins in autophagy vesicles of antigen-presenting cells generates citrullinated peptides recognized by the immune system. Autophagy 2012;8(3):429–30.

20. Raychaudhuri S, Sandor C, Stahl EA, et al. Five amino acids in three HLA proteins explain most of the association between MHC and seropositive rheumatoid arthritis. Nat Genet 2012;44(3):291–6.

21. Scally SW, Petersen J, Law SC, et al. A molecular basis for the association of the HLA-DRB1 locus, citrullination, and rheumatoid arthritis. J Exp Med 2013; 210(12):2569–82.

22. Martin E, O'Sullivan B, Low P, et al. Antigen-specific suppression of a primed immune response by dendritic cells mediated by regulatory T cells secreting interleukin-10. Immunity 2003;18(1):155–67.

23. Kenna TJ, Thomas R, Steptoe RJ. Steady-state dendritic cells expressing cognate antigen terminate memory CD8+ T-cell responses. Blood 2008;111(4):2091–100.

24. Daniel C, Nolting J, von Boehmer H. Mechanisms of self-nonself discrimination and possible clinical relevance. Immunotherapy 2009;1(4):631–44.

25. Thomas R, Turner M, Cope AP. High avidity autoreactive T cells with a low signalling capacity through the T-cell receptor: central to rheumatoid arthritis pathogenesis? Arthritis Res Ther 2008;10(4):210.

26. Viatte S, Plant D, Raychaudhuri S. Genetics and epigenetics of rheumatoid arthritis. Nature reviews. Rheumatology 2013;9(3):141–53.

27. Lemaitre F, Viguier M, Cho MS, et al. Detection of low-frequency human antigen-specific CD4(+) T cells using MHC class II multimer bead sorting and immunoscope analysis. Eur J Immunol 2004;34(10):2941–9.

28. Bacher P, Scheffold A. Flow-cytometric analysis of rare antigen-specific T cells. Cytometry A 2013;83(8):692–701.

29. Altman JD, Moss PA, Goulder PJ, et al. Phenotypic analysis of antigen-specific T lymphocytes. Science 1996;274(5284):94–6.

30. Mallone R, Kochik SA, Reijonen H, et al. Functional avidity directs T-cell fate in autoreactive CD4+ T cells. Blood 2005;106(8):2798–805.

31. Reijonen H, Kwok WW, Nepom GT. Detection of CD4+ autoreactive T cells in T1D using HLA class II tetramers. Ann N Y Acad Sci 2003;1005:82–7.

32. Broughton SE, Petersen J, Theodossis A, et al. Biased T cell receptor usage directed against human leukocyte antigen DQ8-restricted gliadin peptides is associated with celiac disease. Immunity 2012;37(4):611–21.

33. Qiao SW, Raki M, Gunnarsen KS, et al. Posttranslational modification of gluten shapes TCR usage in celiac disease. J Immunol 2011;187(6):3064–71.

34. Su LF, Kidd BA, Han A, et al. Virus-specific CD4(+) memory-phenotype T cells are abundant in unexposed adults. Immunity 2013;38(2):373–83.

35. Gras S, Burrows SR, Turner SJ, et al. A structural voyage toward an understanding of the MHC-I-restricted immune response: lessons learned and much to be learned. Immunol Rev 2012;250(1):61–81.

36. Valitutti S, Muller S, Cella M, et al. Serial triggering of many T-cell receptors by a few peptide-MHC complexes. Nature 1995;375(6527):148–51.

37. Coppieters KT, Dotta F, Amirian N, et al. Demonstration of islet-autoreactive CD8 T cells in insulitic lesions from recent onset and long-term type 1 diabetes patients. J Exp Med 2012;209(1):51–60.

38. De Vries IJ, Bernsen MR, van Geloof WL, et al. In situ detection of antigen-specific T cells in cryo-sections using MHC class I tetramers after dendritic cell vaccination of melanoma patients. Cancer Immunol Immunother 2007; 56(10):1667–76.

39. Moon JJ, Chu HH, Pepper M, et al. Naive CD4(+) T cell frequency varies for different epitopes and predicts repertoire diversity and response magnitude. Immunity 2007;27(2):203–13.

40. Macdonald WA, Chen Z, Gras S, et al. T cell allorecognition via molecular mimicry. Immunity 2009;31(6):897–908.

41. Reinherz EL, Tan K, Tang L, et al. The crystal structure of a T cell receptor in complex with peptide and MHC class II. Science 1999;286(5446):1913–21.

42. Colf LA, Bankovich AJ, Hanick NA, et al. How a single T cell receptor recognizes both self and foreign MHC. Cell 2007;129(1):135–46.

43. Ye M, Kasey S, Khurana S, et al. MHC class II tetramers containing influenza hemagglutinin and EBV EBNA1 epitopes detect reliably specific CD4(+) T cells in healthy volunteers. Hum Immunol 2004;65(5):507–13.

44. Nepom GT. MHC class II tetramers. J Immunol 2012;188(6):2477–82.

45. Novak EJ, Liu AW, Gebe JA, et al. Tetramer-guided epitope mapping: rapid identification and characterization of immunodominant CD4+ T cell epitopes from complex antigens. J Immunol 2001;166(11):6665–70.
46. Birnbaum ME, Mendoza JL, Sethi DK, et al. Deconstructing the peptide-MHC specificity of T cell recognition. Cell 2014;157(5):1073–87.
47. Klenerman P, Cerundolo V, Dunbar PR. Tracking T cells with tetramers: new tales from new tools. Nat Rev Immunol 2002;2(4):263–72.
48. Borchers S, Ogonek J, Varanasi PR, et al. Multimer monitoring of CMV-specific T cells in research and in clinical applications. Diagn Microbiol Infect Dis 2014; 78(3):201–12.
49. Trudeau JD, Kelly-Smith C, Verchere CB, et al. Prediction of spontaneous autoimmune diabetes in NOD mice by quantification of autoreactive T cells in peripheral blood. J Clin Invest 2003;111(2):217–23.
50. Sarikonda G, Pettus J, Phatak S, et al. CD8 T-cell reactivity to islet antigens is unique to type 1 while CD4 T-cell reactivity exists in both type 1 and type 2 diabetes. J Autoimmun 2014;50:77–82.
51. Velthuis JH, Unger WW, Abreu JR, et al. Simultaneous detection of circulating autoreactive CD8+ T-cells specific for different islet cell-associated epitopes using combinatorial MHC multimers. Diabetes 2010;59(7):1721–30.
52. Cernea S, Herold KC. Monitoring of antigen-specific CD8 T cells in patients with type 1 diabetes treated with antiCD3 monoclonal antibodies. Clin Immunol 2010; 134(2):121–9.
53. Liu CP, Jiang K, Wu CH, et al. Detection of glutamic acid decarboxylase-activated T cells with I-Ag7 tetramers. Proc Natl Acad Sci U S A 2000;97(26):14596–601.
54. Reijonen H, Novak EJ, Kochik S, et al. Detection of GAD65-specific T-cells by major histocompatibility complex class II tetramers in type 1 diabetic patients and at-risk subjects. Diabetes 2002;51(5):1375–82.
55. Wong FS, Karttunen J, Dumont C, et al. Identification of an MHC class I-restricted autoantigen in type 1 diabetes by screening an organ-specific cDNA library. Nat Med 1999;5(9):1026–31.
56. Amrani A, Verdaguer J, Serra P, et al. Progression of autoimmune diabetes driven by avidity maturation of a T-cell population. Nature 2000;406(6797):739–42.
57. Martinuzzi E, Novelli G, Scotto M, et al. The frequency and immunodominance of islet-specific CD8+ T-cell responses change after type 1 diabetes diagnosis and treatment. Diabetes 2008;57(5):1312–20.
58. Vollers SS, Stern LJ. Class II major histocompatibility complex tetramer staining: progress, problems, and prospects. Immunology 2008;123(3):305–13.
59. Lissina A, Ladell K, Skowera A, et al. Protein kinase inhibitors substantially improve the physical detection of T-cells with peptide-MHC tetramers. J Immunol Methods 2009;340(1):11–24.
60. Henderson KN, Tye-Din JA, Reid HH, et al. A structural and immunological basis for the role of human leukocyte antigen DQ8 in celiac disease. Immunity 2007; 27(1):23–34.
61. Mallone R, Nepom GT. MHC Class II tetramers and the pursuit of antigen-specific T cells: define, deviate, delete. Clin Immunol 2004;110(3):232–42.
62. Palmer JP, Asplin CM, Clemons P, et al. Insulin antibodies in insulin-dependent diabetics before insulin treatment. Science 1983;222(4630):1337–9.
63. Bingley PJ, Christie MR, Bonifacio E, et al. Combined analysis of autoantibodies improves prediction of IDDM in islet cell antibody-positive relatives. Diabetes 1994;43(11):1304–10.

64. Oling V, Marttila J, Ilonen J, et al. GAD65- and proinsulin-specific CD4+ T-cells detected by MHC class II tetramers in peripheral blood of type 1 diabetes patients and at-risk subjects. J Autoimmun 2005;25(3):235–43.
65. Reijonen H, Mallone R, Heninger AK, et al. GAD65-specific CD4+ T-cells with high antigen avidity are prevalent in peripheral blood of patients with type 1 diabetes. Diabetes 2004;53(8):1987–94.
66. Standifer NE, Burwell EA, Gersuk VH, et al. Changes in autoreactive T cell avidity during type 1 diabetes development. Clin Immunol 2009;132(3):312–20.
67. van den Boorn JG, Le Poole IC, Luiten RM. T-cell avidity and tuning: the flexible connection between tolerance and autoimmunity. Int Rev Immunol 2006; 25(3–4):235–58.
68. Savage PA, Boniface JJ, Davis MM. A kinetic basis for T cell receptor repertoire selection during an immune response. Immunity 1999;10(4):485–92.
69. Fasso M, Anandasabapathy N, Crawford F, et al. T cell receptor (TCR)-mediated repertoire selection and loss of TCR vbeta diversity during the initiation of a CD4(+) T cell response in vivo. J Exp Med 2000;192(12):1719–30.
70. van Gaalen F, Ioan-Facsinay A, Huizinga TW, et al. The devil in the details: the emerging role of anticitrulline autoimmunity in rheumatoid arthritis. J Immunol 2005;175(9):5575–80.
71. Osorio F, Tavernier SJ, Hoffmann E, et al. The unfolded-protein-response sensor IRE-1alpha regulates the function of CD8alpha dendritic cells. Nat Immunol 2014;15:248–57.
72. Fischer DC, Opalka B, Hoffmann A, et al. Limited heterogeneity of rearranged T cell receptor V alpha and V beta transcripts in synovial fluid T cells in early stages of rheumatoid arthritis. Arthritis Rheum 1996;39(3):454–62.
73. Sottini A, Imberti L, Gorla R, et al. Restricted expression of T cell receptor V beta but not V alpha genes in rheumatoid arthritis. Eur J Immunol 1991;21(2):461–6.
74. Striebich CC, Falta MT, Wang Y, et al. Selective accumulation of related CD4+ T cell clones in the synovial fluid of patients with rheumatoid arthritis. J Immunol 1998;161(8):4428–36.
75. Svendsen P, Andersen CB, Willcox N, et al. Tracking of proinflammatory collagen-specific T cells in early and late collagen-induced arthritis in humanized mice. J Immunol 2004;173(11):7037–45.
76. Bischof F, Hofmann M, Schumacher TN, et al. Analysis of autoreactive CD4 T cells in experimental autoimmune encephalomyelitis after primary and secondary challenge using MHC class II tetramers. J Immunol 2004;172(5):2878–84.
77. Stratmann T, Martin-Orozco N, Mallet-Designe V, et al. Susceptible MHC alleles, not background genes, select an autoimmune T cell reactivity. J Clin Invest 2003;112(6):902–14.
78. Qian Z, Latham KA, Whittington KB, et al. An autoantigen-specific, highly restricted T cell repertoire infiltrates the arthritic joints of mice in an HLA-DR1 humanized mouse model of autoimmune arthritis. J Immunol 2010;185(1):110–8.
79. Deane KD, El-Gabalawy H. Pathogenesis and prevention of rheumatic disease: focus on preclinical RA and SLE. Nat Rev Rheumatol 2014;10(4):212–28.

Prediction of Future Rheumatoid Arthritis

Samina A. Turk, MD*,1, Marian H. van Beers-Tas, MD1,
Dirkjan van Schaardenburg, MD, PhD

KEYWORDS

- Rheumatoid arthritis • Prediction • Risk factors • Environmental • Autoantibodies
- Biomarkers • Arthralgia

KEY POINTS

- Risk factors for rheumatoid arthritis (RA) include family history, birth weight, smoking, silica, alcohol nonuse, obesity, diabetes mellitus, autoantibodies, and genetic variants.
- Symptoms, antibodies, and inflammatory biomarkers can be useful in late at-risk stages, and genetic scores plus environmental factors more useful in early at-risk stages.
- Prediction models of RA can help to select candidates for intervention studies.
- The best target populations for screening are relatives of patients with RA and (seropositive) patients with arthralgia. However, only a minority of persons at risk can thus be recognized.
- Screening for RA risk is still experimental, because there is no validated screening tool and no proven therapy to prevent disease.

INTRODUCTION

Rheumatoid arthritis (RA) on average becomes clinically manifest around the age of 55 years. During the healthy part of life, the risk of future RA is determined by genetic, reproductive and environmental factors (**Fig. 1**, green bar). Over time, people at risk for RA may pass through a phase of autoimmunity, accompanied by subclinical inflammation,[1] followed by a symptomatic phase, which may last a few months to several years. In the symptomatic phase, markers of autoimmunity and inflammation increase before the onset of clinical arthritis.[2] Therefore, prediction can be based on different characteristics in the asymptomatic phase and in the symptomatic phase.

The expectation that intervening in the preclinical phase of RA could be beneficial is based on the success of treatment of RA within 1 to 2 years after onset of clinical

Disclosures: None.
Department of Rheumatology, Jan van Breemen Research Institute/Reade, Doctor Jan van Breemenstraat 2, 1056 AB Amsterdam, The Netherlands
1 S.A. Turk and M.H. van Beers-Tas contributed equally to this work.
* Corresponding author. Department of Rheumatology, Jan van Breemen Research Institute/Reade, PO Box 58271, 1040 HG Amsterdam, The Netherlands.
E-mail address: s.turk@reade.nl

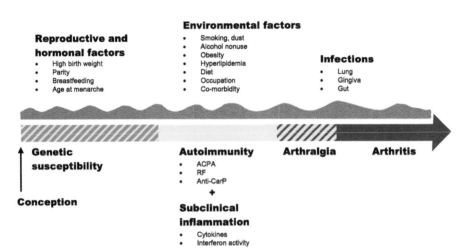

Fig. 1. The evolution of RA from health to disease. ACPA, anti–citrullinated protein antibody; RF, rheumatoid factor. anti-CarP, anti-carbamylated protein antibodies.

disease.[3,4] The new criteria for RA from 2010 with a focus on early signs such as involvement of even only a few small joints together with serology and acute phase reactants facilitate treatment in the earliest clinical phase,[5,6] and the further characterization of the preclinical phase offers new opportunities for intervention studies even before clinically apparent arthritis occurs. Because RA is the most prevalent inflammatory rheumatic disease, with a high burden for the patient and society, it seems the ideal candidate rheumatic disease for screening and intervention programs. However, a lot of steps need to be taken before such programs can be offered to persons at risk.

This article summarizes the present knowledge on risk factors for RA, including genetic, reproductive, and hormonal factors; environmental exposures; biomarkers; personal characteristics and symptoms; and how these can be combined in risk models attempting to increase the accuracy of the prediction of RA. Genetic risk and gene-environmental interactions are dealt with elsewhere in this issue and are only mentioned here in relation to their roles in prediction models. Risk scores from such models require further validation, but could be used to select candidates for intervention studies.

METHODS

We searched the PubMed database on January 29, 2014, for the terms risk, prediction, and development in relation to RA. After excluding articles not directly related to prediction of RA, such as studies on prevalence, diagnosis, treatment, outcome, or comorbidities of RA, more than 200 articles remained on this topic after screening 2000 abstracts. Additional articles were added that were found after the search date until May 1, 2014, by screening rheumatologic journals.

RISK FACTORS: THE BUILDING BLOCKS OF PREDICTION

The current evidence on risk factors for RA is summarized in **Table 1**. Besides the factors reported in the table, many others have been investigated for their association with the risk of RA, but these studies have led to negative, inconclusive, or conflicting results. Among these are variables such as silicone implants[7–9]; consumption of coffee, tea,[10–13] or red meat[13–16]; geographic area[17–22]; and socioeconomic status.[23–28]

Table 1
Overview of evidence on risk factors for the development of RA

Risk Factor	Comments
Family history	Risk increases with number of affected family members[30–33] The longer the disease duration and the higher the age of the proband, the higher the risk[32] Some studies did not find an association between relatives with RA and risk of RA[31,34,35]
Genetic factors	Around 60 risk loci for RA are known, explaining 16% of total susceptibility[36] 65% of RA risk is thought to be heritable[36]
Reproductive and hormonal factors	Risk is 2–4 times higher in women[37,38] A protective effect of oral contraceptives is suggested[38–43] High birth weight (more than 4 kg) increases risk[25,39] Lower risk during pregnancy, compensated by an increased risk in the first postpartum year[40,41] Complications during pregnancy may be related to a higher risk[42] Inconclusive or conflicting results for breastfeeding,[29,43–47] age at menarche, irregular menstrual cycles and age at menopause, postmenopausal hormone use,[43,44,48–50] lower testosterone levels,[37,51–53] parity, age at first childbirth,[29,40–44,50,54,55] low birth weight, and being small for gestational age[54,56,57]
Environmental factors	Smoking is the most established risk factor[58–61] Smoking interacts with the strongest genetic risk factor (HLA-SE) in a dose-dependent manner to increase the risk of seropositive RA[62] Alcohol consumption (even in small quantities) protects[63–65] High consumption of olive oil and fish (oil) protects[66–73] Inconclusive results were found for vitamin D intake and ultraviolet B exposure,[74–78] antioxidant and trace element intake,[16,68,70,71,79–87] and exposure to toxic elements[86,87]
Occupations and occupational exposures	Farmers, blue collar workers, and hairdressers are at increased risk[88–92] Silica exposure gives increased risk[90,93] Exposures that could not be related to RA: asbestos, mineral oil, organic dust, herbicides, insecticides, carbamates, organophosphates, carbaryl, glyphosate, malathion,[94–97] and ambient air pollution[98–100]
Infections and vaccinations	Frequent infections may predispose[54,55] One study reported increased risk after influenza vaccination[101] Risks could not be quantified for: Ebstein-Barr virus infection,[102] hepatitis C,[103,104] HIV,[105] Yersinia enterocolitica,[106] mycoplasma,[107] or Porphyromonas gingivalis infection of the gums,[108,109] and for immunization (other than influenza)[101,110–114]
Comorbidities	Diabetes types 1 and 2[29,115] and inflammatory lung disorders[88,116–118] increase risk Schizophrenia is protective[119] Obesity and the related condition obstructive sleep apnea syndrome increase the risk[13,120–124] Dyslipidemia is present before RA and predicts RA[125–129] Other associations, such as for thyroid disease, are inconclusive[130]
Autoantibodies	Status and levels of (isotypes of) RF and ACPA associate with RA risk[131–143] Higher levels and the combination of RF and ACPA confer a higher risk[144,145] Additional predictive ability independent of RF and ACPA was shown for anti–carbamylated protein antibodies[146] and anti–peptidyl arginine deiminase type 4 antibodies[147]

(continued on next page)

Table 1 (continued)	
Risk Factor	**Comments**
Other biomarkers in blood	Several acute phase reactants and cytokines are increased in pre-RA or at-risk cohorts[1,148–162]
	TNF (receptor), cartilage oligomeric matrix protein, and a high interferon gene score are quantified risk factors[163,164]
Imaging	Ultrasonography abnormalities (mainly power Doppler signal) in seropositive patients with arthralgia were predictive of arthritis at the joint level in 1 study[165] and at the patient level in another study[166]
	Technetium bone scintigraphy is predictive of RA in patients with arthralgia[167] and can exclude inflammatory joint disease[168]
	Macrophage-targeted positron emission tomography predicts arthritis in ACPA-positive patients with arthralgia[169]
	The predictive capacity of MRI in arthralgia is not yet clear[170,171]
Symptoms	Predictive symptoms in combination with the presence of autoantibodies: duration <12 mo, intermittent symptoms, arthralgia in upper and lower extremities, morning stiffness $\geq$1 h, self-reported joint swelling,[145] tenderness of hand or foot joints, and morning stiffness $\geq$30 min[166]

Abbreviations: ACPA, anti–citrullinated protein antibody; HIV, human immunodeficiency virus; MRI, magnetic resonance imaging; RF, rheumatoid factor; TNF, tumor necrosis factor.

In contrast, some of the factors that have statistically significant associations with RA show opposite directions of risk in different studies. Examples of such cases are age at menarche, breastfeeding, and parity. This uncertainty makes the value of such variables questionable, even if they have been included in prediction models, as is the case with parity and breastfeeding in the model by Lahiri and colleagues.[29]

In conclusion, there are not many risk factors with strong and confirmed associations with RA. Among these are family history of RA, high birth weight, smoking, silica exposure, alcohol nonuse, obesity, diabetes mellitus, rheumatoid factor (RF), anti–citrullinated protein antibody (ACPA), and genetic variants such as the shared epitope (SE) and protein tyrosine phosphatase nonreceptor type 22 (PTPN22).

PREDICTION RULES: PUTTING THE BLOCKS TOGETHER

In a manner similar to the way clinical characteristics, signs, and symptoms can be combined to diagnose a disease in a patient, the potential risk factors for a given disease can be combined by statistical modeling of variables measured in an at-risk population in order to produce prediction rules. The advantage of such models is that they clarify the relative impact of the individual variables and quantify the overall risk for individuals coming from that population. The validity of these models can then be further confirmed by testing them in other populations.

Recently, several prediction models have been published that attempt to quantify progression to RA (**Table 2**). Two of these models were based on large population studies, of which 1 was designed for investigating other diseases as well. One of these used clinical characteristics to predict either seropositive or seronegative RA,[29] the other used the combination of clinical characteristics, autoantibodies, and a genetic risk score containing multiple genes (see **Table 2** for the variables in the models).[172] Both studies achieve good prediction. However, it is uncertain whether these values can be reproduced in smaller populations.

Three other studies investigated the development of RA in ACPA-positive and/or RF-positive patients with arthralgia.[121,145,166] The patients were partly recruited in primary care, and partly in the rheumatology clinic. The models were based on clinical characteristics, symptoms, and antibody characteristics, in 1 study supplemented by ultrasonographic power Doppler signal (see **Table 2**).[166] All 3 models provide good discrimination between persons who do or do not develop RA. However, they require ongoing validation as other studies select and follow such cohorts of people at risk for RA. Similar studies from North America designed to predict RA in first-degree relatives of patients with RA are underway but have not yet gathered enough arthritis cases to enable the construction of prediction models.[149,173] These studies are hampered by the low frequency of autoantibodies or of increased biomarkers in relatives of patients with RA.

Measuring the risk of RA is also a matter of timing. During the early at-risk stage, before the onset of autoimmunity, clinicians can only measure genetic susceptibility and environmental factors (see the left part of **Fig. 1**). The predictive capability of models in this situation is becoming good, with areas under the curve of 72% to 77% for the prediction of ACPA-positive RA.[174] However, the measured risk is a life-time risk, which makes it an abstract figure for the individual person at risk. Prediction including a time frame becomes possible nearer to the onset of clinical RA, when the aspects of symptoms, autoimmunity, and inflammation can be taken into account. In the Amsterdam risk model, points can be gathered for clinical characteristics, symptoms, and serology, with more points for high levels of ACPA or positivity for both ACPA and RF.[145] The more points, the higher the risk and the sooner the onset of arthritis can be expected (**Fig. 2**). This prediction reflects studies in pre-RA blood donors, in which autoantibody levels increase during the 1 to 3 years before the onset of clinical arthritis.[2,138] In an US cohort of 81 patients with clinical RA from whom stored serum was available from 1 to 12 years before disease onset, a biomarker profile including autoantibodies and cytokines was identified that predicts the imminent onset of clinical arthritis within 2 years.[160] Autoantibody epitope spreading by itself in the preclinical phase also predicts progression to classifiable RA.[143]

SCREENING STRATEGIES

Many medical, ethical, and economic issues need to be addressed before screening for risk of future RA can be offered to certain categories of unaffected persons. Basic requirements for screening groups of people to predict a disease are (1) a defined population to test; (2) the existence of an asymptomatic (or nonspecific symptomatic) phase; (3) the availability of a test with good accuracy, low rates of side effects, and low cost; and (4) the availability of a cost-effective intervention in the at-risk phase. Only the second requirement of an asymptomatic phase is clearly fulfilled at present. Regarding items 3 and 4, no single test can identify those at risk for RA and no intervention exists with proven efficacy in the at-risk situation.[175,176] All efforts to predict RA and treat persons with an increased risk for RA are therefore currently regarded as investigational. The test for RA will eventually be a validated, cost-effective, and accurate prediction rule that is easy to apply. For comparison, consider the screening programs for colonic cancer, which have recently been established in several countries. All persons more than a certain age are offered screening, which leads to huge numbers of colonoscopies. The high cost of this procedure and the possibility of serious side effects need to be weighed against the benefit of removing polyps that would cause a high morbidity and mortality if left unnoticed.

Table 2
Prediction models of RA

First Author and Year (Ref.)	Cohort; Variables	Numbers	Results
Van de Stadt et al,[145] 2013	Seropositive patients with arthralgia. Prediction rule variables: alcohol consumption, family history, symptoms <12 mo, intermittent, in upper and lower extremities, VAS ≥ 50, morning stiffness ≥1 h, swollen joints reported by patient, autoantibody status	Arthralgia: 374 (131 developed arthritis)	Prediction rule: AUC 0.82 (CI 0.75–0.89) Intermediate-risk vs low-risk group: HR 4.52 (CI 2.42–8.77) High-risk vs low-risk group: HR 14.86 (CI 8.40–28)
de Hair et al,[121] 2013	Seropositive patients with arthralgia. Predictive variables: smoking and BMI	Arthralgia: 55 (15 developed arthritis)	Smoking (ever vs never) and risk of RA: HR 9.6 (CI 1.3–73) Obesity (BMI ≥ 25 vs <25) and risk of RA: HR 5.6 (CI 1.3–25)
Lahiri et al,[29] 2014	European Prospective Investigation of Cancer, Norfolk, United Kingdom 40–79 y. Prediction rule variables: alcohol consumption, smoking, occupation, BMI, diabetes mellitus, parity	Total participants: 25,455 (184 developed IP, 138 developed RA)	Pack-years smoking in men and risk of IP: HR 1.21 (CI 1.08–1.37) Seropositive in men and risk of IP: HR 1.24 (CI 1.10–1.41) Having DM (I or II) and risk of IP: HR 2.54 (CI 1.26–5.09) Alcohol and risk of IP (per unit/d): HR 0.36 (CI 0.15–0.89) Overweight vs normal-weight and risk of seronegative IP: HR 2.75 (CI 1.39–5.46) Parity ≥2 vs no children and risk of IP: HR 2.81 (CI 1.37–5.76) Breastfeeding for every 52 wk and risk of IP: HR 0.66 (CI 0.46–0.94)

Sparks et al,[172] 2014	NHS, United States, women 30–55 y EIRA, Sweden, 18–70 y Prediction rule variables: family history, alcohol consumption, smoking, BMI, parity, autoantibody status, genetic risk score	RA cases: 1625 Controls: 1381	NHS seropositive RA (model family history, epidemiologic, genetic): AUC 0.74 (CI 0.70–0.78) NHS seropositive RA and positive family history: AUC 0.82 (CI 0.74–0.90) EIRA ACPA-positive RA (model family history, epidemiologic, genetic): AUC 0.77 (CI 0.75–0.80) EIRA ACPA-positive RA and positive family history: AUC 0.83 (CI 0.76–0.91) EIRA ACPA-positive RA and positive family history, high genetic susceptibility, smoking, and increased BMI: OR 21.73 (CI 10–44)
Rakieh et al,[166] 2014	Yorkshire, United Kingdom ACPA-positive patients with arthralgia Prediction rule variables: joint tenderness, morning stiffness ≥30 min, high positive autoantibodies, positive ultrasonographic power Doppler signal	Arthralgia: 100 (50 developed RA)	Power Doppler model: Harrell C 0.67 (CI 0.59–0.74) Progression to IA: Low risk (0 points) 0% Moderate risk (1–2 points) 31% High risk (≥3 points) 62%

Abbreviations: AUC, area under the receiver operating characteristic curve; BMI, body mass index; CI, confidence interval; DM, diabetes mellitus; EIRA, Epidemiological Investigation of RA; HR, hazard ratio; IA, inflammatory arthritis; IP, inflammatory polyarthritis; NHS, Nurses Health Study; OR, odds ratio; VAS, visual analogue scale.

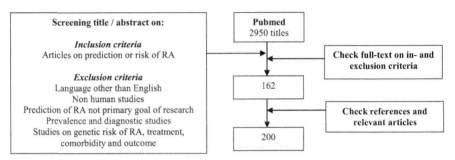

Fig. 2. Flowchart search strategy.

Regarding item 1, careful consideration is needed to decide which population(s) should be screened or tested. The choices from general to specific are general population, relatives of patients with RA, persons with musculoskeletal symptoms, or persons with RA-specific autoimmunity. Because RA is not highly prevalent in most populations, with the possible exception of North American native peoples,[177,178] at this time it is not practical to test the general population for RA. Two recognizable target groups then remain: relatives of patients with RA and persons with musculoskeletal symptoms. The latter are found both in general practice and in rheumatology clinics. After history taking and physical examination, it must be decided which patients should proceed to further testing for RA risk, and which test to use. At present most clinicians use the RF and/or ACPA test, which are widely available and easy to perform. Except for patients with only RF positivity just above the reference range, the results give useful information. The question of who to test in general practice cannot accurately be answered at this time. This question requires structured longitudinal follow-up of patients in general practice, or the following of cohorts with clinically suspect arthralgia in rheumatology clinics.

SUMMARY

There is a trend toward increasingly sophisticated prediction models for RA in different stages of risk. However, further work is needed to combine patient-level information with the published promising biomarkers into more robust models. For example, models for relatives of patients with RA, reflecting the early at-risk stage, depend largely on personal characteristics and genetic risk, whereas models for patients with arthralgia that reflect the late at-risk stage need to include patient-related and symptom characteristics in combination with biomarkers of autoimmunity and inflammation. In view of the vague and unspecific first symptoms of many patients who later develop RA, it will be necessary to better characterize and measure these symptoms in future models.[179]

However, because much is known about the risks for developing RA, it is already possible to use this information to design preventive interventions in persons at high risk for RA. At least in the late preclinical stage, several such interventions are currently being tested or planned.[180]

REFERENCES

1. Nielen MM, van SD, Reesink HW, et al. Simultaneous development of acute phase response and autoantibodies in preclinical rheumatoid arthritis. Ann Rheum Dis 2006;65(4):535–7.

2. van de Stadt LA, de Koning MH, van de Stadt RJ, et al. Development of the anti-citrullinated protein antibody repertoire prior to the onset of rheumatoid arthritis. Arthritis Rheum 2011;63(11):3226–33.
3. Boers M, Verhoeven AC, Markusse HM, et al. Randomised comparison of combined step-down prednisolone, methotrexate and sulphasalazine with sulphasalazine alone in early rheumatoid arthritis. Lancet 1997;350(9074):309–18.
4. Goekoop-Ruiterman YP, de Vries-Bouwstra JK, Allaart CF, et al. Clinical and radiographic outcomes of four different treatment strategies in patients with early rheumatoid arthritis (the BeSt study): a randomized, controlled trial. Arthritis Rheum 2008;58(2 Suppl):S126–35.
5. Aletaha D, Neogi T, Silman AJ, et al. 2010 Rheumatoid arthritis classification criteria: an American College of Rheumatology/European League Against Rheumatism collaborative initiative. Ann Rheum Dis 2010;69(9):1580–8.
6. Britsemmer K, Ursum J, Gerritsen M, et al. Validation of the 2010 ACR/EULAR classification criteria for rheumatoid arthritis: slight improvement over the 1987 ACR criteria. Ann Rheum Dis 2011;70(8):1468–70.
7. Janowsky EC, Kupper LL, Hulka BS. Meta-analyses of the relation between silicone breast implants and the risk of connective-tissue diseases. N Engl J Med 2000;342(11):781–90.
8. Perkins LL, Clark BD, Klein PJ, et al. A meta-analysis of breast implants and connective tissue disease. Ann Plast Surg 1995;35(6):561–70.
9. Wong O. A critical assessment of the relationship between silicone breast implants and connective tissue diseases. Regul Toxicol Pharmacol 1996;23(1 Pt 1):74–85.
10. Heliovaara M, Aho K, Knekt P, et al. Coffee consumption, rheumatoid factor, and the risk of rheumatoid arthritis. Ann Rheum Dis 2000;59(8):631–5.
11. Karlson EW, Mandl LA, Aweh GN, et al. Coffee consumption and risk of rheumatoid arthritis. Arthritis Rheum 2003;48(11):3055–60.
12. Mikuls TR, Cerhan JR, Criswell LA, et al. Coffee, tea, and caffeine consumption and risk of rheumatoid arthritis: results from the Iowa Women's Health Study. Arthritis Rheum 2002;46(1):83–91.
13. Pedersen M, Jacobsen S, Klarlund M, et al. Environmental risk factors differ between rheumatoid arthritis with and without auto-antibodies against cyclic citrullinated peptides. Arthritis Res Ther 2006;8(4):R133.
14. Benito-Garcia E, Feskanich D, Hu FB, et al. Protein, iron, and meat consumption and risk for rheumatoid arthritis: a prospective cohort study. Arthritis Res Ther 2007;9(1):R16.
15. Grant WB. The role of meat in the expression of rheumatoid arthritis. Br J Nutr 2000;84(5):589–95.
16. Pattison DJ, Symmons DP, Lunt M, et al. Dietary risk factors for the development of inflammatory polyarthritis: evidence for a role of high level of red meat consumption. Arthritis Rheum 2004;50(12):3804–12.
17. Alamanos Y, Voulgari PV, Drosos AA. Incidence and prevalence of rheumatoid arthritis, based on the 1987 American College of Rheumatology criteria: a systematic review. Semin Arthritis Rheum 2006;36(3):182–8.
18. Costenbader KH, Chang SC, Laden F, et al. Geographic variation in rheumatoid arthritis incidence among women in the United States. Arch Intern Med 2008; 168(15):1664–70.
19. Kallberg H, Vieira V, Holmqvist M, et al. Regional differences regarding risk of developing rheumatoid arthritis in Stockholm County, Sweden: results from the Swedish Epidemiological Investigation of Rheumatoid Arthritis (EIRA) study. Scand J Rheumatol 2013;42(5):337–43.

20. Li X, Sundquist J, Sundquist K. Risks of rheumatic diseases in first- and second-generation immigrants in Sweden: a nationwide followup study. Arthritis Rheum 2009;60(6):1588–96.
21. Silman A, Bankhead C, Rowlingson B, et al. Do new cases of rheumatoid arthritis cluster in time or in space? Int J Epidemiol 1997;26(3):628–34.
22. Silman A, Harrison B, Barrett E, et al. The existence of geographical clusters of cases of inflammatory polyarthritis in a primary care based register. Ann Rheum Dis 2000;59(2):152–4.
23. Bankhead C, Silman A, Barrett B, et al. Incidence of rheumatoid arthritis is not related to indicators of socioeconomic deprivation. J Rheumatol 1996;23(12):2039–42.
24. Bengtsson C, Nordmark B, Klareskog L, et al. Socioeconomic status and the risk of developing rheumatoid arthritis: results from the Swedish EIRA study. Ann Rheum Dis 2005;64(11):1588–94.
25. Jacobsson LT, Jacobsson ME, Askling J, et al. Perinatal characteristics and risk of rheumatoid arthritis. BMJ 2003;326(7398):1068–9.
26. Olsson AR, Skogh T, Wingren G. Aetiological factors of importance for the development of rheumatoid arthritis. Scand J Rheumatol 2004;33(5):300–6.
27. Pedersen M, Jacobsen S, Klarlund M, et al. Socioeconomic status and risk of rheumatoid arthritis: a Danish case-control study. J Rheumatol 2006;33(6):1069–74.
28. Uhlig T, Hagen KB, Kvien TK. Current tobacco smoking, formal education, and the risk of rheumatoid arthritis. J Rheumatol 1999;26(1):47–54.
29. Lahiri M, Luben RN, Morgan C, et al. Using lifestyle factors to identify individuals at higher risk of inflammatory polyarthritis (results from the European Prospective Investigation of Cancer-Norfolk and the Norfolk Arthritis Register–the EPIC-2-NOAR Study). Ann Rheum Dis 2014;73(1):219–26.
30. Koumantaki Y, Giziaki E, Linos A, et al. Family history as a risk factor for rheumatoid arthritis: a case-control study. J Rheumatol 1997;24(8):1522–6.
31. Svendsen AJ, Holm NV, Kyvik K, et al. Relative importance of genetic effects in rheumatoid arthritis: historical cohort study of Danish nationwide twin population. BMJ 2002;324(7332):264–6.
32. Deighton CM, Roberts DF, Walker DJ. Effect of disease severity on rheumatoid arthritis concordance in same sexed siblings. Ann Rheum Dis 1992;51(8):943–5.
33. Hemminki K, Li X, Sundquist J, et al. Familial associations of rheumatoid arthritis with autoimmune diseases and related conditions. Arthritis Rheum 2009;60(3):661–8.
34. Larkin JG. Family history of rheumatoid arthritis–a non-predictor of inflammatory disease? Rheumatology (Oxford) 2010;49(3):608–9.
35. Jones MA, Silman AJ, Whiting S, et al. Occurrence of rheumatoid arthritis is not increased in the first degree relatives of a population based inception cohort of inflammatory polyarthritis. Ann Rheum Dis 1996;55(2):89–93.
36. Viatte S, Plant D, Raychaudhuri S. Genetics and epigenetics of rheumatoid arthritis. Nat Rev Rheumatol 2013;9(3):141–53.
37. Karlson EW, Chibnik LB, McGrath M, et al. A prospective study of androgen levels, hormone-related genes and risk of rheumatoid arthritis. Arthritis Res Ther 2009;11(3):R97.
38. Colebatch AN, Edwards CJ. The influence of early life factors on the risk of developing rheumatoid arthritis. Clin Exp Immunol 2011;163(1):11–6.
39. Mandl LA, Costenbader KH, Simard JF, et al. Is birthweight associated with risk of rheumatoid arthritis? Data from a large cohort study. Ann Rheum Dis 2009;68(4):514–8.

40. Peschken CA, Robinson DB, Hitchon CA, et al. Pregnancy and the risk of rheumatoid arthritis in a highly predisposed North American Native population. J Rheumatol 2012;39(12):2253–60.
41. Spector TD, Roman E, Silman AJ. The pill, parity, and rheumatoid arthritis. Arthritis Rheum 1990;33(6):782–9.
42. Jorgensen KT, Pedersen BV, Jacobsen S, et al. National cohort study of reproductive risk factors for rheumatoid arthritis in Denmark: a role for hyperemesis, gestational hypertension and pre-eclampsia? Ann Rheum Dis 2010;69(2): 358–63.
43. Karlson EW, Mandl LA, Hankinson SE, et al. Do breast-feeding and other reproductive factors influence future risk of rheumatoid arthritis? Results from the Nurses' Health Study. Arthritis Rheum 2004;50(11):3458–67.
44. Pikwer M, Bergstrom U, Nilsson JA, et al. Early menopause is an independent predictor of rheumatoid arthritis. Ann Rheum Dis 2012;71(3):378–81.
45. Berglin E, Kokkonen H, Einarsdottir E, et al. Influence of female hormonal factors, in relation to autoantibodies and genetic markers, on the development of rheumatoid arthritis in northern Sweden: a case-control study. Scand J Rheumatol 2010;39(6):454–60.
46. Pikwer M, Bergstrom U, Nilsson JA, et al. Breast feeding, but not use of oral contraceptives, is associated with a reduced risk of rheumatoid arthritis. Ann Rheum Dis 2009;68(4):526–30.
47. Brennan P, Silman A. Breast-feeding and the onset of rheumatoid arthritis. Arthritis Rheum 1994;37(6):808–13.
48. Carette S, Marcoux S, Gingras S. Postmenopausal hormones and the incidence of rheumatoid arthritis. J Rheumatol 1989;16(7):911–3.
49. Deighton CM, Sykes H, Walker DJ. Rheumatoid arthritis, HLA identity, and age at menarche. Ann Rheum Dis 1993;52(5):322–6.
50. Hernandez AM, Liang MH, Willett WC, et al. Reproductive factors, smoking, and the risk for rheumatoid arthritis. Epidemiology 1990;1(4):285–91.
51. Heikkila R, Aho K, Heliovaara M, et al. Serum androgen-anabolic hormones and the risk of rheumatoid arthritis. Ann Rheum Dis 1998;57(5):281–5.
52. Pikwer M, Giwercman A, Bergstrom U, et al. Association between testosterone levels and risk of future rheumatoid arthritis in men: a population-based case-control study. Ann Rheum Dis 2014;73(3):573–9.
53. Masi AT, Aldag JC, Chatterton RT. Sex hormones and risks of rheumatoid arthritis and developmental or environmental influences. Ann N Y Acad Sci 2006;1069:223–35.
54. Carlens C, Jacobsson L, Brandt L, et al. Perinatal characteristics, early life infections and later risk of rheumatoid arthritis and juvenile idiopathic arthritis. Ann Rheum Dis 2009;68(7):1159–64.
55. Rogers MA, Levine DA, Blumberg N, et al. Antigenic challenge in the etiology of autoimmune disease in women. J Autoimmun 2012;38(2–3):J97–102.
56. Ma KK, Nelson JL, Guthrie KA, et al. Adverse pregnancy outcomes and risk of subsequent rheumatoid arthritis. Arthritis Rheumatol 2014;66(3):508–12.
57. Simard JF, Costenbader KH, Hernan MA, et al. Early life factors and adult-onset rheumatoid arthritis. J Rheumatol 2010;37(1):32–7.
58. Carlens C, Hergens MP, Grunewald J, et al. Smoking, use of moist snuff, and risk of chronic inflammatory diseases. Am J Respir Crit Care Med 2010; 181(11):1217–22.
59. Di GD, Discacciati A, Orsini N, et al. Cigarette smoking and risk of rheumatoid arthritis: a dose-response meta-analysis. Arthritis Res Ther 2014;16(2):R61.

60. Kallberg H, Ding B, Padyukov L, et al. Smoking is a major preventable risk factor for rheumatoid arthritis: estimations of risks after various exposures to cigarette smoke. Ann Rheum Dis 2011;70(3):508–11.

61. Sugiyama D, Nishimura K, Tamaki K, et al. Impact of smoking as a risk factor for developing rheumatoid arthritis: a meta-analysis of observational studies. Ann Rheum Dis 2010;69(1):70–81.

62. Klareskog L, Stolt P, Lundberg K, et al. A new model for an etiology of rheumatoid arthritis: smoking may trigger HLA-DR (shared epitope)-restricted immune reactions to autoantigens modified by citrullination. Arthritis Rheum 2006;54(1):38–46.

63. Jin Z, Xiang C, Cai Q, et al. Alcohol consumption as a preventive factor for developing rheumatoid arthritis: a dose-response meta-analysis of prospective studies. Ann Rheum Dis 2013. [Epub ahead of print].

64. Scott IC, Tan R, Stahl D, et al. The protective effect of alcohol on developing rheumatoid arthritis: a systematic review and meta-analysis. Rheumatology (Oxford) 2013;52(5):856–67.

65. van de Stadt LA, van SD. Alcohol consumption protects against arthritis development in seropositive arthralgia patients. Ann Rheum Dis 2012;71(8):1431–2.

66. Di GD, Wallin A, Bottai M, et al. Long-term intake of dietary long-chain n-3 polyunsaturated fatty acids and risk of rheumatoid arthritis: a prospective cohort study of women. Ann Rheum Dis 2013. [Epub ahead of print].

67. Linos A, Kaklamanis E, Kontomerkos A, et al. The effect of olive oil and fish consumption on rheumatoid arthritis–a case control study. Scand J Rheumatol 1991;20(6):419–26.

68. Linos A, Kaklamani VG, Kaklamani E, et al. Dietary factors in relation to rheumatoid arthritis: a role for olive oil and cooked vegetables? Am J Clin Nutr 1999; 70(6):1077–82.

69. Oliver JE, Silman AJ. Risk factors for the development of rheumatoid arthritis. Scand J Rheumatol 2006;35(3):169–74.

70. Pattison DJ, Harrison RA, Symmons DP. The role of diet in susceptibility to rheumatoid arthritis: a systematic review. J Rheumatol 2004;31(7):1310–9.

71. Pedersen M, Stripp C, Klarlund M, et al. Diet and risk of rheumatoid arthritis in a prospective cohort. J Rheumatol 2005;32(7):1249–52.

72. Rosell M, Wesley AM, Rydin K, et al. Dietary fish and fish oil and the risk of rheumatoid arthritis. Epidemiology 2009;20(6):896–901.

73. Shapiro JA, Koepsell TD, Voigt LF, et al. Diet and rheumatoid arthritis in women: a possible protective effect of fish consumption. Epidemiology 1996;7(3): 256–63.

74. Song GG, Bae SC, Lee YH. Association between vitamin D intake and the risk of rheumatoid arthritis: a meta-analysis. Clin Rheumatol 2012;31(12):1733–9.

75. Nielen MM, van SD, Lems WF, et al. Vitamin D deficiency does not increase the risk of rheumatoid arthritis: comment on the article by Merlino, et al. Arthritis Rheum 2006;54(11):3719–20.

76. Feser M, Derber LA, Deane KD, et al. Plasma 25,OH vitamin D concentrations are not associated with rheumatoid arthritis (RA)-related autoantibodies in individuals at elevated risk for RA. J Rheumatol 2009;36(5):943–6.

77. Hiraki LT, Munger KL, Costenbader KH, et al. Dietary intake of vitamin D during adolescence and risk of adult-onset systemic lupus erythematosus and rheumatoid arthritis. Arthritis Care Res (Hoboken) 2012;64(12):1829–36.

78. Arkema EV, Hart JE, Bertrand KA, et al. Exposure to ultraviolet-B and risk of developing rheumatoid arthritis among women in the Nurses' Health Study. Ann Rheum Dis 2013;72(4):506–11.

79. Cerhan JR, Saag KG, Merlino LA, et al. Antioxidant micronutrients and risk of rheumatoid arthritis in a cohort of older women. Am J Epidemiol 2003;157(4): 345–54.
80. Comstock GW, Burke AE, Hoffman SC, et al. Serum concentrations of alpha tocopherol, beta carotene, and retinol preceding the diagnosis of rheumatoid arthritis and systemic lupus erythematosus. Ann Rheum Dis 1997;56(5):323–5.
81. Heliovaara M, Knekt P, Aho K, et al. Serum antioxidants and risk of rheumatoid arthritis. Ann Rheum Dis 1994;53(1):51–3.
82. Knekt P, Heliovaara M, Aho K, et al. Serum selenium, serum alpha-tocopherol, and the risk of rheumatoid arthritis. Epidemiology 2000;11(4):402–5.
83. Pattison DJ, Silman AJ, Goodson NJ, et al. Vitamin C and the risk of developing inflammatory polyarthritis: prospective nested case-control study. Ann Rheum Dis 2004;63(7):843–7.
84. Costenbader KH, Kang JH, Karlson EW. Antioxidant intake and risks of rheumatoid arthritis and systemic lupus erythematosus in women. Am J Epidemiol 2010;172(2):205–16.
85. Pattison DJ, Symmons DP, Lunt M, et al. Dietary beta-cryptoxanthin and inflammatory polyarthritis: results from a population-based prospective study. Am J Clin Nutr 2005;82(2):451–5.
86. Afridi HI, Kazi TG, Brabazon D, et al. Association between essential trace and toxic elements in scalp hair samples of smokers rheumatoid arthritis subjects. Sci Total Environ 2011;412–413:93–100.
87. Afridi HI, Kazi TG, Brabazon D, et al. Interaction between zinc, cadmium, and lead in scalp hair samples of Pakistani and Irish smokers rheumatoid arthritis subjects in relation to controls. Biol Trace Elem Res 2012;148(2):139–47.
88. Bergstrom U, Jacobsson LT, Nilsson JA, et al. Pulmonary dysfunction, smoking, socioeconomic status and the risk of developing rheumatoid arthritis. Rheumatology (Oxford) 2011;50(11):2005–13.
89. Cooper GS, Miller FW, Germolec DR. Occupational exposures and autoimmune diseases. Int Immunopharmacol 2002;2(2–3):303–13.
90. Khuder SA, Peshimam AZ, Agraharam S. Environmental risk factors for rheumatoid arthritis. Rev Environ Health 2002;17(4):307–15.
91. Olsson AR, Skogh T, Wingren G. Occupational determinants for rheumatoid arthritis. Scand J Work Environ Health 2000;26(3):243–9.
92. Turner S, Cherry N. Rheumatoid arthritis in workers exposed to silica in the pottery industry. Occup Environ Med 2000;57(7):443–7.
93. Stolt P, Yahya A, Bengtsson C, et al. Silica exposure among male current smokers is associated with a high risk of developing ACPA-positive rheumatoid arthritis. Ann Rheum Dis 2010;69(6):1072–6.
94. De Roos AJ, Cooper GS, Alavanja MC, et al. Rheumatoid arthritis among women in the Agricultural Health Study: risk associated with farming activities and exposures. Ann Epidemiol 2005;15(10):762–70.
95. Olsson AR, Skogh T, Axelson O, et al. Occupations and exposures in the work environment as determinants for rheumatoid arthritis. Occup Environ Med 2004; 61(3):233–8.
96. Sverdrup B, Kallberg H, Bengtsson C, et al. Association between occupational exposure to mineral oil and rheumatoid arthritis: results from the Swedish EIRA case-control study. Arthritis Res Ther 2005;7(6):R1296–303.
97. Stolt P, Kallberg H, Lundberg I, et al. Silica exposure is associated with increased risk of developing rheumatoid arthritis: results from the Swedish EIRA study. Ann Rheum Dis 2005;64(4):582–6.

98. Gan RW, Deane KD, Zerbe GO, et al. Relationship between air pollution and positivity of RA-related autoantibodies in individuals without established RA: a report on SERA. Ann Rheum Dis 2013;72(12):2002–5.

99. Hart JE, Kallberg H, Laden F, et al. Ambient air pollution exposures and risk of rheumatoid arthritis. Arthritis Care Res (Hoboken) 2013;65(7):1190–6.

100. Hart JE, Kallberg H, Laden F, et al. Ambient air pollution exposures and risk of rheumatoid arthritis: results from the Swedish EIRA case-control study. Ann Rheum Dis 2013;72(6):888–94.

101. Ray P, Black S, Shinefield H, et al. Risk of rheumatoid arthritis following vaccination with tetanus, influenza and hepatitis B vaccines among persons 15-59 years of age. Vaccine 2011;29(38):6592–7.

102. Blaschke S, Schwarz G, Moneke D, et al. Epstein-Barr virus infection in peripheral blood mononuclear cells, synovial fluid cells, and synovial membranes of patients with rheumatoid arthritis. J Rheumatol 2000;27(4):866–73.

103. Buskila D, Shnaider A, Neumann L, et al. Musculoskeletal manifestations and autoantibody profile in 90 hepatitis C virus infected Israeli patients. Semin Arthritis Rheum 1998;28(2):107–13.

104. Sawada T, Hirohata S, Inoue T, et al. Development of rheumatoid arthritis after hepatitis C virus infection. Arthritis Rheum 1991;34(12):1620–1.

105. Medina-Rodriguez F, Guzman C, Jara LJ, et al. Rheumatic manifestations in human immunodeficiency virus positive and negative individuals: a study of 2 populations with similar risk factors. J Rheumatol 1993;20(11):1880–4.

106. Saebo A, Lassen J. Yersinia enterocolitica: an inducer of chronic inflammation. Int J Tissue React 1994;16(2):51–7.

107. Schaeverbeke T, Vernhes JP, Lequen L, et al. Mycoplasmas and arthritides. Rev Rhum Engl Ed 1997;64(2):120–8.

108. Hitchon CA, Chandad F, Ferucci ED, et al. Antibodies to Porphyromonas gingivalis are associated with anticitrullinated protein antibodies in patients with rheumatoid arthritis and their relatives. J Rheumatol 2010;37(6):1105–12.

109. Mikuls TR, Thiele GM, Deane KD, et al. Porphyromonas gingivalis and disease-related autoantibodies in individuals at increased risk of rheumatoid arthritis. Arthritis Rheum 2012;64(11):3522–30.

110. Bengtsson C, Kapetanovic MC, Kallberg H, et al. Common vaccinations among adults do not increase the risk of developing rheumatoid arthritis: results from the Swedish EIRA study. Ann Rheum Dis 2010;69(10):1831–3.

111. Cohen AD, Shoenfeld Y. Vaccine-induced autoimmunity. J Autoimmun 1996; 9(6):699–703.

112. Schattner A. Consequence or coincidence? The occurrence, pathogenesis and significance of autoimmune manifestations after viral vaccines. Vaccine 2005; 23(30):3876–86.

113. Shoenfeld Y, Aron-Maor A. Vaccination and autoimmunity-'vaccinosis': a dangerous liaison? J Autoimmun 2000;14(1):1–10.

114. Symmons DP, Chakravarty K. Can immunisation trigger rheumatoid arthritis? Ann Rheum Dis 1993;52(12):843–4.

115. Boyer JF, Gourraud PA, Cantagrel A, et al. Traditional cardiovascular risk factors in rheumatoid arthritis: a meta-analysis. Joint Bone Spine 2011;78(2):179–83.

116. Reynisdottir G, Karimi R, Joshua V, et al. Structural changes and antibody enrichment in the lungs are early features of anti-citrullinated protein antibody-positive rheumatoid arthritis. Arthritis Rheumatol 2014;66(1):31–9.

117. Verstappen SM, Lunt M, Luben RN, et al. Demographic and disease-related predictors of abnormal lung function in patients with established inflammatory

polyarthritis and a comparison with the general population. Ann Rheum Dis 2013;72(9):1517–23.

118. Demoruelle MK, Weisman MH, Simonian PL, et al. Brief report: airways abnormalities and rheumatoid arthritis-related autoantibodies in subjects without arthritis: early injury or initiating site of autoimmunity? Arthritis Rheum 2012; 64(6):1756–61.

119. Oken RJ, Schulzer M. At issue: schizophrenia and rheumatoid arthritis: the negative association revisited. Schizophr Bull 1999;25(4):625–38.

120. Crowson CS, Matteson EL, Davis JM III, et al. Contribution of obesity to the rise in incidence of rheumatoid arthritis. Arthritis Care Res (Hoboken) 2013;65(1): 71–7.

121. de Hair MJ, Landewe RB, van de Sande MG, et al. Smoking and overweight determine the likelihood of developing rheumatoid arthritis. Ann Rheum Dis 2013;72(10):1654–8.

122. Symmons DP, Bankhead CR, Harrison BJ, et al. Blood transfusion, smoking, and obesity as risk factors for the development of rheumatoid arthritis: results from a primary care-based incident case-control study in Norfolk, England. Arthritis Rheum 1997;40(11):1955–61.

123. Wesley A, Bengtsson C, Elkan AC, et al. Association between body mass index and anti-citrullinated protein antibody-positive and anti-citrullinated protein antibody-negative rheumatoid arthritis: results from a population-based case-control study. Arthritis Care Res (Hoboken) 2013;65(1):107–12.

124. Kang JH, Lin HC. Obstructive sleep apnea and the risk of autoimmune diseases: a longitudinal population-based study. Sleep Med 2012;13(6):583–8.

125. Maki-Petaja KM, Booth AD, Hall FC, et al. Ezetimibe and simvastatin reduce inflammation, disease activity, and aortic stiffness and improve endothelial function in rheumatoid arthritis. J Am Coll Cardiol 2007;50(9):852–8.

126. Steiner G, Urowitz MB. Lipid profiles in patients with rheumatoid arthritis: mechanisms and the impact of treatment. Semin Arthritis Rheum 2009;38(5):372–81.

127. van de Stadt LA, van Sijl AM, van SD, et al. Dyslipidaemia in patients with seropositive arthralgia predicts the development of arthritis. Ann Rheum Dis 2012; 71(11):1915–6.

128. van Halm VP, Nielen MM, Nurmohamed MT, et al. Lipids and inflammation: serial measurements of the lipid profile of blood donors who later developed rheumatoid arthritis. Ann Rheum Dis 2007;66(2):184–8.

129. Myasoedova E, Crowson CS, Kremers HM, et al. Total cholesterol and LDL levels decrease before rheumatoid arthritis. Ann Rheum Dis 2010;69(7):1310–4.

130. Dobson R, Giovannoni G. Autoimmune disease in people with multiple sclerosis and their relatives: a systematic review and meta-analysis. J Neurol 2013; 260(5):1272–85.

131. Avouac J, Gossec L, Dougados M. Diagnostic and predictive value of anti-cyclic citrullinated protein antibodies in rheumatoid arthritis: a systematic literature review. Ann Rheum Dis 2006;65(7):845–51.

132. Berglin E, Padyukov L, Sundin U, et al. A combination of autoantibodies to cyclic citrullinated peptide (CCP) and HLA-DRB1 locus antigens is strongly associated with future onset of rheumatoid arthritis. Arthritis Res Ther 2004;6(4):R303–8.

133. Brink M, Hansson M, Mathsson L, et al. Multiplex analyses of antibodies against citrullinated peptides in individuals prior to development of rheumatoid arthritis. Arthritis Rheum 2013;65(4):899–910.

134. Dorner T, Hansen A. Autoantibodies in normals–the value of predicting rheumatoid arthritis. Arthritis Res Ther 2004;6(6):282–4.

135. Kokkonen H, Mullazehi M, Berglin E, et al. Antibodies of IgG, IgA and IgM isotypes against cyclic citrullinated peptide precede the development of rheumatoid arthritis. Arthritis Res Ther 2011;13(1):R13.

136. Majka DS, Holers VM. Can we accurately predict the development of rheumatoid arthritis in the preclinical phase? Arthritis Rheum 2003;48(10):2701–5.

137. Nielen MM, van SD, Reesink HW, et al. Specific autoantibodies precede the symptoms of rheumatoid arthritis: a study of serial measurements in blood donors. Arthritis Rheum 2004;50(2):380–6.

138. Rantapaa-Dahlqvist S, de Jong BA, Berglin E, et al. Antibodies against cyclic citrullinated peptide and IgA rheumatoid factor predict the development of rheumatoid arthritis. Arthritis Rheum 2003;48(10):2741–9.

139. Saraux A, Berthelot JM, Chales G, et al. Value of laboratory tests in early prediction of rheumatoid arthritis. Arthritis Rheum 2002;47(2):155–65.

140. Scofield RH. Autoantibodies as predictors of disease. Lancet 2004;363(9420):1544–6.

141. Koivula MK, Heliovaara M, Rissanen H, et al. Antibodies binding to citrullinated telopeptides of type I and type II collagens and to mutated citrullinated vimentin synergistically predict the development of seropositive rheumatoid arthritis. Ann Rheum Dis 2012;71(10):1666–70.

142. Nielsen SF, Bojesen SE, Schnohr P, et al. Elevated rheumatoid factor and long term risk of rheumatoid arthritis: a prospective cohort study. BMJ 2012;345:e5244.

143. van de Stadt LA, van der Horst AR, de Koning MH, et al. The extent of the anti-citrullinated protein antibody repertoire is associated with arthritis development in patients with seropositive arthralgia. Ann Rheum Dis 2011;70(1):128–33.

144. Bos WH, Wolbink GJ, Boers M, et al. Arthritis development in patients with arthralgia is strongly associated with anti-citrullinated protein antibody status: a prospective cohort study. Ann Rheum Dis 2010;69(3):490–4.

145. van de Stadt LA, Witte BI, Bos WH, et al. A prediction rule for the development of arthritis in seropositive arthralgia patients. Ann Rheum Dis 2013;72(12):1920–6.

146. Shi J, van de Stadt LA, Levarht EW, et al. Anti-carbamylated protein antibodies are present in arthralgia patients and predict the development of rheumatoid arthritis. Arthritis Rheum 2013;65(4):911–5.

147. Kolfenbach JR, Deane KD, Derber LA, et al. Autoimmunity to peptidyl arginine deiminase type 4 precedes clinical onset of rheumatoid arthritis. Arthritis Rheum 2010;62(9):2633–9.

148. Aho K, Palosuo T, Knekt P, et al. Serum C-reactive protein does not predict rheumatoid arthritis. J Rheumatol 2000;27(5):1136–8.

149. Barra L, Summers K, Bell D, et al. Serum cytokine profile of unaffected first-degree relatives of patients with rheumatoid arthritis. J Rheumatol 2014;41(2):280–5.

150. Deane KD, O'Donnell CI, Hueber W, et al. The number of elevated cytokines and chemokines in preclinical seropositive rheumatoid arthritis predicts time to diagnosis in an age-dependent manner. Arthritis Rheum 2010;62(11):3161–72.

151. Edwards CJ, Cooper C. Early environmental factors and rheumatoid arthritis. Clin Exp Immunol 2006;143(1):1–5.

152. El-Gabalawy HS, Robinson DB, Smolik I, et al. Familial clustering of the serum cytokine profile in the relatives of rheumatoid arthritis patients. Arthritis Rheum 2012;64(6):1720–9.

153. Hughes-Austin JM, Deane KD, Derber LA, et al. Multiple cytokines and chemokines are associated with rheumatoid arthritis-related autoimmunity in first-degree relatives without rheumatoid arthritis: studies of the Aetiology of Rheumatoid Arthritis (SERA). Ann Rheum Dis 2013;72(6):901–7.

154. Jorgensen KT, Wiik A, Pedersen M, et al. Cytokines, autoantibodies and viral antibodies in premorbid and postdiagnostic sera from patients with rheumatoid arthritis: case-control study nested in a cohort of Norwegian blood donors. Ann Rheum Dis 2008;67(6):860–6.

155. Karlson EW, Chibnik LB, Tworoger SS, et al. Biomarkers of inflammation and development of rheumatoid arthritis in women from two prospective cohort studies. Arthritis Rheum 2009;60(3):641–52.

156. Limper M, van de Stadt L, Bos W, et al. The acute-phase response is not predictive for the development of arthritis in seropositive arthralgia - a prospective cohort study. J Rheumatol 2012;39(10):1914–7.

157. Masi AT, Aldag JC, Sipes J. Do elevated levels of serum C-reactive protein predict rheumatoid arthritis in men: correlations with pre-RA status and baseline positive rheumatoid factors. J Rheumatol 2001;28(10):2359–61.

158. Nielen MM, van SD, Reesink HW, et al. Increased levels of C-reactive protein in serum from blood donors before the onset of rheumatoid arthritis. Arthritis Rheum 2004;50(8):2423–7.

159. Rantapaa-Dahlqvist S, Boman K, Tarkowski A, et al. Up regulation of monocyte chemoattractant protein-1 expression in anti-citrulline antibody and immunoglobulin M rheumatoid factor positive subjects precedes onset of inflammatory response and development of overt rheumatoid arthritis. Ann Rheum Dis 2007; 66(1):121–3.

160. Sokolove J, Bromberg R, Deane KD, et al. Autoantibody epitope spreading in the pre-clinical phase predicts progression to rheumatoid arthritis. PLoS One 2012;7(5):e35296.

161. Turesson C, Bergstrom U, Jacobsson LT, et al. Increased cartilage turnover and circulating autoantibodies in different subsets before the clinical onset of rheumatoid arthritis. Ann Rheum Dis 2011;70(3):520–2.

162. Woolf AD, Hall ND, Goulding NJ, et al. Predictors of the long-term outcome of early synovitis: a 5-year follow-up study. Br J Rheumatol 1991;30(4):251–4.

163. van Baarsen LG, Wijbrandts CA, Timmer TC, et al. Synovial tissue heterogeneity in rheumatoid arthritis in relation to disease activity and biomarkers in peripheral blood. Arthritis Rheum 2010;62(6):1602–7.

164. Lubbers J, Brink M, van de Stadt LA, et al. The type I IFN signature as a biomarker of preclinical rheumatoid arthritis. Ann Rheum Dis 2013;72(5):776–80.

165. van de Stadt LA, Bos WH, Meursinge RM, et al. The value of ultrasonography in predicting arthritis in auto-antibody positive arthralgia patients: a prospective cohort study. Arthritis Res Ther 2010;12(3):R98.

166. Rakieh C, Nam JL, Hunt L, et al. Predicting the development of clinical arthritis in anti-CCP positive individuals with non-specific musculoskeletal symptoms: a prospective observational cohort study. Ann Rheum Dis 2014. [Epub ahead of print].

167. de Bois MH, Arndt JW, Speyer I, et al. Technetium-99m labelled human immunoglobulin scintigraphy predicts rheumatoid arthritis in patients with arthralgia. Scand J Rheumatol 1996;25(3):155–8.

168. Shearman J, Esdaile J, Hawkins D, et al. Predictive value of radionuclide joint scintigrams. Arthritis Rheum 1982;25(1):83–6.

169. Gent YY, Voskuyl AE, Kloet RW, et al. Macrophage positron emission tomography imaging as a biomarker for preclinical rheumatoid arthritis: findings of a prospective pilot study. Arthritis Rheum 2012;64(1):62–6.

170. van Steenbergen HW, van Nies JA, Huizinga TW, et al. Characterising arthralgia in the preclinical phase of rheumatoid arthritis using MRI. Ann Rheum Dis 2014. [Epub ahead of print].

171. van Steenbergen HW, van Nies JA, Huizinga TW, et al. Subclinical inflammation on MRI of hand and foot of anti-citrullinated peptide antibody-negative arthralgia patients at risk for rheumatoid arthritis. Arthritis Res Ther 2014;16(2):R92.

172. Sparks JA, Chen CY, Jiang X, et al. Improved performance of epidemiologic and genetic risk models for rheumatoid arthritis serologic phenotypes using family history. Ann Rheum Dis 2014. [Epub ahead of print].

173. Young KA, Deane KD, Derber LA, et al. Relatives without rheumatoid arthritis show reactivity to anti-citrullinated protein/peptide antibodies that are associated with arthritis-related traits: studies of the etiology of rheumatoid arthritis. Arthritis Rheum 2013;65(8):1995–2004.

174. Karlson EW, Ding B, Keenan BT, et al. Association of environmental and genetic factors and gene-environment interactions with risk of developing rheumatoid arthritis. Arthritis Care Res (Hoboken) 2013;65(7):1147–56.

175. Bos WH, Dijkmans BA, Boers M, et al. Effect of dexamethasone on autoantibody levels and arthritis development in patients with arthralgia: a randomised trial. Ann Rheum Dis 2010;69(3):571–4.

176. Karlson EW, Shadick NA, Cook NR, et al. Vitamin E in the primary prevention of rheumatoid arthritis: the Women's Health Study. Arthritis Rheum 2008;59(11): 1589–95.

177. del PA, Knowler WC, Pettitt DJ, et al. The incidence of rheumatoid arthritis is predicted by rheumatoid factor titer in a longitudinal population study. Arthritis Rheum 1988;31(10):1239–44.

178. Peschken CA, Hitchon CA, Robinson DB, et al. Rheumatoid arthritis in a North American native population: longitudinal followup and comparison with a white population. J Rheumatol 2010;37(8):1589–95.

179. Stack RJ, Sahni M, Mallen CD, et al. Symptom complexes at the earliest phases of rheumatoid arthritis: a synthesis of the qualitative literature. Arthritis Care Res (Hoboken) 2013;65(12):1916–26.

180. Available at: http://www.trialregister.nl/trialreg/admin/rctsearch.asp?Term=prairi. Accessed on June 20, 2014.

Prevention of Rheumatic Diseases

Strategies, Caveats, and Future Directions

Axel Finckh, MD[a], Kevin D. Deane, MD, PhD[b],*

KEYWORDS

- Prevention • Rheumatic diseases • Prediction

KEY POINTS

- A growing understanding of a preclinical period of many rheumatic diseases suggests that they could be approached in a preventive fashion.
- Prevention of rheumatic diseases may be through primary prevention of initial autoimmunity or tissue injury, or through secondary prevention to halt progression of autoimmunity and/or tissue injury while subjects are still in an asymptomatic or minimally symptomatic phase.
- Prevention may be approached through combinations of risk-factor modification, induction of tolerance, or pharmacologic interventions.
- Additional research is needed to identify effective biological targets and methods for prevention of rheumatic diseases, as well as to learn how to apply effective screening and prevention strategies that are able to improve public health in a cost-effective fashion.

INTRODUCTION

Across the multiple fields of medicine there is increasing interest in preventive approaches to disease. To help guide preventive approaches to disease, in the 1960s, the World Health Organization (WHO) put forward recommendations for disease screening and prevention, as listed in **Box 1.**[1] Overall, these recommendations suggest that diseases targeted for screening and prevention should have an important impact on health, an identifiable asymptomatic (or minimally symptomatic) period

Grant support: Dr K.D. Deane's work was supported by the National Institutes of Health (AI103023 and AI110503), the Rheumatology Research Foundation, and the Walter S. and Lucienne Driskill Foundation. Dr A. Finckh's work was supported by the Swiss National Science Foundation (SNSF 32003B_120639) and by a grant from the Geneva University Hospital.
Conflicts of interest: The investigators declare no relevant conflicts of interest.
[a] Division of Rheumatology, University Hospital of Geneva, Rue Gabrielle-Perret-Gentil 4, Genève 1205, Switzerland; [b] Division of Rheumatology, University of Colorado School of Medicine, 12605 East 16th Avenue, Aurora, CO 80045, USA
* Corresponding author.
E-mail address: kevin.deane@ucdenver.edu

Box 1
WHO recommendations regarding screening and prevention for a disease

- The disease should represent an important health problem
- A treatment should be available for the disease
- Facilities for diagnosis and treatment of the disorder should be available
- A latent (preclinical) stage of the disease should be detectable
- A test or examination for the condition should exist
- The screening test should be acceptable to the general population
- The natural history of the disease should be adequately understood
- An agreed policy on whom to treat is required
- The total cost of identifying a case among the population should be economically balanced in relation to medical expenditure as a whole
- Case finding should be a continuous process, necessitating regular repeat testing, and not just a once-and-for-all project

Adapted from Wilson JMG, Jungner G. Principles and practice of screening for disease. WHO Public Health Papers 1968;34:1–163.

---

during which individuals at high risk for future disease can accurately be identified, and that there be available an effective means for preventing the further evolution of disease. Screening and prevention approaches that follow these guidelines are in action for many diseases. For example, across the globe there is considerable effort put into to screening and preventing adverse outcomes from cardiovascular disease and many types of cancer, as well as programs to prevent many infectious diseases.

Although most rheumatologists agree that rheumatic diseases are important health problems and meet several of the other WHO criteria for screening, many key questions regarding prevention of rheumatic diseases are still unanswered. However, given the growing understanding of the causes of rheumatic disease, and, as discussed herein, a growing awareness that many rheumatic diseases have a period of largely asymptomatic disease development during which there are abnormalities of biomarkers that can be used to predict future risk for disease,[2] there is hope that rheumatic diseases may join the list of preventable diseases.

This article discusses some general principles of disease prevention applicable to rheumatic disease, and outlines a potential research strategy for the development of effective preventive strategies that will be able to reduce the adverse impact of these diseases.

GENERAL STRATEGIES FOR DISEASE PREVENTION

Prevention strategies are typically categorized into primary, secondary, or tertiary interventions (**Fig. 1**).[3,4] The aim of primary prevention is to avoid the development of disease by eliminating specific risk factors or increasing an individual's resistance to the condition. An example of this type of approach is vaccines against infections. The aim of secondary prevention is to reduce the progression from a latent or asymptomatic phase of disease to symptomatic disease. Thus a secondary preventive intervention attempts to interrupt the mechanisms of disease development before they evolve into an apparent illness. Examples of this type of approach include early identification of cancers through programs such as mammograms and colonoscopies.

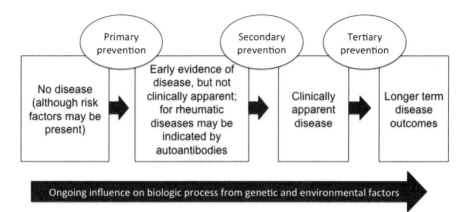

Fig. 1. Natural history of rheumatic disease and possibilities for prevention. The natural history of rheumatic disease begins on the left with no disease, although genetic and environmental factors may be present. Over time, there is early evidence of disease that is not clinically apparent. Examples of this are autoantibodies, increased uric acid, or early cartilage injury. Later, clinically apparent disease develops that may be classifiable as a specific rheumatic disease. Once disease is clinically manifest, longer-term outcomes include issues such as response to therapy and disability. Throughout disease evolution, there are ongoing influences from genetic and environmental factors. Progression of rheumatic disease may be prevented at several points: before development of asymptomatic disease (primary prevention), during asymptomatic disease (secondary prevention), and after clinically apparent disease has developed (tertiary prevention).

The aim of tertiary prevention is to delay or to limit the impact of an established disease.[5] Most rheumatic diseases are currently treated at this stage, and rheumatologists typically perform tertiary prevention by attempting to prevent progression of disease to disability or premature death after patient presents with clinically apparent disease (eg, swollen joints in rheumatoid arthritis [RA], or skin rash in systemic lupus erythematosus [SLE]). However, rheumatologists are less used to performing primary or secondary preventive interventions for rheumatic diseases. As knowledge of the risk factors for rheumatic diseases grows (eg, smoking for RA),[6] primary prevention may become more of a priority for rheumatic diseases.

POTENTIAL PRIMARY PREVENTIVE STRATEGIES

Environmental risk factors are of great interest for preventive strategies for rheumatic diseases, because they are potentially modifiable. In particular, lifestyle modifications are a common request from at-risk populations; specifically, when individuals at high risk for RA were interviewed about potential preventive interventions, most of them primarily mentioned lifestyle adjustments as approaches with which they would be comfortable.[7]

Multiple environmental and lifestyle factors have been identified for rheumatic diseases. In RA, tobacco smoking is the best-established risk factor and is responsible for 1 in every 4 to 6 cases of RA (population attributable risk).[8] The effect of tobacco is dose dependent and larger in shared-epitope–positive individuals.[8,9] Other inhaled pollutants have also been implicated in the development of RA, such as silica dusts, factory dusts, or exposure to traffic pollution.[10,11] Reproductive and hormonal factors also play a role in the development of RA and several other autoimmune diseases. Sex hormones have immunomodulatory effects, but the complex interactions among hormones are not fully understood. Oral contraceptive and hormone replacement therapy have been associated with a lower RA risk, but not all studies have confirmed these findings. Several studies have found an increased risk of RA with obesity and with lower social class.[12,13] Dietary factors have generally given inconclusive results, but recently high intake of soda and salt have been associated with an increased risk of RA.[14,15] In contrast, a moderate alcohol consumption has consistently been associated with a decreased risk of RA.[16] In a similar way, tobacco smoking, occupational exposure to silica dust, and exposure to sunlight have also been associated with an increased risk of SLE, whereas moderate alcohol intake seems to decrease the risk.[17] In some cases, specific disease triggers such as toxic oil, certain medications, or possibly exposure to certain mycotoxins may provide information on the pathophysiology of specific rheumatic diseases such as eosinophilic disease, drug-induced autoimmune syndromes, and potentially certain forms of osteoarthritis (OA) such as Kashin-Beck disease.[18–21] Emerging data also suggest that microorganisms, such as Epstein-Barr Virus in SLE[22] or bacterial organisms in RA, may be implicated in the development of certain rheumatic diseases.[23–25] If the infectious cause for rheumatic diseases is confirmed, it could allow the development of preventive strategies involving vaccines against the causative organisms.

Risk factors for other rheumatic diseases are also known. For example, diet-related metabolic effects such as central obesity and diabetes as well as alcohol intake have been shown to be related to increased risk for gout.[26] In addition, prior injury, obesity, and abnormal joint mechanics are risk factors for OA.[27] Many more environmental risk factors for rheumatic diseases exist, although more research is warranted to elucidate the complex interactions between genetics and the environment, both to understand the cause of these diseases and to initiate preventive interventions.

Although there are many environmental factors that have been associated with the development of rheumatic diseases, few of the identified environmental triggers for rheumatic diseases have enough supportive evidence and strong enough effect sizes overall to warrant altering a specific environmental risk factor on a population level. Even tobacco smoke, which as discussed earlier is one of the best-established environmental risk factor for RA, still only explains ~30% of seropositive disease.[28,29] However, the effect of environmental risk factors may be much stronger in individuals with a certain genetic makeup.[9,30]

An interesting approach to identify individuals for whom environmental factor(s) or and/or lifestyle modifications may be most effective is to combine several environmental risk factors to identify individuals at very high risk for rheumatic disease. For example, a British study has proposed a risk score for inflammatory polyarthritis based solely on easily ascertained lifestyle factors.[31] This lifestyle risk score combines pack-years of smoking (every 10 pack-years), alcohol consumption (units/d), occupational class (professional, manual, neither), obesity (body mass index >30), presence of diabetes, parity ($\geq$2), and duration of breastfeeding in women (years). Based on a summation of these lifestyle factors, this risk score can identify individuals who have up to a 6 times higher risk of developing polyarthritis. In addition, using the United States–based Nurses Health Study, Karlson and colleagues[32] used a combination of family history, genetic factors, and environmental factors to predict future risk for RA, with area under the curve of greater than 0.8 for their best predictive models for RA.[33] Although targeting single environmental factors in the general population may not be a feasible strategy for uncommon diseases, approaches combining genetic and environmental risk factors may be useful to detect specific individuals in whom a preventive intervention designed to modify lifestyle factors is most indicated.

IDENTIFICATION OF PRECLINICAL PHASES OF RHEUMATIC DISEASE

Because of the difficulty in identifying specific environmental risk factors for most rheumatic diseases as well as the weak effect sizes of known environmental risk factors when applied on a population basis,[6] a more feasible approach to rheumatic disease prevention may be to focus on interventions in individuals who are at a very early phase of rheumatic disease development before the development of significant tissue injury. This concept has gained traction over the past few years in large part because of a growing understanding of the natural history of rheumatic diseases. Many autoimmune rheumatic diseases are currently thought to result from multistep processes, whereby an environmental trigger (or triggers) induces an immune reaction in genetically susceptible individuals (**Fig. 1**). The genetic susceptibility may be assessed through a careful family history of disease or may be measured with specific genetic markers.[2,9,34] Furthermore, in many rheumatic diseases, including SLE,[35] RA,[36–40] and antineutrophil cytoplasmic antibody–positive vasculitis,[41,42] disease-specific autoantibodies may precede by several years the clinically apparent manifestations of disease, often termed preclinical disease. Other rheumatic diseases, such as gout and OA, also have preclinical phases with abnormal biomarkers (eg, uric acids[43]) or early structural changes (eg, hip dysplasia[44]), in the absence of significant clinical symptoms. Thus, a high-risk population could be identified either by identifying genetically susceptible individuals (ie, genetic screening using genetic risk scores, or using a family history of autoimmune disorders as a proxy),[45] by detecting the presence of specific biomarkers (eg, autoantibodies), or by recognizing a set of highly relevant environmental exposures.[31]

POTENTIAL SECONDARY PREVENTION STRATEGIES

Although many rheumatic diseases may be identified in their preclinical phases, it is not clear how to safely and effectively prevent either the initiation of early autoimmunity or the progression of early autoimmunity or other rheumatic disease mechanisms (eg, high uric acid in gout, or early cartilage damage in OA) while the disease is in an asymptomatic state. As discussed above, there are multiple environmental risk factors associated with rheumatic diseases, and as such is possible that environmental risk-factor modification could be effective to halt initiation of autoimmunity, or even progression of early autoimmunity to clinically apparent disease. However, there is still a lack of knowledge of which factors act to initiate and propagate autoimmunity once it develops. Furthermore, modulating an environmental risk factor or factors may be effective to prevent the development and/or progression of rheumatic disease but it may be difficult to measure its effect because the time between an intervention and the potential clinical benefit may be long. For example, using data from the Nurses' Health Study, Karlson and colleagues found that risk of RA remained increased until 20+ years after smoking cessation[46]; such an effect would be difficult to measure in a clinical trial to show benefit in an evidence-based fashion. Tolerance-inducing regimens could also be an attractive approach for altering progression of autoimmunity; however, this approach is difficult to use unless specific antigen targets and immune regulatory pathways are well understood.

Given the difficulties of modulating environmental risk factors to prevent rheumatic disease, perhaps pharmacologic intervention using agents known to be effective for the treatment of established rheumatic diseases would be the best approach to prevent the progression of autoimmunity. In support of this approach, in animal models of autoimmune diseases, early therapeutic interventions are capable of averting the development of the clinical disease.[47] However, to date, only indirect evidence supporting this hypothesis is available in humans: in the early stages of RA, a therapeutic window of opportunity seems to exist in which early antirheumatic therapy seems to modify and improve the disease permanently in some patients.[48–53] Furthermore, in the Dutch probable rheumatoid arthritis: methotrexate versus placebo (PROMPT) study, a limited course of methotrexate in patients with early undifferentiated arthritis initially delayed or prevented the onset of classifiable RA in a proportion of patients, especially those with seropositivity for antibodies to citrullinated proteins,[49] although the effects of this intervention seemed to wane after 5 years of follow-up.[50] The exact mechanism for improved long-term outcomes is unclear, although several observations suggest that in the early stages of the disease process the immune system might still be amendable to immunologic reprogramming. It has also been suggested that early intervention prevents the recruitment and/or evolution of effector cells such as synovial fibroblasts to a more pathogenic phenotype.[51]

Based on these findings, drugs already known to be effective in clinically apparent rheumatic diseases could be applied in the preclinical phase to halt progression to a more damaging phase of disease. For example, in individuals who are at risk for RA or SLE, drugs such as hydroxychloroquine or methotrexate could be applied in the preclinical phase of disease development. Furthermore, interventions at this early phase of disease may be more effective at altering autoimmunity because of less development of more persistent immune and inflammatory responses.

There is already limited evidence that such approaches may be effective in some rheumatic and other autoimmune diseases. In uncontrolled trials, use of hydroxychloroquine seems to reduce rates of progression from palindromic rheumatism (which may be a form of preclinical RA) to persistent inflammatory arthritis[52–54]; in addition, in uncontrolled studies of SLE, early use of hydroxychloroquine seemed to delay the fulfillment of classification criteria for SLE and reduce the expansion of autoantibodies.[55] Furthermore, a small trial tested a limited preventive intervention in postpartum women with presumed preclinical Graves disease based on high titers of thyroid antibodies, and suggested that a short-term course of prednisolone may prevent the development of postpartum hypothyroidism.[56] In addition, a clinical trial in The Netherlands is examining the efficacy and safety of rituximab to prevent the progression from systemic autoimmunity associated with RA (autoantibody-positive individuals) to clinically classifiable RA.[57] The results of this study could be highly informative about potential preventive approaches to RA, which could be applied to other rheumatic diseases as well.

CAVEATS TO PREVENTION

Although alterations of environmental factors or pharmacologic approaches to prevention of rheumatic diseases are attractive, there are many caveats. Perhaps most importantly, a careful balance is needed between determining the risk of future disease and the potential adverse impact from screening and preventive interventions.

In terms of identifying individuals at risk for future rheumatic disease, there are several possibilities. Importantly, any approach to identifying those at risk for future rheumatic disease needs to have sufficiently high predictive values for future disease that would allow the balancing of risks for developing disease and the potential benefit of prevention against the risks of preventive interventions, potential adverse effects from the test, which could include emotional and physical harms, as well as inappropriate health care costs that may arise from false positivity. Autoantibodies are known to be present before clinically apparent SLE and RA, and in some studies have high (>90%) positive predictive values (PPVs) for future disease. For example, in case-control studies of RA-related autoantibodies, positivity for antibodies to citrullinated proteins in combination with rheumatoid factor were highly specific for RA, and had a PPV of close to 100%.[39,40] However, when the diagnostic accuracy of these autoantibodies is compared with population rates of RA of ~1%, PPVs decrease to ~16%.[39] If these autoantibodies were used in broad screening programs to identify individuals at high risk for future onset of disease, the absolute risk predicted by certain biomarkers may need to be higher in order to justify use of a potentially toxic medication. For diseases such as gout, high levels of uric acid may predict the future onset of clinically apparent gouty arthritis[58]; however, is the risk of disease that can be estimated from an increased level of uric acid high enough to justify the use of a medication such as allopurinol that has a low but real risk of serious adverse effects?[59]

In addition, screening strategies for rheumatic diseases should allow for the prediction of an individual's likelihood of developing future disease (ie, will a person develop the disease?), as well as timing (ie, when will they develop disease?), which is important both for an individual, when contemplating preventive interventions, as well as for prevention trials, in which it is important to identify the number of expected outcomes within a temporally limited period. In RA, several studies have found that a combination of autoantibodies and specific cytokines and chemokines predicted the likelihood and timing of future RA.[60,61] A Dutch study showed that a combination of these factors can be used in individuals with arthralgias, but without inflammatory arthritis, to predict the likelihood and the timing of future RA.[62]

Another caveat to prevention of rheumatic diseases is that the mechanisms at play in the earliest phases of development of rheumatic diseases are largely unknown. An agent, such as anti–tumor necrosis factor (TNF) alpha may not be effective in the preclinical phase of disease, in which TNF may not yet be a major pathogenic factor. If this is the case, then the use of such an agent may not offer any preventive benefit, but only potential harm. In addition, the duration of a pharmacologic intervention in the preclinical phase to prevent progression to disease is unknown. Could a short-term intervention reset the immune system and lead to permanent reduction of future risk for clinically apparent rheumatic disease, or would an intervention need to be continued indefinitely in order to prevent tissue injury? A Dutch trial using 2 doses of intramuscular corticosteroids was unsuccessful in preventing progression to clinically classifiable RA.[63] This trial may not have used the correct pharmacologic agent, or the duration of therapy may have been inadequate, but these results highlight that these issues need to be addressed in carefully designed clinical trials.

In addition, identifying and measuring important outcomes in prevention is a difficult issue. Should the goal of prevention be to prevent the clinical onset of classifiable disease? To that end, are currently available classification schemes for rheumatic diseases adequate outcome measures for disease prevention? What if individuals participating in rheumatic disease prevention had improvements of symptoms or findings that did not meet standardized classification criteria for disease? For example, in RA prevention, what if a patient had improved arthralgias from a preventive therapy for RA even in the absence of developing clinically apparent synovitis? Are current systems for measuring such outcomes adequate for robust determination of effectiveness of preventive strategies? Furthermore, would other outcomes such as alterations of biomarkers be acceptable? Rheumatologists may think that an intervention that made a specific autoantibody disappear is worthwhile, but unless this results in meaningful improvement in clinical outcomes it may be less attractive to regulatory agencies or even individuals participating in prevention strategies.

Although there are caveats to prevention of rheumatic diseases, it must also be considered that the potential benefits of prevention approaches may extend beyond the disease they are addressing. For example, perhaps strategies for RA prevention will prevent joint damage but also prevent cardiovascular disease associated with autoimmunity.[64–67] Perhaps decreasing uric acid with an agent such as allopurinol will prevent gouty arthritis but also improve cardiovascular disease risk and all-cause mortality, as emerging data suggest that it might.[68–70] These issues are difficult to define, but they need to be considered when assessing the risks and potential benefits of preventive approaches in rheumatic diseases.

PERSONALIZING APPROACHES TO PREVENTION

Any preventive intervention for rheumatic disease involves an individual choosing to participate in screening and preventive activities. The factors that may influence this choice to participate in screening and prevention include perceived personal risk for disease, familiarity with the illness, and the expected personal benefit.[7,71] The characteristics of the preventive approach (administration mode, duration of the preventive therapy, adverse event profile) may modulate the decision to participate in prevention.[47]

An individual's perception of personal risk may be based on numbers that are provided to individuals by the health care community regarding risk (eg, PPV of a test), but may also involve personal characteristics such as underlying tendency to trust health care information or acknowledge personal risk for a disease.[72] In addition, familiarity with the disease may further influence an individual's decision to participate in preventive strategies. For example, an individual whose mother had severe RA, or whose father had severe gout, may approach prevention differently than someone who has never known anyone with the disease. The perceived benefits of a preventive intervention may also be difficult to ascertain and explain to individuals. For example, someone who is asymptomatic but at risk for future rheumatic disease may have special requirements to convince them to participate in a strategy that will prevent an adverse health outcome in the distant future.[73] These issues are important because individuals are less likely to be compliant with a therapeutic approach if they do not gain any perceived benefit.[74] Moreover, the benefits of prevention need to be explained carefully to patients, because the perceived harm of many rheumatic diseases is decreasing with modern therapies. Using RA as an example, it may not be fair to scare someone into participating in disease prevention based on their knowledge of a patient with very severe joint damage that developed in an era before effective disease-modifying therapy.

Furthermore, although the potential harms of pharmacologic agents may be readily ascertainable based on known side effect profiles, other possible preventive interventions, such as smoking cessation (RA) or weight loss (OA), may seem beneficial overall but be intolerable or very difficult for some individuals. As an example, a youth with mild valgus deformity of the knee that increases his risk for future OA[75] may not be willing to avoid risky but enjoyable behaviors, such as playing soccer, in order to avoid potential future symptomatic knee OA. Because these issues differ between diseases, acceptability of a preventive intervention needs to be appraised in each target population.

Highlighting some of these issues, in one of the possible target populations for a preventive strategy of RA, namely first-degree relatives of patients with the condition, a qualitative study suggested that preventive interventions could meet the expectations of this population, given that the screening procedure used to identify at-risk individuals is reliable and that the potential preventive therapy has only minimal constraints and a good safety profile.[7] The theoretic risk of developing RA in the next 5 years had to more than 30% before most of the target population would consider taking a prophylactic treatment (**Fig. 2**). Another study examined the factors that persons at risk consider before taking a preventive treatment. As expected, participants were more likely to consider taking a preventive treatment when the risk of developing the disease increased. The efficacy of the preventive intervention and the risk of serious adverse events were the most important attributes for choosing a preventive treatment of RA. It is noteworthy that individuals at risk of RA request considerable effectiveness from a potential preventive treatment before they consider taking such a therapy.[76]

Even if the future development of autoimmune disorders could adequately be predicted, not everyone wants to find out about their risk of future disease. In a prospective cohort study of first-degree relatives of patients with RA,[77] participants could receive the results of their genetic and immunologic tests. Although most participants wanted to know, a significant proportion of participants opted not to receive the results of their biomarkers (Axel Finckh, personal communication).

The potential harms of screening have been largely debated in the oncology literature, in particular for breast cancer screening and the related risk of overtreatment.[15] Thus, in breast cancer, the trend is moving away from organized population screening programs toward a more personalized, risk-based approach.[78] The ethical issues may become even harder with the advent of genetic testing, as clinicians move away from conventional screening, designed to detect early-stage diseases, to probabilistic approaches. If this is applied to rheumatic diseases, clinicians will have to interpret results of potential screening tests for rheumatic diseases in light of the individual's probability of disease.[79] Furthermore, screening for disease before a valid treatment option becomes available may not be ethical, because no preventive treatment can be offered to patients identified at very high risk,[80,81] although to develop preventive strategies there will need to be some initial steps to test interventions without knowing

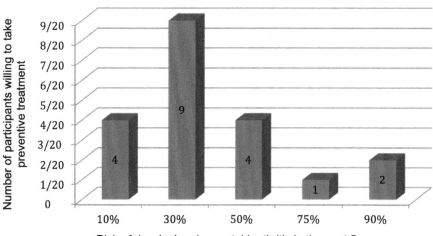

Fig. 2. Theoretic 5-year risk of developing RA above which persons at risk are willing to take preventive medicine. At a 30% hypothetical risk of developing RA within the next 5 years, most first-degree relatives of patients with RA were willing to take a limited preventive treatment. (*Adapted from* Novotny F, Haeny S, Hudelson P, et al. Primary prevention of rheumatoid arthritis: a qualitative study in a high-risk population. Joint Bone Spine 2013;80(6):673–4; with permission.)

their full effects. For rheumatologists, the coming era of prevention will require considerable counseling talents and communication skills, because probabilities are often not well understood by patients and the issues are complex.[82]

THE PUBLIC HEALTH IMPACT OF PREVENTION

In terms of potential impact, prevention of rheumatic diseases has a great potential for public health benefit, given the burden of these conditions in terms of disability and lost productivity. However, in spite of their impact, prevention of rheumatic diseases has not been a priority in most countries, possibly because these conditions are not immediately lethal. However, if rheumatic diseases are evaluated in aggregate, their overall impact on public health should make addressing preventive strategies a top priority for authorities.

If prevention of rheumatic conditions is to gain acceptance, it needs to meet certain criteria for primary prevention established by public health agencies. As mentioned earlier, as well as in the article by Dr Ned Calonge elsewhere in this issue, the WHO has presented guidelines for disease screening and prevention (see **Box 1**) that apply to preventive approaches to rheumatic diseases. Any such approaches require understanding of the natural history of these condition from their asymptomatic phases to their clinically apparent phases. At present, of the rheumatic diseases, few meet these requirements, with the exception of osteoporosis, and potentially rheumatic fever, for which treating patients with low bone density and streptococcal pharyngeal infection, respectively, has shown benefits.[83,84] As for preventive strategies for other rheumatic diseases, the study of RA pathogenesis is probably the most advanced; its high prevalence in relation to other autoimmune rheumatic diseases makes it an attractive first target for a preventive intervention. However, although identifying preclinical RA has become a major scientific priority, it still needs study before curing or preventing can become a reality. However, if success is met in one rheumatic disease, it could set a precedent for preventive approaches for a host of immune-mediated conditions, ultimately leading to substantial benefits to public health.

SUMMARY AND FUTURE DIRECTIONS

Rheumatic diseases affect a large number of individuals and lead to significant morbidity, in some cases increased mortality, and high health care costs and loss of productivity. A growing understanding of the natural history of many of these diseases suggests that they could be approached in a preventive fashion either to stop the initial development of disease or to halt progression to disease during its preclinical phase. A better understanding of disease pathogenesis may lead to effective screening and prevention strategies for a broad range of rheumatic diseases in the near future. Furthermore, studies of disease pathogenesis need to be paralleled by studies of the cost-effectiveness, feasibility, and ethics of prevention strategies as well as subject-related factors that can influence participation in prevention.

REFERENCES

1. Wilson JM, Jungner YG. Principles and practice of mass screening for disease. Bol Oficina Sanit Panam 1968;65(4):281–393 [in Spanish].
2. Deane KD, El-Gabalawy H. Pathogenesis and prevention of rheumatic disease: focus on preclinical RA and SLE. Nat Rev Rheumatol 2014;10(4):212–28. http://dx.doi.org/10.1038/nrrheum.2014.6.

3. Public health measures in disease prevention. Science 2012;337(6101): 1468–70. http://dx.doi.org/10.1126/science.337.6101.1468-b.
4. Ash C, Kiberstis P, Marshall E, et al. Disease prevention. It takes more than an apple a day. Introduction. Science 2012;337(6101):1466–7. http://dx.doi.org/10. 1126/science.337.6101.1466.
5. Katz DL, Ali A. Preventive medicine, integrative medicine & the health of the public. Commissioned for the IOM summit on integrative medicine and the health of the public. Washington, DC: Institute of Medicine (IOM); 2009.
6. Karlson EW, Deane K. Environmental and gene-environment interactions and risk of rheumatoid arthritis. Rheum Dis Clin North Am 2012;38(2):405–26. http://dx.doi.org/10.1016/j.rdc.2012.04.002.
7. Novotny F, Haeny S, Hudelson P, et al. Primary prevention of rheumatoid arthritis: a qualitative study in a high-risk population. Joint Bone Spine 2013; 80(6):673–4. http://dx.doi.org/10.1016/j.jbspin.2013.05.005.
8. Kallberg H, Ding B, Padyukov L, et al. Smoking is a major preventable risk factor for rheumatoid arthritis: estimations of risks after various exposures to cigarette smoke. Ann Rheum Dis 2011;70(3):508–11. http://dx.doi.org/10.1136/ard.2009.120899.
9. Klareskog L, Stolt P, Lundberg K, et al. A new model for an etiology of rheumatoid arthritis: smoking may trigger HLA-DR (shared epitope)-restricted immune reactions to autoantigens modified by citrullination. Arthritis Rheum 2006;54(1):38–46.
10. Stolt P, Yahya A, Bengtsson C, et al. Silica exposure among male current smokers is associated with a high risk of developing ACPA-positive rheumatoid arthritis. Ann Rheum Dis 2010;69(6):1072–6.
11. Hart JE, Laden F, Puett RC, et al. Exposure to traffic pollution and increased risk of rheumatoid arthritis. Environ Health Perspect 2009;117(7):1065–9.
12. Symmons DP, Bankhead CR, Harrison BJ, et al. Blood transfusion, smoking, and obesity as risk factors for the development of rheumatoid arthritis: results from a primary care-based incident case-control study in Norfolk, England. Arthritis Rheum 1997;40(11):1955–61.
13. Bengtsson C, Nordmark B, Klareskog L, et al. Socioeconomic status and the risk of developing rheumatoid arthritis: results from the Swedish EIRA study. Ann Rheum Dis 2005;64(11):1588–94. http://dx.doi.org/10.1136/ard.2004.031666.
14. Yang H, Costenbader KH, Hu F, et al, editors. Sugar-sweetened soft drink consumption and risk of developing rheumatoid arthritis. American College of Rheumatology 2013 annual meeting. San Diego (CA): Arthritis Rheum; 2013.
15. Sundström B, Johansson I, Rantapää Dahlqvist S, editors. Dietary sodium increases the risk for rheumatoid arthritis among smokers – results from a nested case-control study. American College of Rheumatology 2013 annual meeting. San Diego (CA): Arthritis Rheum; 2013.
16. Maxwell JR, Gowers IR, Moore DJ, et al. Alcohol consumption is inversely associated with risk and severity of rheumatoid arthritis. Rheumatology (Oxford) 2010;49(11):2140–6.
17. Takvorian S, Merola J, Costenbader K. Cigarette smoking, alcohol consumption and risk of systemic lupus erythematosus. Lupus 2014;23(6):537–44. http://dx. doi.org/10.1177/0961203313501400.
18. Patterson R, Germolec D. Review article toxic oil syndrome: review of immune aspects of the disease. J Immunotoxicol 2005;2(1):51–8. http://dx.doi.org/10. 1080/15476910590960143.
19. Perez-Alvarez R, Perez-de-Lis M, Ramos-Casals M, BIOGEAS study group. Biologics-induced autoimmune diseases. Curr Opin Rheumatol 2013;25(1):56–64. http://dx.doi.org/10.1097/BOR.0b013e32835b1366.

20. Sudre P, Mathieu F. Kashin-Beck disease: from etiology to prevention or from prevention to etiology? Int Orthop 2001;25(3):175–9.
21. van Steensel MA. Why minocycline can cause systemic lupus - a hypothesis and suggestions for therapeutic interventions based on it. Med Hypotheses 2004;63(1):31–4. http://dx.doi.org/10.1016/j.mehy.2003.12.040.
22. James JA, Robertson JM. Lupus and Epstein-Barr. Curr Opin Rheumatol 2012; 24(4):383–8. http://dx.doi.org/10.1097/BOR.0b013e3283535801.
23. Ebringer A. Rheumatoid arthritis and proteus. London: Springer-Verlag; 2012.
24. Scher JU, Abramson SB. Periodontal disease, *Porphyromonas gingivalis*, and rheumatoid arthritis: what triggers autoimmunity and clinical disease? Arthritis Res Ther 2013;15(5):122. http://dx.doi.org/10.1186/ar4360.
25. Scher JU, Sczesnak A, Longman RS, et al. Expansion of intestinal *Prevotella copri* correlates with enhanced susceptibility to arthritis. Elife (Cambridge) 2013;2: e01202. http://dx.doi.org/10.7554/eLife.01202.
26. Roddy E, Choi HK. Epidemiology of gout. Rheum Dis Clin North Am 2014;40(2): 155–75. http://dx.doi.org/10.1016/j.rdc.2014.01.001.
27. Arden NK, Leyland KM. Osteoarthritis year 2013 in review: clinical. Osteoarthritis Cartilage 2013;21(10):1409–13. http://dx.doi.org/10.1016/j.joca.2013.06.021.
28. Sugiyama D, Nishimura K, Tamaki K, et al. Impact of smoking as a risk factor for developing rheumatoid arthritis: a meta-analysis of observational studies. Ann Rheum Dis 2010;69(1):70–81. http://dx.doi.org/10.1136/ard.2008.096487.
29. Costenbader KH, Kim DJ, Peerzada J, et al. Cigarette smoking and the risk of systemic lupus erythematosus: a meta-analysis. Arthritis Rheum 2004;50(3): 849–57. http://dx.doi.org/10.1002/art.20049.
30. Keenan BT, Chibnik LB, Cui J, et al. Effect of interactions of glutathione S-transferase T1, M1, and P1 and HMOX1 gene promoter polymorphisms with heavy smoking on the risk of rheumatoid arthritis. Arthritis Rheum 2010;62(11): 3196–210.
31. Lahiri M, Luben RN, Morgan C, et al. Using lifestyle factors to identify individuals at higher risk of inflammatory polyarthritis (results from the European prospective investigation of Cancer-Norfolk and the Norfolk Arthritis Register–the EPIC-2-NOAR Study). Ann Rheum Dis 2013;73(1):219–26.
32. Karlson EW, Ding B, Keenan BT, et al. Association of environmental and genetic factors and gene-environment interactions with risk of developing rheumatoid arthritis. Arthritis Care Res (Hoboken) 2013;65(7):1147–56. http://dx.doi.org/10.1002/acr.22005.
33. Sparks JA, Chen CY, Jiang X, et al. Improved performance of epidemiologic and genetic risk models for rheumatoid arthritis serologic phenotypes using family history. Ann Rheum Dis 2014. http://dx.doi.org/10.1136/annrheumdis-2013-205009.
34. Hemminki K, Li X, Sundquist J, et al. Familial associations of rheumatoid arthritis with autoimmune diseases and related conditions. Arthritis Rheum 2009;60(3): 661–8. http://dx.doi.org/10.1002/art.24328.
35. Arbuckle MR, McClain MT, Rubertone MV, et al. Development of autoantibodies before the clinical onset of systemic lupus erythematosus. N Engl J Med 2003; 349(16):1526–33.
36. Aho K, Palosuo T, Heliovaara M. Predictive significance of rheumatoid factor. J Rheumatol 1995;22(11):2186–7.
37. Aho K, von Essen R, Kurki P, et al. Antikeratin antibody and antiperinuclear factor as markers for subclinical rheumatoid disease process. J Rheumatol 1993; 20(8):1278–81.

38. Del Puente A, Knowler WC, Pettitt DJ, et al. High incidence and prevalence of rheumatoid arthritis in Pima Indians. Am J Epidemiol 1989;129(6):1170–8.

39. Rantapaa-Dahlqvist S, de Jong BA, Berglin E, et al. Antibodies against cyclic citrullinated peptide and IgA rheumatoid factor predict the development of rheumatoid arthritis. Arthritis Rheum 2003;48(10):2741–9.

40. Nielen MM, van Schaardenburg D, Reesink HW, et al. Specific autoantibodies precede the symptoms of rheumatoid arthritis: a study of serial measurements in blood donors. Arthritis Rheum 2004;50(2):380–6.

41. McAdoo SP, Hall A, Levy J, et al. Proteinase-3 antineutrophil cytoplasm antibody positivity in patients without primary systemic vasculitis. J Clin Rheumatol 2012; 18(7):336–40. http://dx.doi.org/10.1097/RHU.0b013e31826d2005.

42. Olson SW, Owshalimpur D, Yuan CM, et al. Relation between asymptomatic proteinase 3 antibodies and future granulomatosis with polyangiitis. Clin J Am Soc Nephrol 2013;8(8):1312–8. http://dx.doi.org/10.2215/CJN.10411012.

43. Chen JH, Pan WH, Hsu CC, et al. Impact of obesity and hypertriglyceridemia on gout development with or without hyperuricemia: a prospective study. Arthritis Care Res (Hoboken) 2013;65(1):133–40. http://dx.doi.org/10.1002/acr.21824.

44. Laborie LB, Engesaeter IO, Lehmann TG, et al. Screening strategies for hip dysplasia: long-term outcome of a randomized controlled trial. Pediatrics 2013;132(3):492–501. http://dx.doi.org/10.1542/peds.2013-0911.

45. Chibnik LB, Keenan BT, Cui J, et al. Genetic risk score predicting risk of rheumatoid arthritis phenotypes and age of symptom onset. PLoS One 2011;6(9): e24380.

46. Costenbader KH, Feskanich D, Mandl LA, et al. Smoking intensity, duration, and cessation, and the risk of rheumatoid arthritis in women. Am J Med 2006;119(6): 503.e1–9. http://dx.doi.org/10.1016/j.amjmed.2005.09.053.

47. Bowman MA, Leiter EH, Atkinson MA. Prevention of diabetes in the NOD mouse: implications for therapeutic intervention in human disease. Immunol Today 1994; 15(3):115–20.

48. Finckh A, Liang MH, van Herckenrode CM, et al. Long-term impact of early treatment on radiographic progression in rheumatoid arthritis: a meta-analysis. Arthritis Rheum 2006;55(6):864–72. http://dx.doi.org/10.1002/art.22353.

49. Van Dongen H, Van Aken J, Lard LR, et al. Efficacy of methotrexate treatment in patients with probable rheumatoid arthritis. A double-blind, randomized, placebo-controlled trial. Arthritis Rheum 2007;56(5):1424–32.

50. van Aken J, Heimans L, Gillet-van Dongen H, et al. Five-year outcomes of probable rheumatoid arthritis treated with methotrexate or placebo during the first year (the PROMPT study). Ann Rheum Dis 2014;73(2):396–400. http://dx.doi.org/10.1136/annrheumdis-2012-202967.

51. Arend WP, Firestein GS. Pre-rheumatoid arthritis: predisposition and transition to clinical synovitis. Nat Rev Rheumatol 2012;8(10):573–86. http://dx.doi.org/10.1038/nrrheum.2012.134.

52. Katz SJ, Russell AS. Palindromic rheumatism: a pre-rheumatoid arthritis state? J Rheumatol 2012;39(10):1912–3. http://dx.doi.org/10.3899/jrheum.120995.

53. Abraham RR. Palindromic rheumatism: strategies to prevent evolution to rheumatoid arthritis. South Med J 2012;105(6):322. http://dx.doi.org/10.1097/SMJ.0b013e318257c53e [author reply: 323].

54. Gonzalez-Lopez L, Gamez-Nava JI, Jhangri G, et al. Decreased progression to rheumatoid arthritis or other connective tissue diseases in patients with palindromic rheumatism treated with antimalarials. J Rheumatol 2000;27(1):41–6.

55. James JA, Kim-Howard XR, Bruner BF, et al. Hydroxychloroquine sulfate treatment is associated with later onset of systemic lupus erythematosus. Lupus 2007;16(6):401–9. http://dx.doi.org/10.1177/0961203307078579.

56. Tada H, Hidaka Y, Izumi Y, et al. A preventive trial of short-term immunosuppressive therapy in postpartum thyroid dysfunction. Int J Endocrinol Metab 2003;2: 48–54.

57. Tak PP. Prevention of clinically manifest rheumatoid arthritis by B cell directed therapy in the earliest phase of the disease (PRAIRI). Nederlands Trials Register [Internet]. 2010. Available at: http://www.trialregister.nl/trialreg/admin/rctview. asp?TC=2442.

58. Singh JA, Reddy SG, Kundukulam J. Risk factors for gout and prevention: a systematic review of the literature. Curr Opin Rheumatol 2011;23(2):192–202. http://dx.doi.org/10.1097/BOR.0b013e3283438e13.

59. Kim SC, Newcomb C, Margolis D, et al. Severe cutaneous reactions requiring hospitalization in allopurinol initiators: a population-based cohort study. Arthritis Care Res (Hoboken) 2013;65(4):578–84. http://dx.doi.org/10.1002/acr.21817.

60. Deane KD, O'Donnell CI, Hueber W, et al. The number of elevated cytokines and chemokines in preclinical seropositive rheumatoid arthritis predicts time to diagnosis in an age-dependent manner. Arthritis Rheum 2010;62(11):3161–72.

61. Sokolove J, Bromberg R, Deane KD, et al. Autoantibody epitope spreading in the pre-clinical phase predicts progression to rheumatoid arthritis. PLoS One 2012;7(5):e35296. http://dx.doi.org/10.1371/journal.pone.0035296.

62. van de Stadt LA, Witte BI, Bos WH, et al. A prediction rule for the development of arthritis in seropositive arthralgia patients. Ann Rheum Dis 2013;72(12):1920–6. http://dx.doi.org/10.1136/annrheumdis-2012-202127.

63. Bos WH, Dijkmans BA, Boers M, et al. Effect of dexamethasone on autoantibody levels and arthritis development in patients with arthralgia: a randomised trial. Ann Rheum Dis 2010;69(3):571–4. http://dx.doi.org/10.1136/ard.2008.105767.

64. Hjeltnes G, Hollan I, Forre O, et al. Anti-CCP and RF IgM: predictors of impaired endothelial function in rheumatoid arthritis patients. Scand J Rheumatol 2011; 40(6):422–7. http://dx.doi.org/10.3109/03009742.2011.585350.

65. Bartoloni E, Alunno A, Bistoni O, et al. How early is the atherosclerotic risk in rheumatoid arthritis? Autoimmun Rev 2010;9(10):701–7. http://dx.doi.org/10. 1016/j.autrev.2010.06.001.

66. Liang KP, Gabriel SE. Autoantibodies: innocent bystander or key player in immunosenescence and atherosclerosis? J Rheumatol 2007;34(6):1203–7.

67. Aho K, Salonen JT, Puska P. Autoantibodies predicting death due to cardiovascular disease. Cardiology 1982;69(3):125–9.

68. Richette P, Perez-Ruiz F, Doherty M, et al. Improving cardiovascular and renal outcomes in gout: what should we target? Nat Rev Rheumatol 2014. [Epub ahead of print].

69. Rodrigues TC, Maahs DM, Johnson RJ, et al. Serum uric acid predicts progression of subclinical coronary atherosclerosis in individuals without renal disease. Diabetes Care 2010;33(11):2471–3.

70. Dubreuil M, Zhu Y, Zhang Y, et al. Allopurinol initiation and all-cause mortality in the general population. Ann Rheum Dis 2014. http://dx.doi.org/10.1136/ annrheumdis-2014-205269.

71. Harmsen CG, Stovring H, Jarbol DE, et al. Medication effectiveness may not be the major reason for accepting cardiovascular preventive medication: a population-based survey. BMC Med Inform Decis Mak 2012;12:89. http://dx. doi.org/10.1186/1472-6947-12-89.

72. Groopman J, Hartzband P. Your medical mind: how to decide what is right for you. New York: Penguin Books; 2011.
73. Hardcastle SJ, Legge E, Laundy CS, et al. Patients' perceptions and experiences of familial hypercholesterolemia, cascade genetic screening and treatment. Int J Behav Med 2014. http://dx.doi.org/10.1007/s12529-014-9402-x.
74. Kucukarslan SN. A review of published studies of patients' illness perceptions and medication adherence: lessons learned and future directions. Research in social & administrative pharmacy. Res Social Adm Pharm 2012;8(5): 371–82. http://dx.doi.org/10.1016/j.sapharm.2011.09.002.
75. Hayashi D, Englund M, Roemer FW, et al. Knee malalignment is associated with an increased risk for incident and enlarging bone marrow lesions in the more loaded compartments: the MOST study. Osteoarthritis Cartilage 2012;20(11): 1227–33. http://dx.doi.org/10.1016/j.joca.2012.07.020.
76. Finckh A, Liang M, Escher M, et al, editors. Factors involved in the decision to take medications to prevent rheumatoid arthritis in first degree relatives of patients with RA. A discrete choice experiment. Annual scientific meeting of the American College of Rheumatology (ACR). Chicago: Arthritis & Rheum; 2011.
77. Finckh A, Müller R, Möller B, et al, editors. A novel screening strategy for preclinical rheumatoid arthritis (RA) in first degree relatives of patients with RA. Annual European Congress of Rheumatology EULAR. London: Ann Rheum Dis; 2011.
78. Vilaprinyo E, Forne C, Carles M, et al, Interval Cancer Study Group. Cost-effectiveness and harm-benefit analyses of risk-based screening strategies for breast cancer. PLoS One 2014;9(2):e86858. http://dx.doi.org/10.1371/journal.pone.0086858.
79. Finckh A, Liang MH. Anti-cyclic citrullinated peptide antibodies in the diagnosis of rheumatoid arthritis: bayes clears the haze. Ann Intern Med 2007;146(11): 816–7.
80. Notkins AL. New predictors of disease. Molecules called predictive autoantibodies appear in the blood years before people show symptoms of various disorders. Tests that detected these molecules could warn of the need to take preventive action. Sci Am 2007;296:72–9.
81. Wilson JMG, Jungner G. Principles and practice of screening for disease. Geneva: WHO Public Health Papers #34; 1968.
82. Smerecnik CM, Mesters I, Verweij E, et al. A systematic review of the impact of genetic counseling on risk perception accuracy. J Genet Couns 2009;18(3): 217–28. http://dx.doi.org/10.1007/s10897-008-9210-z.
83. Cunningham MW. *Streptococcus* and rheumatic fever. Curr Opin Rheumatol 2012;24(4):408–16. http://dx.doi.org/10.1097/BOR.0b013e32835461d3.
84. Cooper C, Reginster JY, Cortet B, et al. Long-term treatment of osteoporosis in postmenopausal women: a review from the European Society for Clinical and Economic Aspects of Osteoporosis and Osteoarthritis (ESCEO) and the International Osteoporosis Foundation (IOF). Curr Med Res Opin 2012;28(3):475–91.

Developing Evidence-Based Screening Recommendations, with Consideration for Rheumatology

Ned Calonge, MD, MPH[a,b,c],*

KEYWORDS

- U.S. Preventive Services Task Force • Rheumatoid arthritis • Screening
- Evidence-based recommendations

KEY POINTS

- Screening for preclinical rheumatic disease may improve health by enabling treatment to start before clinical symptoms occur.
- Potential health harms associated with screening programs, such as the harms associated with false-positive tests and overdiagnosis, must be weighed against health benefits.
- The U.S. Preventive Services Task Force (USPSTF) uses an explicit process to create evidence-based screening recommendations that assess net benefit, or benefits minus harms.
- Screening tests recommended by the USPSTF are provided with first dollar coverage under the Affordable Care Act.

INTRODUCTION

In the clinical prevention world, screening for the early detection of disease is categorized as secondary prevention, involving interventions that are implemented after the asymptomatic onset of biologic disease, but before the progression to symptomatic disease that would be diagnosed through the usual health care approach. Conceptually, intervening early leads to better health outcomes than does waiting until the disease manifests clinically. Good examples of effective screening modalities exist in the chronic disease arena: screening for cervical cancer with cytology can almost eliminate deaths from this cancer,[1] and screening for and treating hypertension

Disclosure: None.
[a] The Colorado Trust, 1600 Sherman Street, Denver, CO 80111, USA; [b] Department of Family Medicine, University of Colorado School of Medicine, Mail Stop F-496, Academic Office 1, 12631 East 17th Avenue, Aurora, CO 80045, USA; [c] Department of Epidemiology, Colorado School of Public Health, Campus Box B119, 13001 E. 17th Place, Aurora, CO 80045, USA
* The Colorado Trust, 1600 Sherman Street, Denver, CO 80111.
E-mail address: ned@coloradotrust.org

Rheum Dis Clin N Am 40 (2014) 787–795
http://dx.doi.org/10.1016/j.rdc.2014.07.016
0889-857X/14/$ – see front matter © 2014 Elsevier Inc. All rights reserved.

rheumatic.theclinics.com

significantly reduces the occurrence of atherosclerotic disease in the coronary and cerebral arteries in nearly all adult age groups.[2] A broader definition of screening, brought to the forefront of medicine by the current interest in genetic testing, involves screening for the risk of disease and intervening even before the biologic onset of a condition. This new technology will continue to bring new challenges for decision making in screening programs.

Screening for asymptomatic or preclinical rheumatic conditions has the potential for providing improved disease outcomes, with the early treatment of disease using safe and effective therapeutics started before symptomatic tissue damage. However, even though screening is conceptually appealing, as it is in other conditions, it has downsides in terms of the potential for harm, which is associated with almost all medical interventions. Screening benefits must be weighed against harms when deciding to offer screening.

The benefits of screening are straightforward: early intervention leads to earlier treatment and better health outcomes. On the other hand, 4 or 5 categories of potential harms exist. A test can be falsely negative, creating false reassurance and the potential to delay the diagnosis of a treatable condition when patients ignore symptoms. The test may be falsely positive, arguably the most important negative outcome, leading to unnecessary and potentially harmful diagnostic tests, treatment, and labeling. The test could overdiagnose disease that does not require treatment. In this scenario, the test result is a true-positive, but detects disease that would not progress, meaning that any treatment is unnecessary. Overdiagnosis is a critical harm associated with screening for prostate cancer, in which most cancers are indolent and would never impact the patient's health,[3] and screening for breast cancer, in which most ductal carcinoma in situ does not benefit from treatment.[4] Finally, the test can be correct, but early detection may have no real benefit, and therefore screening consumes resources, increasing the cost of medical care without health benefit. In addition, harms may be associated with the test itself, such as additional radiation exposure with x-ray screening, which could, over a lifetime of screening, increase the risk of disease, or, in the case of a somewhat invasive test such as colonoscopy, the test may carry the risk of adverse outcomes, including hemorrhage and perforation.

The evidence bar tends to be set high for screening, more so than for other medical interventions, because the population targeted is asymptomatic. If clinicians are going to medically intervene with people who are otherwise well and clinically manifesting no illness, they should only do so based on strong evidence showing that the benefits well outweigh the harms.

FRAMEWORK FOR DISEASE SCREENING

In creating a framework for deciding whether to implement a disease screening program, Wilson and Jungner[5] created a list of critical criteria to assess. Paraphrasing this sentinel article, these criteria include the following queries:

- Is the disease an important health problem (in terms of severity and incidence)?
- Does the disease have a recognizable presymptomatic stage that lasts long enough to allow for screening, diagnosis, and treatment?
- Are acceptable and reliable screening tests available for the presymptomatic stage?
- Does treatment of the disease during the presymptomatic stage result in improved outcomes?
- Do sufficient resources exist for diagnosing and treating the population with positive screening results?

A group of evidence-based medicine researchers reframed these criteria for to-day's evidence-based approach in 2011,[6] stating that the fundamental question to answer when determining whether to screen should be whether the program, if imple-mented under present conditions, would result in sufficient net benefit (benefits minus harms) to justify starting (or continuing) the program given the level of resources required. This determination should include an evidence-based consideration of several factors, including the probability of an adverse health outcome without screening, the degree to which screening identifies all those who would experience the adverse health outcome, and the magnitude of incremental health benefit conferred by earlier treatment initiated as a result of screening. Also important in the assessment of a screening test are the frequency of false-positive tests; the ex-periences of people with false-positive results, including the frequency and severity of workup and treatment; and the frequency and severity of outcomes associated with overdiagnosis.

PROCESS OF THE UNITED STATES PREVENTIVE SERVICES TASK

These considerations guide the process of the U.S. Preventive Services Task Force (USPSTF), an independent panel of nationally recognized, nonfederal experts experi-enced in primary care, disease prevention, evidence-based medicine, and research methods. The USPSTF, which is hosted by the Agency for Health Research and Qual-ity, was created in 1985 and charged by Congress to review the scientific evidence for clinical preventive services and develop evidence-based recommendations for the health care community. Under section 2713(a)(1) of the Affordable Care Act,[7] the rec-ommendations from the USPSTF have taken on greater importance; recommenda-tions that are graded A or B (described in detail later) will involve services covered by all insurers, with no additional out-of-pocket costs to the patient (ie, first dollar coverage).

The USPSTF uses an explicit process[8,9] that can be categorized into specific steps:

1. Define the question about the provision of a preventive service within an analytical framework and using a set of key questions.
2. Define, retrieve, and review the relevant evidence; judge the quality of individual studies; and summarize the evidence for each key question.
3. Synthesize and judge the strength or adequacy of the body of evidence for each, and across all, key questions.
4. Determine the magnitude of net benefit[10] (the balance of benefits and harms).
5. Judge the certainty of net benefit.[10]
6. Link magnitude and certainty of net benefit to a recommendation statement/letter grade.

The steps are implemented in 2 integrated activities, one being a systematic evidence review (SER) that addresses the literature search, study quality rating, and summary of the evidence on the magnitude of benefits and harms. The other process, the recommendation process, takes the SER results, assesses the strength of evi-dence, and determines the magnitude and certainly of net benefit and the correspond-ing letter grade/recommendation statement.

Step 1: Define the Analytical Framework and Key Questions

The analytical framework defines the clinical scenario for the topic—who are you screening, how, for what condition, in what setting, and for what purpose—and creates a set of key questions that guide the SER and decision making. A generic analytical framework for evaluating a screening test is presented in **Fig. 1**, in which the numbers refer to the list of key questions:

1. Does direct evidence show that providing the service improves health outcomes if implemented in a general primary care population? Outside of treatment scenarios, sufficient direct evidence is rarely available. If insufficient evidence is available to answer this question, the remaining framework allows the creation of a chain of evidence to support a recommendation.
2. Can a population at risk and/or at increased risk be identified? Higher-risk populations have a higher rate of disease, and this translates to better screening test performance (specifically, fewer false-positives).
3. Does screening reliably lead to preclinical/earlier detection? This question deals with the screening test utilities of sensitivity, specificity, and predictive values of positive and negative tests.
4. Does treatment of screening-detected disease lead to improvement in important health outcomes, including mortality or morbidity? This critical question was often not satisfactorily addressed before the widespread adoption of some screening tests, as evident with prostate-specific antigen testing for prostate cancer.
5. Are harms associated with specific parts of the screening process, including risk identification, screening itself, confirmatory diagnosis for people with positive tests, and treatment?

Step 2: Find, Review, Judge the Quality of, and Summarize the Available Evidence

Rating the quality of the studies included in the SER requires assessment and judgment based on explicit research design criteria. The USPSTF rates studies as good, fair, or poor, wherein good quality means high internal validity with outcomes confidently assigned to the factors under study; fair quality indicates some minor threats to internal validity; and poor quality indicates major threats to internal validity so that competing hypotheses regarding study outcomes cannot be confidently excluded.

Step 3: Determine the Strength of Evidence

Grading the strength of evidence, which the USPSTF categorizes as inadequate, adequate, or convincing, considers more than just the quality of studies, and requires

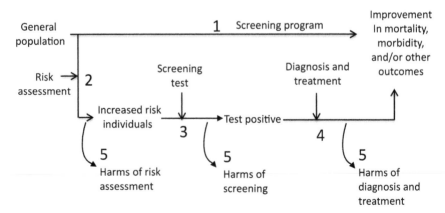

Fig. 1. Generic analytical framework for screening for disease (numbers refer to key questions described in text).

assessment and judgment based on explicit epidemiologic research criteria captured by 6 critical appraisal questions:

1. Do the studies have the appropriate research design to answer the key question?
2. To what extent are the studies of high quality (ie, have good internal validity)?
3. To what extent are the studies generalizable to the US population (ie, have good external validity)?
4. How many studies, and of what size, have been performed to answer the key question (ie, how precise is the evidence)?
5. How consistent are the studies (ie, do they support the same conclusion)?
6. Do additional factors support the conclusions?

If several high-quality studies existed with consistent, logical results generalizable to the United States, the evidence would be convincing. If most but not all criteria are addressed satisfactorily, the evidence is adequate. If the studies are conflicting or are of poor quality, individually or in aggregate, the evidence is inadequate. Note that adequate evidence is not possible with poor-quality studies, but inadequate evidence is possible with fair- or good-quality studies if they have conflicting results that cannot otherwise be explained.

Step 4: Determine the Magnitude of Net Benefit

Determining net benefit involves an assessment of the available evidence on benefits and harms. The magnitude of benefit is based on the effect sizes (results) from studies in the SER. If more than one study is available, the SER process summarizes the effect sizes with meta-analysis. The magnitude of harm is also taken from the SER, although traditionally researchers have focused less on measuring and reporting harms than on reporting benefits.

The magnitude of net benefit is graded as substantial, moderate, small, or zero/net harm by the USPSTF. This grading requires a judgment of the comparison between benefits and harms. For many topics this can be challenging, because the "currency" of benefits and harms is likely to be different, and how different benefits and harms are valued can vary widely. For example, within her lifetime, a woman choosing to begin screening mammography at age 40 years will reduce her risk of dying of breast cancer from approximately 30 in 1000 to 22 in 1000 (the benefit), while accepting a 50% risk of having a false-positive mammogram that will require follow-up testing[11] and around a 20% risk of overdiagnosis and unnecessary treatment (the harms).[4] Depending on personal values and preferences, this tradeoff may be worth it for some women.

Step 5: Determine the Certainty of Net Benefit

Based on the magnitude of net benefit and the strength of evidence assessed, the USPSTF makes a judgment about the certainty of net benefit, determined again using the critical appraisal questions, synthesized across all of the key questions and the entire body of evidence. *Certainty* can be considered the opposite of the risk of making the wrong recommendation: either recommending for a screening test that will not improve overall individual or population health, or recommending against a test that may have important net benefit. A rating of high certainty, which has a low risk of being wrong, must be supported by consistent results from good-quality studies assessing the impact on important health outcomes. The conclusion is unlikely to be affected by future studies. A rating of moderate certainty, based on sufficient evidence, has a somewhat higher risk of being wrong, because the assessment is constrained by issues raised in the critical appraisal; here, additional information from future studies could change the conclusion. In the case of low certainty, the evidence is insufficient to assess the net effects, positive or negative, on health outcomes, and future studies will be needed for further assessment.

Step 6: Assign a Letter Grade/Recommendation

Once the certainty and magnitude of net benefit are determined, the USPSTF links this assessment to a letter grade and a specific recommendation using a matrix presented in **Table 1**. A and B recommendations should be implemented in practice, and clinicians and patients can have confidence that these will improve health. D recommendations should not be implemented, because at least moderate certainty exists that they will have no net health benefit, or that the harms outweigh the benefits. C recommendations require a bit more effort. The net benefit, although positive and real, is small, and the tradeoffs between benefits and harms should be discussed with the patient, taking into account unique patient characteristics, values, and preferences.

The inconclusive evidence letter grade I deserves additional comment. Compared with the other letter grades, it is a conclusion, not a recommendation. It means that evidence of effectiveness is insufficient, not that sufficient evidence shows no effectiveness. Common reasons for a grade of I include a lack of evidence on clinical outcomes, poor quality of existing studies, and good-quality studies with conflicting results. With this conclusion, a possibility of clinically important health benefit remains, but more research is needed.

EVIDENCE-BASED SCREENING RECOMMENDATIONS FOR RHEUMATIC DISEASE

In considering the USPSTF process, rheumatology must address some questions when evaluating potential screening and early treatment for rheumatologic conditions:

- Is the disease sufficiently described, including its natural history (including treatment), to implement effective prevention strategies?
- What is the prevalence of the disease? Can a population at increased risk be determined? For example, the prevalence of rheumatoid arthritis (RA) is known to be higher among American Indians and Alaska Natives[12] and their first-degree relatives,[13] and prevalence drives the population performance of any screening test; therefore, a disease with a low prevalence will generate a large number of false-positive tests, even if the test is highly specific. Conversely, in terms of the predictive value of a positive test, screening performance improves with the increased prevalence in higher-risk populations.
- What important health outcomes could screening improve, and how can these be measured? For example, one could measure joint destruction through imaging and arthritis-related quality of life. Evidence that a screening strategy improves an intermediate clinical outcome, such as a blood test result, may be

Table 1
Recommendation matrix for the U.S. Preventive Services Task Force

Certainty of Net Benefit	Magnitude of Net Benefit (Benefit Minus Harms)			
	Substantial	Moderate	Small	Zero/Negative
High	A	B	C	D
Moderate	B	B	C	D
Low	I			

A & B: recommend use. C: recommend against routine use. D: recommend against use. I: No recommendation; insufficient evidence.

insufficient to support a positive recommendation, unless evidence of a link to an important health outcome (morbidity or mortality) is sufficient.

- Is or could there be supportive evidence from randomized controlled trials (RCTs)? Although a convincing chain of evidence can be created without an RCT, it is still the gold standard of study design and can provide the best support for a recommendation. Regardless of the design, any supportive study must be of good quality; even an RCT must account for harms, lead-time, and length-time bias, and all other sources of bias.

OUTCOMES TABLES

A useful approach to evaluating a potential screening strategy, and one that the USPSTF often uses in estimating net benefit, is the construction of an outcomes table.[4] For example, if 10,000 people are screened for RA, how many will benefit, how many will be harmed, what is the resource consumption, and how does all this compare with not screening? **Fig. 2** presents a simplified approach to creating an outcomes table, using estimates of population prevalence and screening test utilities. The positive predictive value in this example, 34%, indicates that just more than one-third of individuals with positive test results will have RA, whereas two-thirds will have positive results but not have disease. With these estimates in hand, the next step is to determine the potential benefit and harm for each result group (**Table 2**):

- True-positives (n = 252): what are the expected benefits from early intervention (prevention, joint sparing, symptom improvement, quality of life) and how does this compare with waiting for clinical diagnosis? Are there harms associated with treatment that might be increased from a longer duration of treatment?
- False-negatives (n = 13): are there any harms for these individuals? Might these individuals delay seeking diagnosis and treatment because they think they are disease-free?
- False-positives (n = 487): are there any harms for these individuals? What additional testing will be required to determine that their results are in fact negative? What is the risk of unnecessary treatment? Will these individuals experience harm from labeling or increased anxiety?
- Overdiagnosis: can this number be estimated? Are these individuals who will test positive and may never develop symptomatic disease, or who may have a natural history of disease that does not require preventive or other therapeutic intervention?

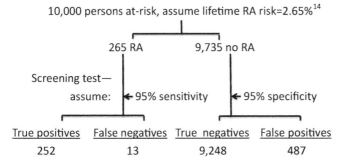

10,000 persons at-risk, assume lifetime RA risk=2.65%[14]

265 RA   9,735 no RA

Screening test—

assume: ← 95% sensitivity   ← 95% specificity

True positives   False negatives   True negatives   False positives
252   13   9,248   487

Positive predictive value (proportion testing positive who have disease) = 34%

Fig. 2. Hypothetical performance of a screening test to detect preclinical rheumatoid arthritis (RA).[14]

Table 2 Hypothetical outcomes table for RA screening		
Outcomes	10,000 People with Usual Care	10,000 People Screened for RA
RA	265 (diagnosed clinically)	265
True-positives		252 people with early detection
True-negatives		9248 reassured they do not have RA
False-positives		487 with incorrect positive tests
False-negatives		13 with incorrect negative tests
Overdiagnosis		# not needing treatment (unknown)

This exercise provides information that a clinician can use to determine whether a given screening process is likely to result in a net health benefit to those screened. It also provides guidance on what research is needed to answer the key questions in an analytical framework designed to create an evidence-based recommendation.

FUTURE CONSIDERATIONS/SUMMARY

Creating evidence-based screening recommendations is a complex process, and the process used by the USPSTF has been codified in the Affordable Care Act to the degree that the conclusions of the USPSTF have major coverage implications for insures, providers, and patients. As ongoing research discovers promising evidence for the potential of preclinical identification of individuals with rheumatologic diseases, understanding the evidence-based process and using simple computational tools, such as outcomes tables, can help rheumatology researchers provide the evidence needed to identify potentially effective screening programs, and help determine when a program may not lead to improvements in individual and population health.

Further information on USPSTF methods and procedures are available on the Task Force's Web site (www.uspreventiveservicestaskforce.org/), as are all of their recommendations and supportive SERs that provide examples of the processes outlined in this article.

REFERENCES

1. U.S. Preventive Services Task Force, Moyer VA. Screening for cervical cancer: U.S. Preventive Services Task Force recommendation statement. Ann Intern Med 2012;156:880–91.
2. James PA, Oparil S, Carter BL, et al. 2014 evidence-based guideline for the management of high blood pressure in adults: report from the panel members appointed to the Eighth Joint National Committee (JNC 8). JAMA 2014;311(5): 507–20.
3. U.S. Preventive Services Task Force, Moyer VA. Screening for prostate cancer: U.S. Preventive Services recommendation statement. Ann Intern Med 2012; 157:120–34.
4. Miller AB, Wall C, Baines CJ, et al. Twenty five year follow-up for breast cancer incidence and mortality of the Canadian National Breast Screening Study: randomised screening trial. BMJ 2014;348:g366.
5. Wilson JMG, Jungner G. Principles and practice of screening for disease. Geneva: World Health Organization; 1968.

6. Harris R, Sawaya GF, Moyer VA, et al. Reconsidering the criteria for evaluating proposed screening programs: reflections from 4 current and former members of the U.S. Preventive Services Task Force. Epidemiol Rev 2011;33(1):20–35.

7. H.R. 3590, One Hundred Eleventh Congress of the United States of America At the Second Session, "An Act Entitled The Patient Protection and Affordable Care Act," United States Government Printing Office, 2010.

8. Guirguis-Blake J, Calonge N, Miller T, et al. Current Processes of the U.S. Preventive Services Task Force: refining evidence-based recommendation development. Ann Intern Med 2007;147:117–22.

9. Barton MB, Miller T, Wolff T, et al. How to read the new recommendation statement: methods update from the U.S. Preventive Services Task Force. Ann Intern Med 2007;147:123–7.

10. Sawaya GF, Guirguis-Blake J, LeFevre M, et al. Update on the methods: estimating certainty and magnitude of net benefit. Ann Intern Med 2007;147:871–5.

11. U.S. Preventive Services Task Force. Screening for breast cancer: U.S. Preventive Services Task Force recommendation statement. Ann Intern Med 2009;151: 716–26.

12. Ferucci ED, Emplin DW, Laneir AP. Rheumatoid arthritis in American Indians and Alaska Natives: a review of the literature. Semin Arthritis Rheum 2005;34(4): 662–7.

13. Smolik I, Robinson DB, Bernstein CN, et al. First-degree relatives of patients with rheumatoid arthritis exhibit high prevalence of joint symptoms. J Rheumatol 2013; 40(6):818–24.

14. Crowson CS, Matteson EL, Myasoedova E, et al. The lifetime risk of adult-onset rheumatoid arthritis and other inflammatory autoimmune rheumatic diseases. Arthritis Rheum 2011;63(3):633–9.

Lessons from Type 1 Diabetes for Understanding Natural History and Prevention of Autoimmune Disease

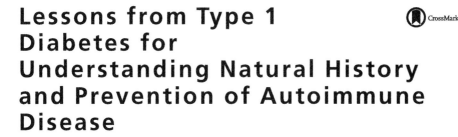

Kimber Simmons, MD, Aaron W. Michels, MD*

KEYWORDS

- Type 1 diabetes • Autoimmunity • Autoantibodies • Prevention • Immune therapies

KEY POINTS

- Type 1 diabetes is a chronic progressive autoimmune disorder with a preclinical phase of disease before clinical onset.
- Type 1 diabetes can be predicted based on the measurement of antibodies directed against islet antigens.
- Large prospective randomized double-blinded placebo-controlled secondary prevention trials for Type 1 diabetes have been completed.
- As rheumatoid arthritis and other rheumatic diseases have a defined preclinical stage of disease, the lessons learned from diabetes prevention efforts can be applied to rheumatic diseases.

INTRODUCTION

Type 1 diabetes mellitus (T1D), the immune-mediated form of diabetes requiring insulin treatment, is a prevalent chronic autoimmune disease affecting both children and adults.[1–3] The incidence of T1D is increasing dramatically, doubling in the past 20 years. The vast majority of T1D cases result from autoimmune-mediated, nonreversible destruction of insulin-producing beta cells within the pancreatic islets. Progressive beta cell destruction and decreased endogenous insulin production occur during a silent preclinical phase in which blood glucose levels remain normal. During

The authors have no conflicts of interest relevant to this article.
Department of Pediatrics, Barbara Davis Center for Childhood Diabetes, University of Colorado School of Medicine, 1775 Aurora Court, Aurora, CO 80045, USA
* Corresponding author. Barbara Davis Center for Childhood Diabetes, University of Colorado Denver, Mail Stop A140, 1775 Aurora Court, Aurora, CO 80045.
E-mail address: Aaron.michels@ucdenver.edu

the preclinical phase of disease, autoantibodies directed toward beta cell–specific antigens can be measured in a patient's blood, and measurement of islet autoantibodies has made T1D a predictable disease. Inflammation and T-cell–mediated destruction of islet beta cells result in the development of clinically apparent disease marked by abnormal glucose homeostasis. With the ability to assess diabetes risk and predict disease onset, many large clinical trials aimed at disease prevention have been completed over the past decade. These studies have not completely prevented disease onset but hold promise for identifying an intervention to slow disease progression. This review focuses on the natural history of T1D, with brief sections on clinical diagnosis and treatment, prevention efforts in preclinical T1D, and a final section applying the lessons learned from diabetes prevention to rheumatic diseases.

EPIDEMIOLOGY

Great strides in understanding the natural history and pathogenesis of T1D have occurred in large part from longitudinal studies following children from birth for the development of islet autoantibodies and diabetes development (DAISY in the United States, EURODIAB in Germany, and the Type 1 Diabetes Prediction and Prevention Trial [DIPP] in Finland).[4–7] T1D incidence has also been well defined through these studies. The incidence of T1D varies greatly by geographic location, with an average annual incidence of 2.3% per year. The incidence among Caucasians in the United States is 17.8/100,000 patient years for children younger than 14 years. Unlike most other autoimmune diseases in which female individuals are affected more than male individuals, male and female individuals are equally affected with T1D. The age of diabetes onset has 2 peaks, 1 in children 5 to 7 years of age and again in adolescents 10 to 14 years old.[8] Adults also develop T1D, with approximately 25% of new T1D cases diagnosed in individuals older than 18 years of age.[3] With few exceptions, the incidence rate for T1D is rising in all age groups between 2.4% and 3.3% per year, with the largest increase among children who are younger than 5 years.[9]

T1D is still the predominant form of diabetes in youth, even though the incidence of type 2 diabetes (T2D) mellitus is increasing. More than 85% of people with T1D or T2D who are younger than 20 years old have T1D.[10] Although most individuals diagnosed with T1D have no family history of T1D, the development is strongly influenced by genetic factors.[11] In the general population, there is a 1 in 300 lifetime risk for developing T1D.[12] Individuals with a first-degree relative with T1D have a 1 in 7 to 1 in 30 lifetime risk of developing the disease depending on the affected relative. Children of mothers with T1D carry an approximately 3% lifetime risk of developing T1D, whereas the risk increases to approximately 5% for a father with diabetes.[11] A recent analysis of monozygotic twins who were initially discordant for T1D showed that by 60 years of age, persistent autoantibody positivity, T1D, or both had occurred in 78% of these individuals.[13]

RISK FACTORS
Genes

T1D is clearly a polygenic disorder, as evidenced by genome-wide association studies, which have identified more than 40 genetic polymorphisms that confer susceptibility to T1D development.[14,15] The HLA antigen class II region on chromosome 6 confers greater than 50% of the genetic susceptibility to T1D.[12] Specific major histocompatibility complex class II alleles can confer both risk and dominant protection. Individuals having a haplotype containing DR4 and DQ8, which are in close linkage disequilibrium, have the highest risk for disease development. Approximately 60% of all T1D patients have this haplotype, whereas 90% of patients have either or both the DR4/DQ8 and DR3/DQ2 haplotypes. Those individuals with a DQ6 allele (DQB1*06:02) are protected from diabetes development with a striking odds ratio of 0.03 for disease development.[16]

Besides the HLA class II genes, non-HLA genes also confer genetic risk for T1D. Of the non-HLA genes, the insulin gene (INS), protein tyrosine phosphatase nonreceptor type 22 (PTPN22), CTLA4, and IL2RA have the greatest association with T1D development.[17] Similar to the class II genes, the insulin gene polymorphisms confer both risk and protection for T1D. Variable number of tandem repeats 5′ of the insulin gene allow for more or less insulin message to be expressed in the thymus. More insulin expressed in the thymus results in central tolerance and increased protection of T1D. On the other hand, less insulin message in the thymus correlates with a lack of negative selection for autoreactive CD4 T cells and risk for T1D development.[18] Many non-HLA genes appear to be markers of generalized autoimmunity, as a number are present in other autoimmune disorders. For example, PTPN22 is associated with rheumatoid arthritis (RA), Crohn disease, Graves disease, and systemic lupus erythematous.[19] PTPN22 is expressed in lymphocytes and is involved in T-cell activation.

Environment

Despite significant research efforts aimed at identifying an environmental trigger that leads to a loss of tolerance and T1D development in genetically susceptible individuals, no clear risk factor has been causally linked to islet autoimmunity (detected by the measurement of serum autoantibodies) or T1D onset. T1D natural history studies indicate that islet autoantibodies can be detected between 9 months and 2 years of age in genetically high-risk newborns, suggesting that the initiating environmental trigger may occur in utero or early in postnatal life. Many viruses have been proposed to break tolerance, initiate the preclinical phase of T1D, and accelerate the onset of clinical T1D. These include coxsackie virus, cytomegalovirus, and enterovirus, with the most recent research focusing on enteroviruses. In the Diabetes Autoimmunity Study in the Young (DAISY) cohort, there was a strong correlation between children who developed autoantibodies and enterovirus in their serum.[20]

Other hypothesized environmental triggers include the hygiene hypothesis, in which a lack of exposure to bacterial pathogens during childhood leads to altered protective immunity and increased risk of autoimmune diseases. The north-south gradient hypothesis postulates that a lack of vitamin A and D early in life triggers the onset of autoimmune disorders, such as T1D and multiple sclerosis. Vitamin D is implicated to have immune modulatory and anti-inflammatory effects, thereby protecting from disease development. Studies suggest that supplementation with vitamin D may have a protective effect on T1D development.[21,22] Another well-studied environmental factor is that the introduction of cow's milk or gluten early in life may trigger islet autoimmunity. Two recent studies found that exposing an infant to gluten before 3 months of age or after 7 months of age is associated with the development of islet autoantibodies.[23,24] There is limited evidence suggesting that other environmental factors, including vaccinations, confer any risk for islet autoimmunity or progression to diabetes. Potential environmental triggers that are under further evaluation include delivery via cesarean, mothers with preeclampsia or advanced maternal age, exposure to nitrosamine compounds, increased body weight, and exposure to rubella virus.

PATHOPHYSIOLOGY AND ISLET AUTOANTIBODY DEVELOPMENT

Three decades ago, it was hypothesized that T1D is a chronic autoimmune disorder that develops in stages. The model combined genetic, immunologic, and metabolic markers for disease development and still remains relevant today.[6] The adapted model in **Fig. 1** proposes that in genetically susceptible individuals there is a precipitating event that leads to the development of preclinical disease where there are overt immunologic abnormalities leading to progressive loss of beta cell mass, reduced insulin release, and intermittent dysglycemia. Serum autoantibodies in the preclinical stage of disease development are present years before metabolic decompensation. The 4 islet autoantibodies are directed against insulin (IAA), glutamic decarboxylase (GAD), tyrosine phosphataselike insulinoma antigen (IA-2), and zinc transporter 8 (ZnT8).[25] These autoantibodies are markers of disease, whereas T-cell–mediated destruction results in beta cell loss. As the disease progresses and there is approximately 10% to 20% of beta cell mass remaining, a patient will become symptomatic and satisfy clinical criteria for T1D diagnosis. At this time, there will be minimal endogenous insulin release and abnormal blood glucose levels.

Multiple antibodies tend to develop simultaneously in an individual, indicating that epitope spreading occurs rapidly. If a single antibody is detected in children, it is most often to insulin. Insulin autoantibody levels directly correlate to T1D progression.[26] In adults who develop T1D, GAD and IA-2 tend to be the most common detected antibodies. The risk of developing T1D is strongly correlated with the number of positive antibodies, and individuals with 2 or more go onto develop T1D with almost 100% certainty.[27] Autoantibodies are most useful in predicting disease when they are present at a young age, in high levels, or in individuals with high-risk HLA genotypes. In general, islet autoantibodies persist until diagnosis and up to several decades

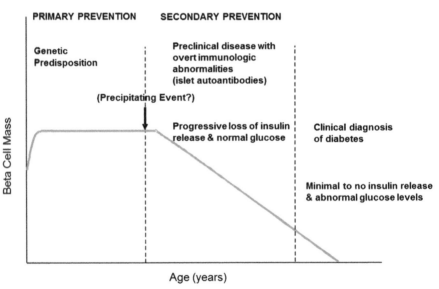

Fig. 1. Hypothetical stages and loss of beta cells in the development of type 1 diabetes. Genetics and the environment play a central role in initiating the loss of beta-cell mass, followed by preclinical disease marked by the presence of islet autoantibodies (insulin, GAD, IA-2, and ZnT8) but normal glucose homeostasis, and finally the development of overt T1D marked by the loss of insulin release and hyperglycemia. The model allows for prevention strategies early in the disease course (primary prevention) and during preclinical disease (secondary prevention). Islet autoantibodies are used to define preclinical disease, as the presence of 2 or more of these antibodies always leads to the development of clinically diagnosed T1D.

thereafter. It is estimated that 5% to 10% of all T1D patients are islet autoantibody negative, indicating that other islet autoantigens may exist.[28]

There are many hypotheses as to how beta-cell autoimmunity is initiated after a precipitating event, none of which are proven. One hypothesis is that the inciting event is an environmental determinant that shares amino acid sequence homology with beta-cell proteins and through molecular mimicry induces autoimmune destruction of beta cells. Another hypothesis proposes genetic susceptibility may lead to abnormal central tolerance (ie, specific HLA alleles do not allow for negative selection of islet antigens) followed by an inciting event that causes acute immune activation and targeting of beta cells when there are higher levels of antigen to be presented to T cells. One final proposal is that beta cells become more sensitive to free-radical or cytokine-activated inflammation that is present following a triggering event.[29] Recent efforts to study pancreata of T1D organ donors, the network for pancreatic organ donors (nPOD), have shed light on the islet infiltrates of T1D patients.[30] In those cases that have mononuclear cell infiltration within the islets (insulitis), there is a reduction of insulin-producing beta cells and an infiltrate consisting of CD8 T cells most frequently along with CD4 T cells, B-lymphocytes, and macrophages.[31]

CLINICAL FEATURES

The classic clinical presentation of T1D consists of a triad of symptoms: polyuria, polydipsia, and weight loss. From the American Diabetes Association (ADA), an individual meets diagnostic criteria for diabetes if he or she has one of the following: (1) a fasting ($\geq$8 hours) plasma glucose $\geq$126 mg/dL; (2) a random plasma glucose $\geq$200 mg/d with symptoms of hyperglycemia; (3) a 2-hour plasma glucose after a standard oral glucose tolerance test $\geq$200 mg/dL; (4) a hemoglobin A1C $\geq$6.5%. In distinguishing which type of diabetes an individual has, the ADA defines T1D as a disease caused by cellular-mediated autoimmune destruction of pancreatic beta cells; autoantibodies against beta-cell antigens (insulin, GAD, IA-2, and ZnT8) are markers of this destruction.[32] Measurement of autoantibodies remains the best way to distinguish T1D from other forms of diabetes at this time.

Studies screening genetically at-risk individuals for islet autoantibodies have identified patients early in the disease course (ie, more remaining beta-cell mass). Hemoglobin A1c values rise 1.0 to 1.5 years before clinically apparent disease, indicating that hyperglycemia occurs before acute disease onset.[33,34] Without an effective treatment to prevent beta-cell destruction, all individuals eventually develop hyperglycemia and T1D. After diagnosis, many patients enter a "honeymoon" period in which there is endogenous insulin production, and they require small amounts of exogenous insulin to maintain good glycemic control. Unfortunately, the destruction of beta cells continues and all individuals eventually become reliant on exogenous insulin to maintain euglycemia. Although intensive insulin therapy decreases the risk for complications in T1D, macrovascular and microvascular complications are still prevalent. Over time, sustained hyperglycemia damages small vessels and leads to nephropathy, retinopathy, and neuropathy. Large vessels also are damaged and cardiovascular events occur 10 times more often in people with T1D than in age-matched controls.[35]

MANAGEMENT

The mainstay of treatment for T1D is the subcutaneous administration of insulin. Currently, there are no Food and Drug Administration–approved therapies that effectively preserve residual beta-cell mass. In large diabetes centers, patients are almost exclusively started on multiple daily injection therapy with a long-acting insulin analogue to counteract basal glucose release from the liver and a short-acting insulin analogue to cover the carbohydrate content of meals and correct for hyperglycemia (ie, basal-bolus therapy). Many patients go on to use insulin pump therapy that provides continuous subcutaneous insulin infusion (CSII).[36] Studies show that CSII has a clear effect on lowering the rate of hypoglycemic events by approximately 70%.[37–39] To dose insulin and keep blood glucoses in target range, T1D patients perform self-monitoring of their blood glucose with a glucometer on average 4 to 6 times daily. Recent advances in technology now provide patients the option of a continuous glucose monitoring system (CGM). With CGM, a subcutaneous sensor is inserted and interstitial blood glucose is continuously measured. A significant amount of research is focused on creating a closed loop system, combining CGM data with algorithms to automatically deliver insulin from an insulin pump, which would function autonomously as an artificial pancreas.[40]

PREVENTION TRIALS

With the incidence and disease burden of T1D increasing, international efforts at delaying or preventing diabetes onset have occurred over the past 15 years. Large clinical trial networks have helped define the natural history of T1D, identify those individuals with preclinical disease, and provide infrastructure for coordinating prevention trials. Both primary and secondary prevention efforts in T1D are reviewed below.

Primary Prevention

Primary prevention trials have been conducted in high-risk individuals who have no islet autoantibodies or metabolic abnormalities. These individuals are generally first-degree relatives of T1D patients and have the presence of high-risk HLA genes. These trials involve infants and young children, necessitating minimal risk, and therefore they have been mostly limited to early in life dietary interventions. A clinical trial completed in Finland enrolled 230 high-risk infants, based on HLA and a first-degree relative with T1D, to receive either a casein hydrolysate formula or a conventional cow's milk formula at the time when breastfeeding was decreased or no longer available within the first 6 to 8 months of life. Casein hydrolysate contains more processed proteins cow's milk or traditional infant formula. Islet autoantibodies were measured periodically over 10 years, and the study showed that individuals who received the casein hydrolysate formula had a decreased incidence of developing positive autoantibodies.[41] Based on these data, the Trial to Reduce Incidence of Diabetes in Genetically at Risk (TRIGR) study was initiated. Enrollment at 77 centers in 15 countries was completed in 2006. In this trial, infants with HLA susceptibility and a first-degree relative with T1D were randomized to casein hydrolysate or conventional formula at birth and were allowed to breastfeed as often as desired. The main outcomes from this trial include islet autoantibody positivity and clinical development of T1D. Although this trial is still ongoing, an interim analysis suggests that hydrolyzed infant formula may lessen the risk of developing a single islet autoantibody and a trend toward developing 2 islet autoantibodies ($P = .07$).[42] Further follow-up is needed to determine if clinical diabetes onset is delayed with this dietary intervention. Another pilot study took place in a similar genetically at-risk population, the Finnish Dietary Intervention Trial for the Prevention of Type 1 Diabetes (FINDIA). The study examined the removal of bovine insulin from whey-based hydrolyzed formula and randomized children to 1 of 3 intervention groups: (1) cow's milk formula, (2) whey-based hydrolyzed formula that contains bovine insulin, or (3) whey-based hydrolyzed formula without bovine insulin. Islet autoantibodies were followed for 3 years and the infants assigned to the whey-based formula without bovine insulin had a lower risk of developing islet autoantibodies.[43]

A final primary prevention trial under way is the TrialNet Nutritional Intervention to Prevent (NIP) Type 1 Diabetes Pilot Trial, which aims to assess the effect of omega-3 fatty acid supplementation on prevention of T1D autoimmunity. Dietary omega-3 fatty acid intake has been shown to reduce the risk of islet autoimmunity in genetically at-risk infants when analyzed retrospectively and is believed to have anti-inflammatory properties.[44] At-risk infants were recruited into the NIP study and received docosahexaenoic acid or placebo for 6 months. Enrollment is now complete and the study is currently in the follow-up phase assessing for islet autoantibody development.

Secondary Prevention

T1D develops in stages, and the preclinical period is readily defined by the presence of 2 or more islet autoantibodies. Many secondary prevention trials are aimed at delaying or preventing the progression to T1D in individuals with islet autoantibodies have been completed (**Table 1**). To conduct these large randomized double-blinded placebo-controlled trials, infrastructure in the form of financial support and a clinical trials network has been necessary. The first T1D clinical trials network emerged in the early 1990s as the National Institutes of Health–sponsored Diabetes Prevention Trial-Type 1 (DPT-1). DPT-1 became known as TrialNet, and conducts clinical intervention trials focused on delaying/preventing T1D onset and identifying therapies to preserve residual beta-cell mass in newly diagnosed T1D patients. TrialNet is an international consortium with 18 clinical centers and an additional 150 affiliated sites.[45] TrialNet has

Table 1
Selected phase II/III secondary prevention trials in T1D

Study	Agent	Number Randomized	Age, y	Comments
DIAPREV-IT	GAD/Alum	50	4–18	Trial in follow-up phase
[a]Abatacept	CTLA-4 Ig	Currently enrolling	6–45	TrialNet sponsored
[a]Teplizumab	Anti-CD3 mAb	Currently enrolling	8–45	TrialNet sponsored
[a]Intranasal Insulin Trial (INIT-II)[52]	Intranasal Insulin	Currently enrolling	4–20	Less-frequent dosing than prior studies
[a]Oral Insulin	Oral Insulin	currently enrolling	3–45	TrialNet sponsored
Diabetes Prevention Trial – Type 1 Study Group (DPT-1)[48,49]	Oral Insulin	372	3–45	Post hoc analysis shows delay to T1D diagnosis in subset of patients
European Nicotinamide Diabetes Intervention Trial (ENDIT)[61]	Nicotinamide	552	3–40	No effect on prevention
Diabetes Prediction and Prevention Trial (DIPP)[53]	Intranasal Insulin	224	1–5	No effect on prevention
Diabetes Prevention Trial–Type 1 Study Group (DPT-1)[47]	Parenteral Insulin	339	4–45	No effect on prevention

Abbreviations: GAD, glutamic decarboxylase; Ig, immunoglobulin; T1D, type 1 diabetes.
[a] Indicates trials currently enrolling at the time of publication.

already completed many studies and provides ongoing support for clinical trials with several prevention trials currently enrolling participants.

Most secondary prevention trials have focused on antigen-specific therapies, mainly using preparations of insulin. Antigen-specific therapies are believed to enhance the function of regulatory T cells, which traffic to the tissue-specific site of the antigen, and potentially protect beta-cell mass from immune-mediated destruction.[46] The first clinical trial sponsored through DPT-1 was a randomized, placebo-controlled study aimed at evaluating the effects of insulin in relatives of patients with T1D. At-risk individuals identified by HLA susceptibility and the presence of one or more islet autoantibodies, were treated with subcutaneous or oral insulin. To enroll both of these insulin-prevention trials, 84,228 individuals were screened for islet cell antibodies and 3152 (3.7%) were positive when the screening was conducted between 1994 and 2000.[47] Participants aged 3 to 45 years who already had signs of abnormal glucose metabolism (n = 339) were given 0.25 U/kg per day of Ultralente insulin twice daily. They also received a continuous intravenous insulin infusion for 4 days at the beginning of the study and then annually. The study showed no effect of low-dose insulin on delaying the progression to T1D diagnosis.[47] Participants in the DPT-1 trial who did not yet have signs of abnormal glucose tolerance were given 7.5 mg/kg of oral insulin daily (n = 372). The primary end point was diagnosis of diabetes, and an oral glucose tolerance test was completed every 6 months during a 6-year follow-up. The study did not show any delay in progression to T1D in the oral insulin group. However, interestingly, a post hoc analysis showed that in participants with persistently high levels of insulin autoantibody (IAA) ($\geq$80 U/mL), there seemed to be a delay in T1D onset.[48] Furthermore, after stopping oral insulin, the rate of progression to T1D onset was faster.[49] Based on these findings, TrialNet is currently recruiting individuals for a larger oral insulin trial to determine if oral insulin can delay the progression to T1D in participants with high IAA levels (NCT00419562).

The Belgian T1D Registry also studied parenteral insulin administration. Participants who were positive for IAAs and did not have a diabetes protective HLA haplotype (presence of a DQB1*06:02 allele) were enrolled in a prospective nonrandomized study and given 2 injections of insulin for 36 months (n = 50). There was no difference in the development of T1D between the participants who were treated with insulin and those who refused treatment or agreed to observation.[50]

Insulin also has been administered nasally, as opposed to parental and oral administration, in an attempt to delay or prevent diabetes onset. Mucosal administration of antigens can induce a protective immune response with regulatory T cells, and it was hypothesized that this may lead to disease prevention.[51] The Intranasal Insulin Trial (INIT-I) was a randomized, double-blinded, crossover pilot study done in Australia in people who were high risk by HLA and had one or more islet autoantibodies present (n = 38). The results indicated that intranasal insulin decreases T-cell responsiveness, arguing for a protective effect on the development of T1D.[52] A larger study, INIT-II, is now enrolling individuals to determine if intranasal insulin can delay or prevent the progression to T1D (NCT 00336674). The DIPP trial in Finland screened infants and siblings of children with T1D for high-risk HLA. Participants who were high risk were then followed for autoantibody development. On developing 2 or more autoantibodies, participants (n = 264) were eligible for randomization and if randomized to the intranasal insulin arm (n = 137), they received 1 U/kg per day of insulin. The trial was stopped early because interim analyses showed no benefit of intranasal insulin in delaying the onset of T1D.[53]

Nicotinamide (vitamin B6) is a water-soluble vitamin that increases nicotinamide adenine dinucleotide, which is believed to consequently reduce beta-cell inflammation, and has inhibited the development of T1D in animal models of autoimmune diabetes.[54–56] Initial pilot trials in first-degree relatives of people with T1D and who were positive for one or more islet cell antibodies have had conflicting results.[57–59] In New Zealand, school-age children were screened for autoantibodies and then treated with nicotinamide in a randomized, non–placebo-controlled trial. Children who received nicotinamide supplementation developed T1D at a much lower rate than eligible children who did not participate in the trial.[60] However, follow-up larger clinical trials failed to validate these findings. The European Nicotinamide Diabetes Intervention Trial was a randomized, placebo-controlled, double-blinded study that enrolled people aged 5 to 40 years from 15 different countries who had a first-degree relative with T1D and one or more islet cell antibodies (n = 552). The participants randomized to receive nicotinamide received 1.2 mg/m^2 for 5 years. There was no difference between the 2 groups in the development of T1D.[61] The German Nicotinamide Diabetes Intervention Study was a randomized, placebo-controlled, double-blinded study that enrolled siblings of children with T1D who were aged 3 to 12 years and had high titers of islet cell autoantibodies. There was no significant difference in the rate of diabetes onset between the 2 groups.[62] There have been several pilot studies completed using other non–autoantigen-specific therapies. These therapies include ketotifen (histamine antagonist), oral cyclosporine, and Bacille Calmette-Guerin (BCG) injections. Although oral cyclosporine showed a slight delay in the development of T1D, none of these studies prevented T1D development.[63–66]

Several trials aimed at modifying the immune system in high-risk individuals are currently under way. CTLA4-Ig (Abatacept) for Prevention of Abnormal Glucose Tolerance and Diabetes in Relatives At-Risk is a multicenter, randomized, controlled, double-blinded trial currently enrolling first-degree relatives of people with T1D aged 6 to 45 years who have developed autoantibodies (NCT 01773707). Participants will receive 14 infusions of either abatacept or normal saline over 1 year. Participants will have an oral glucose tolerance test every 6 months and will be monitored for the development of abnormal glucose tolerance. Anti-CD3 mAb (Teplizumab) for Prevention of Diabetes in Relatives At Risk for Type 1 Diabetes Mellitus is the other TrialNet study, which is enrolling high-risk, autoantibody-positive relatives of people with T1D who are aged 8 to 45 years. Participants will be monitored for the development of T1D. DIAPREV-IT is an ongoing study in children 4 years of age and older who are positive for GAD and one or more additional autoantibodies (NCT 01122446). Participants will receive a GAD/alum vaccine at enrollment and at 30 days; then follow-up for the development of T1D over the ensuing 5 years.

Although none of the secondary prevention studies have yet been able to delay the progression to T1D diagnosis, these trials have confirmed repeatedly that large-scale controlled clinical prevention trials are feasible. Another added benefit of these trials is that close follow-up permits earlier diagnosis of T1D in many individuals. This in turn leads to the decreased incidence of diabetic ketoacidosis at diagnosis and the initiation of insulin therapy while there is still beta cell mass present. Other lessons from these trials are listed in **Box 1**.

APPLICATION TO RHEUMATIC DISEASES

T1D has many similarities to other rheumatic diseases, especially RA and lupus, that have been demonstrated to have preclinical periods marked by autoantibodies in the absence of clinically apparent disease (**Table 2**).[67,68] Using T1D as an example, large randomized double-blinded placebo-controlled trials for prevention can be

---

Box 1
Lessons learned from T1D prevention trials

- It is possible to do large-scale prevention trials as randomized double-blinded placebo-controlled trials.
- The trials have allowed for better understanding of disease natural history, heterogeneity, and biomarker identification.
- The trials validated the prediction and risk assessments in preclinical disease for diabetes development.
- Once the infrastructure for prevention trials is in place, more trials with specific therapies will follow. This is evidenced by the abatacept, teplizumab, intranasal, and oral insulin trials that are currently enrolling.

---

undertaken in these rheumatic diseases. For prevention of a chronic autoimmune disorder several key features are necessary:

1. Ability to assess preclinical disease risk
2. Adequate prevalence of disease
3. Infrastructure for clinical trial support
4. Clinically well-established and easily administered therapies

For both T1D, and in particular RA, both autoimmune diseases are marked by a preclinical phase before clinical manifestations of disease. These preclinical stages are characterized by immunologic markers of underlying autoimmunity, islet autoantibodies in T1D and anti-citrullinated protein antibodies (ACPA) in RA.[69,70] Titers of ACPA antibodies can predict risk of developing clinical RA within 3 years.[71] With biomarkers of preclinical disease and prediction measurements, subjects can now be readily identified for clinical intervention trials for RA prevention. Second, the prevalence of RA in first-degree relatives is similar to that of T1D. The overall prevalence in the general population is estimated to be 1 in 300 for T1D and 1 in 100 for RA.[72] However, when taking into account a first-degree relative, the prevalence for both diseases is approximately 1 in 30. These high rates of disease development make for effective screening efforts.

Table 2
Similarities between T1D and RA for disease prevention

Characteristic	T1D	RA
Prevalence (general population)	~1/300	~1/100
Infrastructure	TrialNet	SERA RAIN FDRs in clinic
Risk	Islet autoantibodies, HLA	CCP, RF, CRP, others
Therapies	Insulin	Hydroxychloroquine Methotrexate Sulfasalazine Leflunomide Azathioprine Biologics Others

Abbreviations: CCP, cyclic citrullinated protein; CRP, C-reactive protein; FDR, first degree relative; RAIN, Rheumatoid Arthritis Investigational Network; RF, rheumatoid factor; SERA, Studies on the Etiology of Rheumatoid Arthritis; T1D, type 1 diabetes.

In T1D, the initial Diabetes Prevention Trial (DPT-1) provided infrastructure and a framework for identifying at-risk relatives and conducting prevention trials for T1D. The DPT investigators reorganized into Type 1 Diabetes TrialNet, which is funded by the National Institutes of Health, and focuses on screening at-risk relatives for islet autoantibodies (TrialNet Natural History Study) and then placing these individuals into clinical intervention trials. At the current time, approximately 25,000 at-risk relatives are screened each year for islet autoantibodies through the TrialNet Natural History Study. In RA, there are several established investigational networks similar to Trial-Net, including Studies on the Etiology of Rheumatoid Arthritis (SERA) and the Rheumatoid Arthritis Investigational Network (RAIN).[73] SERA investigators are identifying at-risk subjects in the preclinical stage of RA, assessing biomarkers, and laying the foundation for RA prevention trials. Furthermore, there is a growing population of first degree relative being identified in the preclinical stage of RA development in clinics worldwide. RAIN investigators have focused on investigator-initiated trials to define better treatments for RA and have pioneered the use of medication combinations for treatment.[74]

In addition to assessing disease risk in a prevalent condition and having the appropriate infrastructure in place, a potential therapy that could delay the onset or prevent progression to clinically apparent disease should be available for testing. In T1D, until very recently, most therapies were limited to various formulations of insulin. Insulin is the mainstay of treatment of all patients with T1D and was a natural choice for a preventive agent with hopes that early administration could lead to immune tolerance to anti-insulin autoimmunity. Currently there are no Food and Drug Administration–approved immune therapies for the treatment of T1D to preserve residual beta cell function after clinical diagnosis. In RA, there are numerous clinically well-established treatments with immunologic targets that could be considered for use in disease prevention.[75] A prevention therapy needs to be safe, easily administered, and affordable, as all participants will not have any clinical symptoms of disease. Hydroxychloroquine (Plaquenil) fulfills these requirements, as it is has been in clinical use for decades, is orally administered, has limited adverse effects, and is not cost prohibitive for treating large numbers of subjects. However, it is our belief that eventually therapies for T1D or RA prevention will need to be tailored to cohorts of individuals based on genetic and immunologic assessments.

T1D and RA are both prevalent chronic autoimmune disorders with readily identifiable preclinical stages of disease. Prediction of disease onset is possible in both diseases and prevention is now a goal. The lessons learned from T1D prevention efforts can be applied to RA and reduce the disease burden by making RA a preventable disease.

ACKNOWLEDGMENTS

This work was supported by grants from the National Institute of Diabetes and Digestive Kidney Diseases (R01 DK032083, K08 DK095995), Juvenile Diabetes Research Foundation, the Children's Diabetes Foundation, and the Brehm Coalition.

REFERENCES

1. Atkinson MA, Eisenbarth GS, Michels AW. Type 1 diabetes. The Lancet 2014; 383(9911):69–82.
2. Karvonen M, Viik-Kajander M, Moltchanova E, et al. Incidence of childhood type 1 diabetes worldwide. Diabetes Mondiale (DiaMond) Project Group. Diabetes Care 2000;23(10):1516–26.

3. Haller MJ, Atkinson MA, Schatz D. Type 1 diabetes mellitus: etiology, presentation, and management. Pediatr Clin North Am 2005;52(6):1553–78.
4. Rewers M, Bugawan TL, Norris JM, et al. Newborn screening for HLA markers associated with IDDM: diabetes autoimmunity study in the young (DAISY). Diabetologia 1996;39(7):807–12.
5. Levy-Marchal C, Patterson CC, Green A, et al, EURODIAB ACE Study Group. Europe and Diabetes. Geographical variation of presentation at diagnosis of type I diabetes in children: the EURODIAB study. European and Diabetes. Diabetologia 2001;44(Suppl 3):B75–80.
6. Eisenbarth GS. Type I diabetes mellitus. A chronic autoimmune disease. N Engl J Med 1986;314(21):1360–8.
7. Group DP. Incidence and trends of childhood type 1 diabetes worldwide 1990-1999. Diabet Med 2006;23(8):857–66.
8. Harjutsalo V, Sjoberg L, Tuomilehto J. Time trends in the incidence of type 1 diabetes in Finnish children: a cohort study. Lancet 2008;371(9626):1777–82.
9. Patterson CC, Dahlquist GG, Gyurus E, et al. Incidence trends for childhood type 1 diabetes in Europe during 1989-2003 and predicted new cases 2005-20: a multicentre prospective registration study. Lancet 2009;373(9680):2027–33.
10. SEARCH for Diabetes in Youth Study Group, Liese AD, D'Agostino RB Jr, Hamman RF, et al. The burden of diabetes mellitus among US youth: prevalence estimates from the SEARCH for Diabetes in Youth Study. Pediatrics 2006;118(4): 1510–8.
11. Hamalainen AM, Knip M. Autoimmunity and familial risk of type 1 diabetes. Curr Diab Rep 2002;2(4):347–53.
12. Redondo MJ, Eisenbarth GS. Genetic control of autoimmunity in Type I diabetes and associated disorders. Diabetologia 2002;45(5):605–22.
13. Redondo MJ, Jeffrey J, Fain PR, et al. Concordance for islet autoimmunity among monozygotic twins. N Engl J Med 2008;359(26):2849–50.
14. Barrett JC, Clayton DG, Concannon P, et al. Genome-wide association study and meta-analysis find that over 40 loci affect risk of type 1 diabetes. Nat Genet 2009;41(6):703–7.
15. Noble JA, Valdes AM, Cook M, et al. The role of HLA class II genes in insulin-dependent diabetes mellitus: molecular analysis of 180 Caucasian, multiplex families. Am J Hum Genet 1996;59(5):1134–48.
16. Erlich H, Valdes AM, Noble J, et al. HLA DR-DQ haplotypes and genotypes and type 1 diabetes risk: analysis of the type 1 diabetes genetics consortium families. Diabetes 2008;57(4):1084–92.
17. Polychronakos C, Li Q. Understanding type 1 diabetes through genetics: advances and prospects. Nat Rev Genet 2011;12(11):781–92.
18. Pugliese A, Zeller M, Fernandez A Jr, et al. The insulin gene is transcribed in the human thymus and transcription levels correlated with allelic variation at the INS VNTR-IDDM2 susceptibility locus for type 1 diabetes. Nat Genet 1997;15(3): 293–7.
19. Lee YH, Bae SC, Choi SJ, et al. The association between the PTPN22 C1858T polymorphism and rheumatoid arthritis: a meta-analysis update. Mol Biol Rep 2012;39(4):3453–60.
20. Stene LC, Oikarinen S, Hyoty H, et al. Enterovirus infection and progression from islet autoimmunity to type 1 diabetes: the Diabetes and Autoimmunity Study in the Young (DAISY). Diabetes 2010;59(12):3174–80.
21. Hypponen E, Laara E, Reunanen A, et al. Intake of vitamin D and risk of type 1 diabetes: a birth-cohort study. Lancet 2001;358(9292):1500–3.

22. Zipitis CS, Akobeng AK. Vitamin D supplementation in early childhood and risk of type 1 diabetes: a systematic review and meta-analysis. Arch Dis Child 2008; 93(6):512–7.
23. Snell-Bergeon JK, Smith J, Dong F, et al. Early childhood infections and the risk of islet autoimmunity: the Diabetes Autoimmunity Study in the Young (DAISY). Diabetes Care 2012;35(12):2553–8.
24. Hummel S, Pfluger M, Hummel M, et al. Primary dietary intervention study to reduce the risk of islet autoimmunity in children at increased risk for type 1 diabetes: the BABYDIET study. Diabetes Care 2011;34(6):1301–5.
25. Watkins RA, Evans-Molina C, Blum JS, et al. Established and emerging biomarkers for the prediction of type 1 diabetes: a systematic review. Transl Res 2014;164(2):110–21.
26. Steck AK, Johnson K, Barriga KJ, et al. Age of islet autoantibody appearance and mean levels of insulin, but not GAD or IA-2 autoantibodies, predict age of diagnosis of type 1 diabetes: diabetes autoimmunity study in the young. Diabetes Care 2011;34(6):1397–9.
27. Ziegler AG, Rewers M, Simell O, et al. Seroconversion to multiple islet autoantibodies and risk of progression to diabetes in children. JAMA 2013;309(23): 2473–9.
28. Bingley PJ. Clinical applications of diabetes antibody testing. J Clin Endocrinol Metab 2010;95(1):25–33.
29. Padgett LE, Broniowska KA, Hansen PA, et al. The role of reactive oxygen species and proinflammatory cytokines in type 1 diabetes pathogenesis. Ann N Y Acad Sci 2013;1281:16–35.
30. Pugliese A, Yang M, Kusmarteva I, et al. The Juvenile Diabetes Research Foundation Network for Pancreatic Organ Donors with Diabetes (nPOD) Program: goals, operational model and emerging findings. Pediatr Diabetes 2014;15(1):1–9.
31. Spencer J, Peakman M. Post-mortem analysis of islet pathology in type 1 diabetes illuminates the life and death of the beta cell. Clin Exp Immunol 2009; 155(2):125–7.
32. American Diabetes Association. Standards of medical care in diabetes–2013. Diabetes Care 2013;36(Suppl 1):S11–66.
33. Sosenko JM, Skyler JS, Krischer JP, et al. Glucose excursions between states of glycemia with progression to type 1 diabetes in the diabetes prevention trial-type 1 (DPT-1). Diabetes 2010;59(10):2386–9.
34. Ferrannini E, Mari A, Nofrate V, et al. Progression to diabetes in relatives of type 1 diabetic patients: mechanisms and mode of onset. Diabetes 2010;59(3):679–85.
35. Orchard TJ, Costacou T, Kretowski A, et al. Type 1 diabetes and coronary artery disease. Diabetes Care 2006;29(11):2528–38.
36. Norgaard K. A nationwide study of continuous subcutaneous insulin infusion (CSII) in Denmark. Diabet Med 2003;20(4):307–11.
37. Pickup J, Keen H. Continuous subcutaneous insulin infusion at 25 years: evidence base for the expanding use of insulin pump therapy in type 1 diabetes. Diabetes Care 2002;25(3):593–8.
38. Bode BW, Steed RD, Davidson PC. Reduction in severe hypoglycemia with long-term continuous subcutaneous insulin infusion in type I diabetes. Diabetes Care 1996;19(4):324–7.
39. Boland EA, Grey M, Oesterle A, et al. Continuous subcutaneous insulin infusion. A new way to lower risk of severe hypoglycemia, improve metabolic control, and enhance coping in adolescents with type 1 diabetes. Diabetes Care 1999; 22(11):1779–84.

40. Peyser T, Dassau E, Breton M, et al. The artificial pancreas: current status and future prospects in the management of diabetes. Ann N Y Acad Sci 2014; 1311(1):102–23.

41. Akerblom HK, Virtanen SM, Ilonen J, et al. Dietary manipulation of beta cell autoimmunity in infants at increased risk of type 1 diabetes: a pilot study. Diabetologia 2005;48(5):829–37.

42. Knip M, Virtanen SM, Seppa K, et al. Dietary intervention in infancy and later signs of beta-cell autoimmunity. N Engl J Med 2010;363(20):1900–8.

43. Vaarala O, Ilonen J, Ruohtula T, et al. Removal of bovine insulin from cow's milk formula and early initiation of beta-cell autoimmunity in the FINDIA Pilot Study. Arch Pediatr Adolesc Med 2012;166(7):608–14.

44. Norris JM, Yin X, Lamb MM, et al. Omega-3 polyunsaturated fatty acid intake and islet autoimmunity in children at increased risk for type 1 diabetes. JAMA 2007;298(12):1420–8.

45. Skyler JS, Greenbaum CJ, Lachin JM, et al. Type 1 Diabetes TrialNet–an international collaborative clinical trials network. Ann N Y Acad Sci 2008;1150:14–24.

46. Michels AW, von Herrath M. 2011 Update: antigen-specific therapy in type 1 diabetes. Curr Opin Endocrinol Diabetes Obes 2011;18(4):235–40.

47. Diabetes Prevention Trial–Type 1 Diabetes Study Group. Effects of insulin in relatives of patients with type 1 diabetes mellitus. N Engl J Med 2002;346(22): 1685–91.

48. Skyler JS, Krischer JP, Wolfsdorf J, et al. Effects of oral insulin in relatives of patients with type 1 diabetes: the diabetes prevention trial–type 1. Diabetes Care 2005;28(5):1068–76.

49. Vehik K, Cuthbertson D, Ruhlig H, et al. Long-term outcome of individuals treated with oral insulin: diabetes prevention trial-type 1 (DPT-1) oral insulin trial. Diabetes Care 2011;34(7):1585–90.

50. Vandemeulebroucke E, Gorus FK, Decochez K, et al. Insulin treatment in IA-2A-positive relatives of type 1 diabetic patients. Diabetes Metab 2009;35(4): 319–27.

51. Martinez NR, Augstein P, Moustakas AK, et al. Disabling an integral CTL epitope allows suppression of autoimmune diabetes by intranasal proinsulin peptide. J Clin Invest 2003;111(9):1365–71.

52. Harrison LC, Honeyman MC, Steele CE, et al. Pancreatic beta-cell function and immune responses to insulin after administration of intranasal insulin to humans at risk for type 1 diabetes. Diabetes Care 2004;27(10):2348–55.

53. Nanto-Salonen K, Kupila A, Simell S, et al. Nasal insulin to prevent type 1 diabetes in children with HLA genotypes and autoantibodies conferring increased risk of disease: a double-blind, randomised controlled trial. Lancet 2008; 372(9651):1746–55.

54. Dulin WE, Wyse BM. Reversal of streptozotocin diabetes with nicotinamide. Proc Soc Exp Biol Med 1969;130(3):992–4.

55. Yamada K, Nonaka K, Hanafusa T, et al. Preventive and therapeutic effects of large-dose nicotinamide injections on diabetes associated with insulitis. An observation in nonobese diabetic (NOD) mice. Diabetes 1982;31(9):749–53.

56. Lazarow A. Protection against alloxan diabetes. Anat Rec 1947;97(3):353.

57. Herskowitz RD, Jackson RA, Soeldner JS, et al. Pilot trial to prevent type I diabetes: progression to overt IDDM despite oral nicotinamide. J Autoimmun 1989; 2(5):733–7.

58. Elliott RB, Chase HP. Prevention or delay of type 1 (insulin-dependent) diabetes mellitus in children using nicotinamide. Diabetologia 1991;34(5):362–5.

59. Manna R, Migliore A, Martin LS, et al. Nicotinamide treatment in subjects at high risk of developing IDDM improves insulin secretion. Br J Clin Pract 1992;46(3): 177–9.

60. Elliott RB, Pilcher CC, Stewart A, et al. The use of nicotinamide in the prevention of type 1 diabetes. Ann N Y Acad Sci 1993;696:333–41.

61. Gale EA, Bingley PJ, Emmett CL, et al, European Nicotinamide Diabetes Intervention Trial Group. European Nicotinamide Diabetes Intervention Trial (ENDIT): a randomised controlled trial of intervention before the onset of type 1 diabetes. Lancet 2004;363(9413):925–31.

62. Lampeter EF, Scherbaum WA, Henize E, et al. The Deutsche Nicotinamide Intervention Study: an attempt to prevent type 1 diabetes. DENIS Group. Diabetes Care 1998;47:980–4.

63. Bohmer KP, Kolb H, Kuglin B, et al. Linear loss of insulin secretory capacity during the last six months preceding IDDM. No effect of antiedematous therapy with ketotifen. Diabetes Care 1994;17(2):138–41.

64. Carel JC, Boltard C, Eisenbarth G, et al. Cyclosporine delays but does not prevent clinical onset in glucose intolerant pre-type 1 diabetic children. J Autoimmun 1996;9:739–45.

65. Huppmann M, Baumgarten A, Ziegler AG, et al. Neonatal Bacille Calmette-Guerin vaccination and type 1 diabetes. Diabetes Care 2005;28(5):1204–6.

66. Ziegler AG, Schmid S, Huber D, et al. Early infant feeding and risk of developing type 1 diabetes-associated autoantibodies. JAMA 2003;290(13):1721–8.

67. Deane KD, El-Gabalawy H. Pathogenesis and prevention of rheumatic disease: focus on preclinical RA and SLE. Nat Rev Rheumatol 2014;10(4):212–28.

68. Arbuckle MR, McClain MT, Rubertone MV, et al. Development of autoantibodies before the clinical onset of systemic lupus erythematosus. N Engl J Med 2003; 349(16):1526–33.

69. Demoruelle MK, Parish MC, Derber LA, et al. Performance of anti-cyclic citrullinated peptide assays differs in subjects at increased risk of rheumatoid arthritis and subjects with established disease. Arthritis Rheum 2013;65(9):2243–52.

70. Young KA, Deane KD, Derber LA, et al. Relatives without rheumatoid arthritis show reactivity to anti-citrullinated protein/peptide antibodies that are associated with arthritis-related traits: studies of the etiology of rheumatoid arthritis. Arthritis Rheum 2013;65(8):1995–2004.

71. Majka DS, Deane KD, Parrish LA, et al. Duration of preclinical rheumatoid arthritis-related autoantibody positivity increases in subjects with older age at time of disease diagnosis. Ann Rheum Dis 2008;67(6):801–7.

72. Scott DL, Wolfe F, Huizinga TW. Rheumatoid arthritis. Lancet 2010;376(9746): 1094–108.

73. Kolfenbach JR, Deane KD, Derber LA, et al. A prospective approach to investigating the natural history of preclinical rheumatoid arthritis (RA) using first-degree relatives of probands with RA. Arthritis Rheum 2009;61(12):1735–42.

74. O'Dell JR, Mikuls TR, Taylor TH, et al. Therapies for active rheumatoid arthritis after methotrexate failure. N Engl J Med 2013;369(4):307–18.

75. Smolen JS, Aletaha D, Koeller M, et al. New therapies for treatment of rheumatoid arthritis. Lancet 2007;370(9602):1861–74.

Index

Note: Page numbers of article titles are in **boldface** type.

Rheum Dis Clin N Am 40 (2014) 813–822
http://dx.doi.org/10.1016/S0889-857X(14)00087-8
0889-857X/14/$ – see front matter © 2014 Elsevier Inc. All rights reserved.

rheumatic.theclinics.com

United States Postal Service

Statement of Ownership, Management, and Circulation
(All Periodicals Publications Except Requestor Publications)

1. Publication Title	2. Publication Number	3. Filing Date
Rheumatic Disease Clinics of North America	0 0 6 - 2 7 2	9/14/14

4. Issue Frequency	5. Number of Issues Published Annually	6. Annual Subscription Price
Feb, May, Aug, Nov	4	$335.00

7. Complete Mailing Address of Known Office of Publication (Not printer) (Street, city, county, state, and ZIP+4®)

Elsevier Inc.
360 Park Avenue South
New York, NY 10010-1710

Contact Person
Stephen R. Bushing

Telephone (Include area code)
215-239-3688

8. Complete Mailing Address of Headquarters or General Business Office of Publisher (Not printer)

Elsevier Inc., 360 Park Avenue South, New York, NY 10010-1710

9. Full Names and Complete Mailing Addresses of Publisher, Editor, and Managing Editor (Do not leave blank)

Publisher (Name and complete mailing address)

Linda Belfus, Elsevier, Inc., 1600 John F. Kennedy Blvd. Suite 1800, Philadelphia, PA 19103-2899

Editor (Name and complete mailing address)

Jennifer Flynn-Briggs, Elsevier, Inc., 1600 John F. Kennedy Blvd. Suite 1800, Philadelphia, PA 19103-2899

Managing Editor (Name and complete mailing address)

Adrianne Brigido, Elsevier, Inc., 1600 John F. Kennedy Blvd. Suite 1800, Philadelphia, PA 19103-2899

10. Owner (Do not leave blank. If the publication is owned by a corporation, give the name and address of the corporation immediately followed by the names and addresses of all stockholders owning or holding 1 percent or more of the total amount of stock. If not owned by a corporation, give the names and addresses of the individual owners. If owned by a partnership or other unincorporated firm, give its name and address as well as those of each individual owner. If the publication is published by a nonprofit organization, give its name and address.)

Full Name	Complete Mailing Address
Wholly owned subsidiary of	1600 John F. Kennedy Blvd, Ste. 1800
Reed/Elsevier, US holdings	Philadelphia, PA 19103-2899

11. Known Bondholders, Mortgagees, and Other Security Holders Owning or Holding 1 Percent or More of Total Amount of Bonds, Mortgages, or Other Securities. If none, check box ☐ None

Full Name	Complete Mailing Address
N/A	

12. Tax Status (For completion by nonprofit organizations authorized to mail at nonprofit rates) (Check one)
The purpose, function, and nonprofit status of this organization and the exempt status for Federal income tax purposes
☐ Has Not Changed During Preceding 12 Months
☐ Has Changed During Preceding 12 Months (Publisher must submit explanation of change with this statement)

PS Form 3526, August 2012 (Page 1 of 3 (Instructions Page 3)) PSN 7530-01-000-9931 PRIVACY NOTICE: See our Privacy policy in www.usps.com

---

13. Publication Title	14. Issue Date for Circulation Data Below
Rheumatic Disease Clinics of North America	August 2014

15. Extent and Nature of Circulation		Average No. Copies Each Issue During Preceding 12 Months	No. Copies of Single Issue Published Nearest to Filing Date
a. Total Number of Copies (Net press run)		683	683
b. Paid Circulation (By Mail and Outside the Mail)	(1) Mailed Outside-County Paid Subscriptions Stated on PS Form 3541. (Include paid distribution above nominal rate, advertiser's proof copies, and exchange copies)	330	319
	(2) Mailed In-County Paid Subscriptions Stated on PS Form 3541 (Include paid distribution above nominal rate, advertiser's proof copies, and exchange copies)		
	(3) Paid Distribution Outside the Mails Including Sales Through Dealers and Carriers, Street Vendors, Counter Sales, and Other Paid Distribution Outside USPS®	127	141
	(4) Paid Distribution by Other Classes Mailed Through the USPS (e.g. First-Class Mail®)		
c. Total Paid Distribution (Sum of 15b (1), (2), (3), and (4))	►	457	460
d. Free or Nominal Rate Distribution (By Mail and Outside the Mail)	(1) Free or Nominal Rate Outside-County Copies Included on PS Form 3541	92	88
	(2) Free or Nominal Rate In-County Copies Included on PS Form 3541		
	(3) Free or Nominal Rate Copies Mailed at Other Classes Through the USPS (e.g. First-Class Mail)		
	(4) Free or Nominal Rate Distribution Outside the Mail (Carriers or other means)		
e. Total Free or Nominal Rate Distribution (Sum of 15d (1), (2), (3) and (4))	►	92	88
f. Total Distribution (Sum of 15c and 15e)	►	549	548
g. Copies not Distributed (See instructions to publishers #4 (page #3))	►	134	135
h. Total (Sum of 15f and g)	►	683	683
i. Percent Paid (15c divided by 15f times 100)	►	83.24%	83.94%

16. Total circulation includes electronic copies. Report circulation on PS Form 3526-X worksheet.

17. Publication of Statement of Ownership.
If the publication is a general publication, publication of this statement is required. Will be printed in the November 2014 issue of this publication.

18. Signature and Title of Editor, Publisher, Business Manager, or Owner

[signature]

Stephen R. Bushing – Inventory Distribution Coordinator

Date
September 14, 2014

I certify that all information furnished on this form is true and complete. I understand that anyone who furnishes false or misleading information on this form or who omits material or information requested on the form may be subject to criminal sanctions (including fines and imprisonment) and/or civil sanctions (including civil penalties).

PS Form 3526, August 2012 (Page 2 of 3)

Moving?

Make sure your subscription moves with you!

To notify us of your new address, find your **Clinics Account Number** (located on your mailing label above your name), and contact customer service at:

Email: journalscustomerservice-usa@elsevier.com

800-654-2452 (subscribers in the U.S. & Canada)
314-447-8871 (subscribers outside of the U.S. & Canada)

Fax number: 314-447-8029

Elsevier Health Sciences Division
Subscription Customer Service
3251 Riverport Lane
Maryland Heights, MO 63043

*To ensure uninterrupted delivery of your subscription, please notify us at least 4 weeks in advance of move.

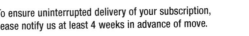